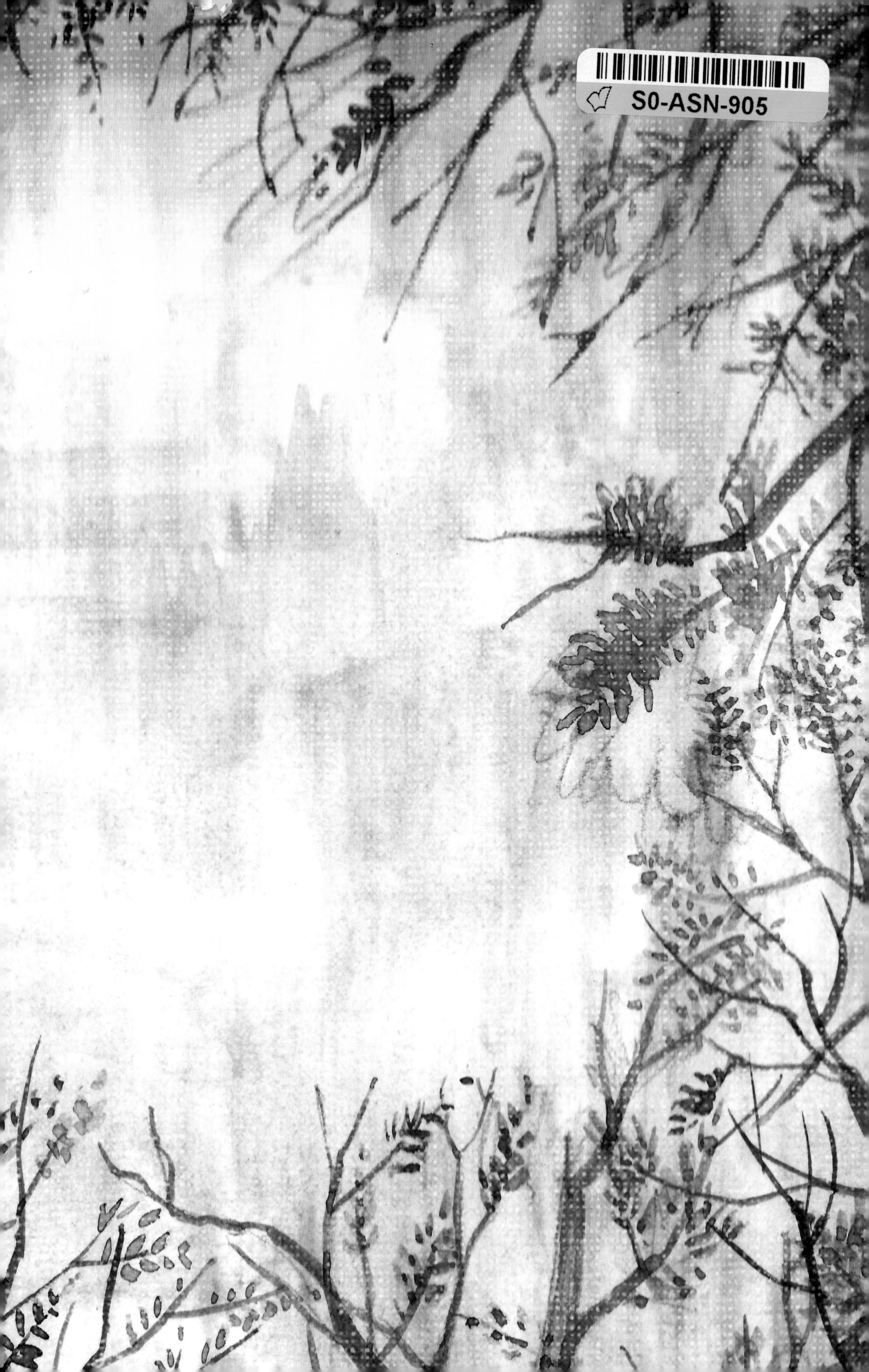

First published in 2017 by Educational Resources Ltd.
PO Box 6628, Wellington 6141, New Zealand
www.edresources.co.nz

National Library of New Zealand Cataloguing-in-Publication Data

Williams, Brent, 1958-
Out of the woods : a journey through depression and anxiety /
Brent Williams ; illustrator, Korkut Öztekin.
ISBN 978-0-473-39006-8
1. Williams, Brent, 1958- —Mental health—Comic books, strips, etc.
2. Depression, Mental—Comic books, strips, etc. 3. Anxiety—
Comic books, strips, etc. I. Öztekin, Korkut. II. Title.
616.8527—dc 23

Author: Brent Williams
Illustrator: Korkut Öztekin
Editor: James McLean
Lettering: Pippa Keel & Tom Barclay
Cover design: Cato Brand Partners
Cover illustrations: Korkut Öztekin
Copy editor: Mitch Marks
Author photo: Emily Fawkner
Illustrator photo: Mehmet Kostumoglu

Printed by Everbest Printing Investment Limited, China

OUT OF THE
WOODS

A Journey Through
Depression and Anxiety

Brent Williams

Illustrated by Korkut Öztekin

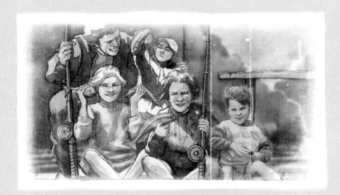

Dedicated to my children
Helen, Joe, Henry and Sam

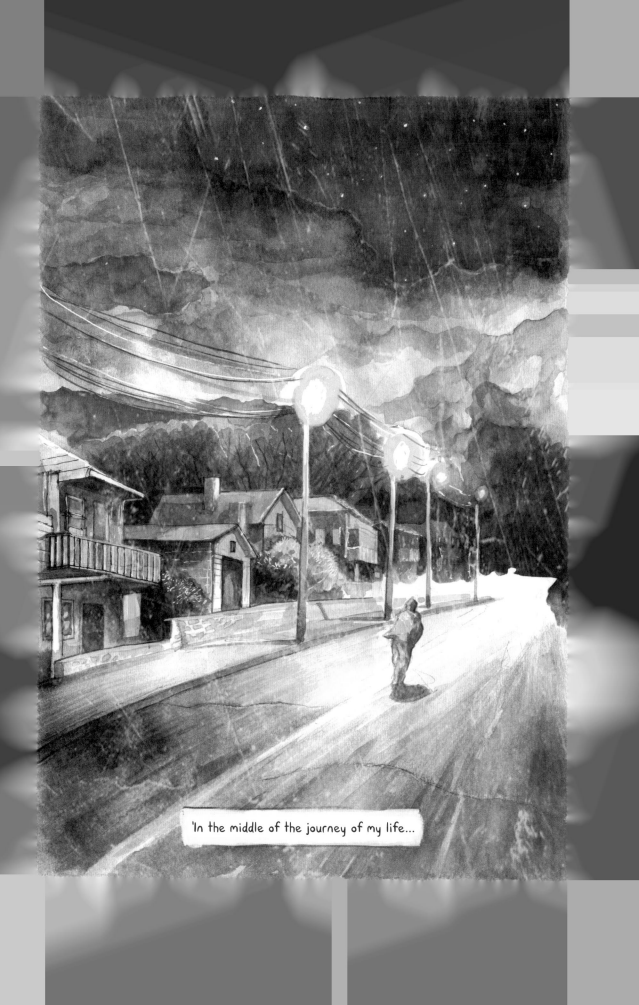

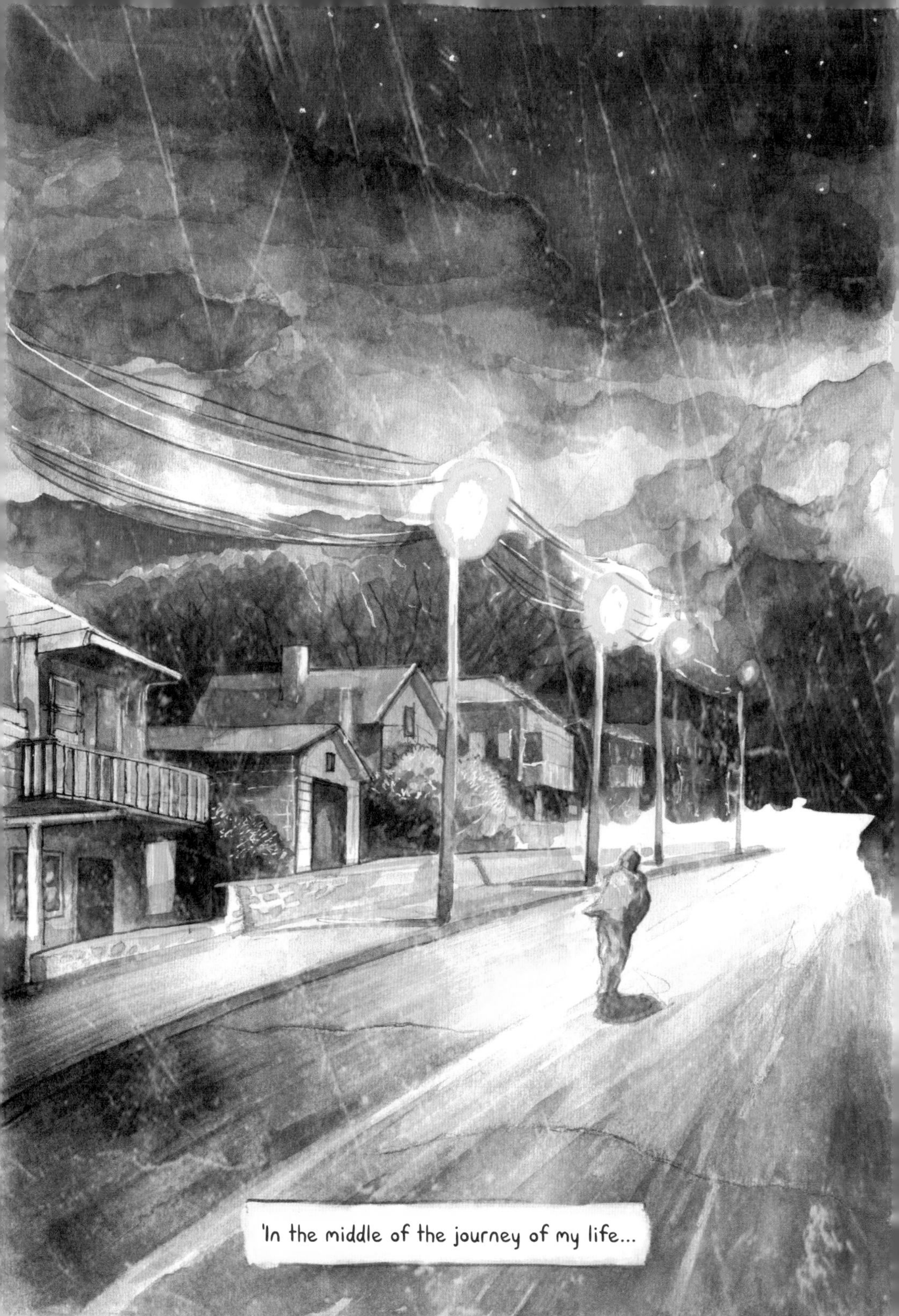
'In the middle of the journey of my life...

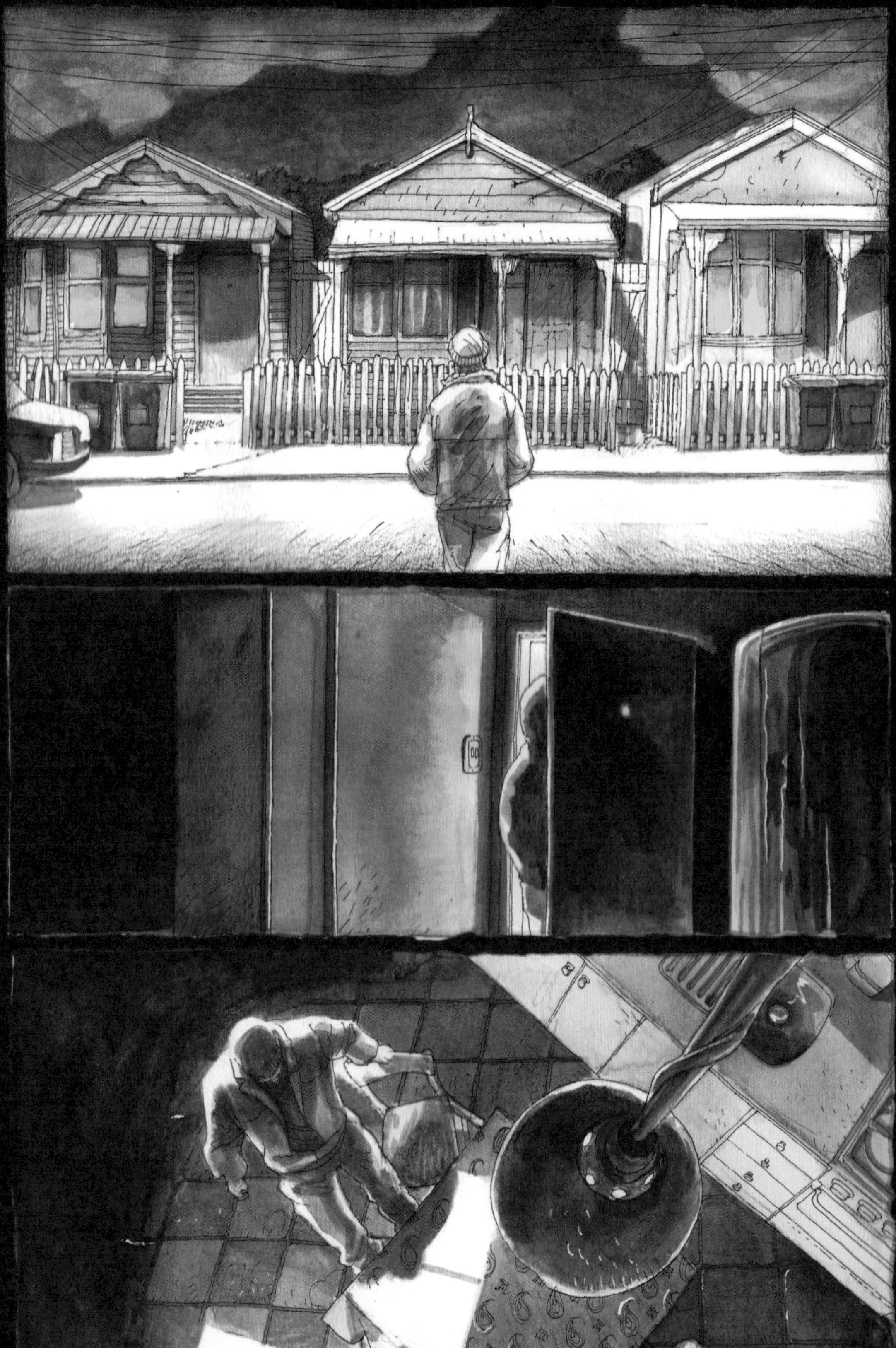

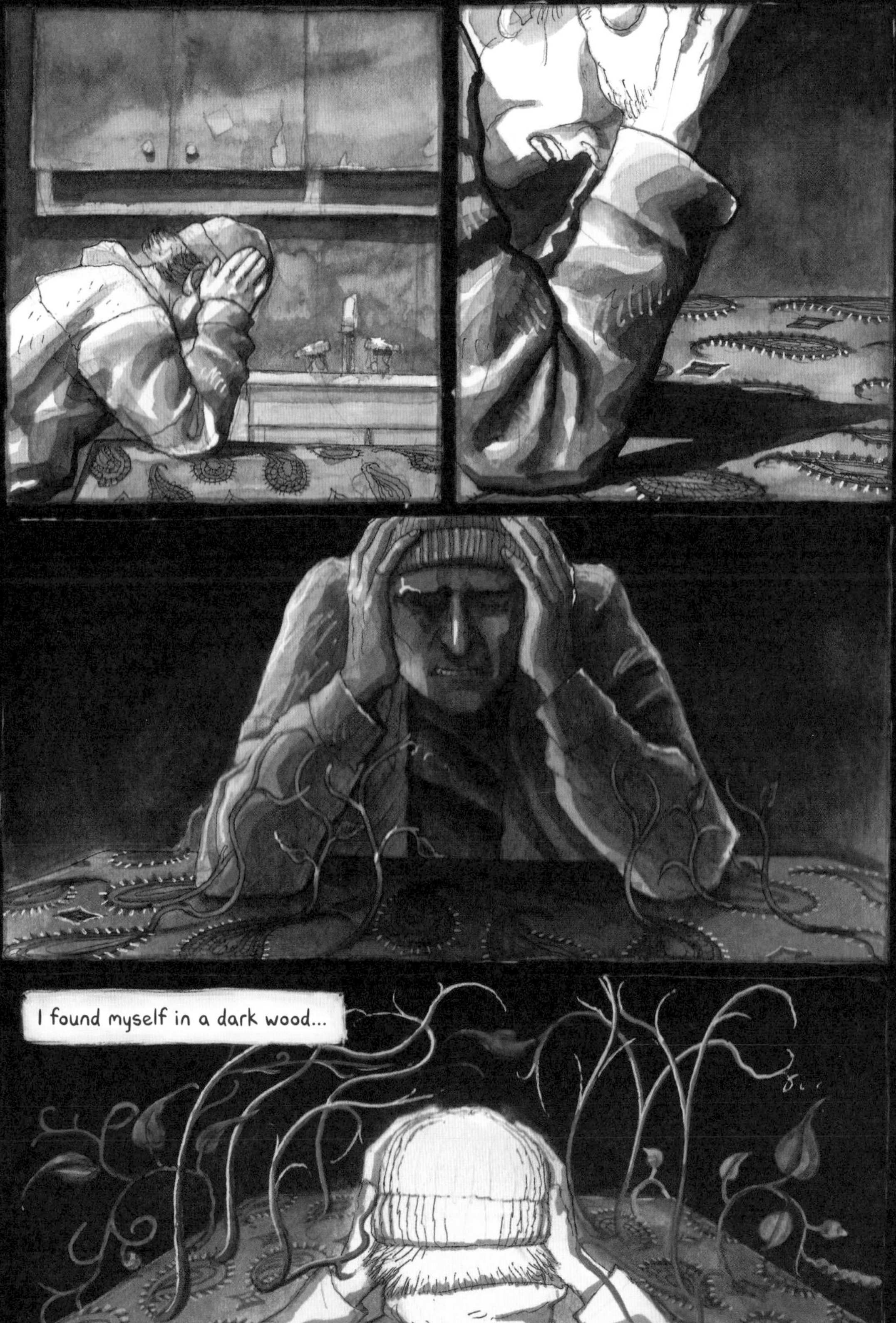
I found myself in a dark wood...

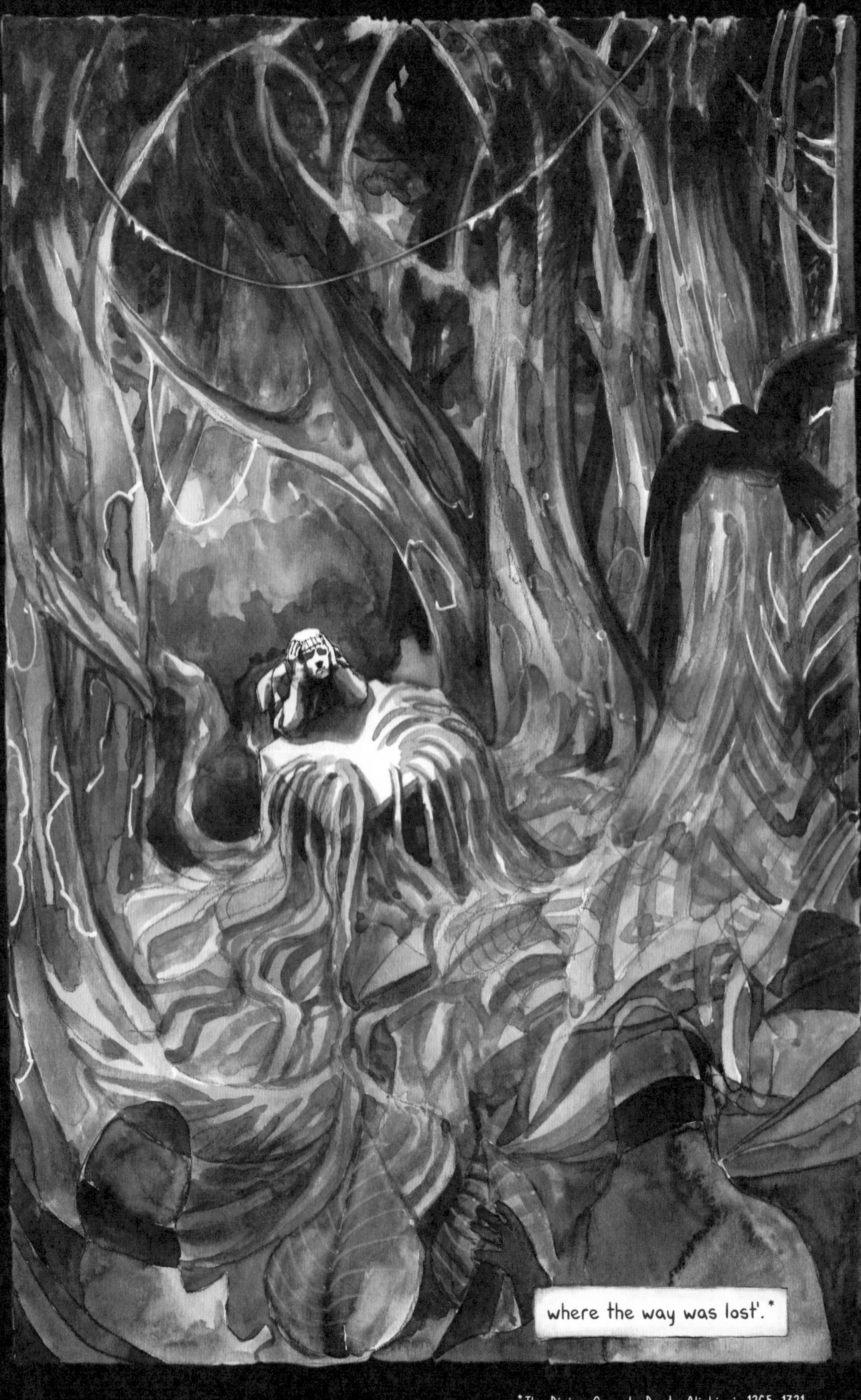
where the way was lost'.*

*The Divine Comedy, Dante Alighieri 1265-1321

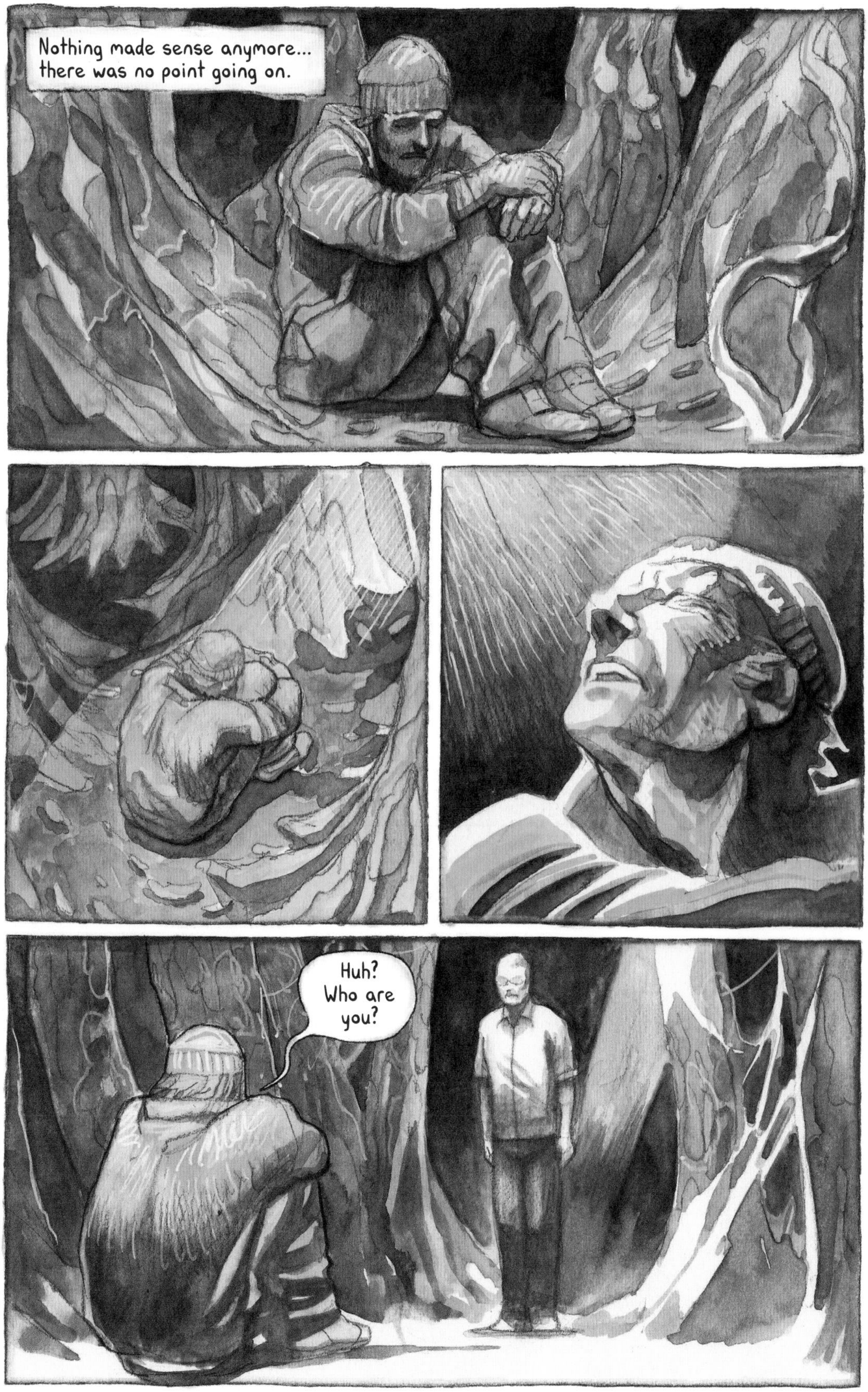
Nothing made sense anymore...
there was no point going on.
Huh?
Who are
you?

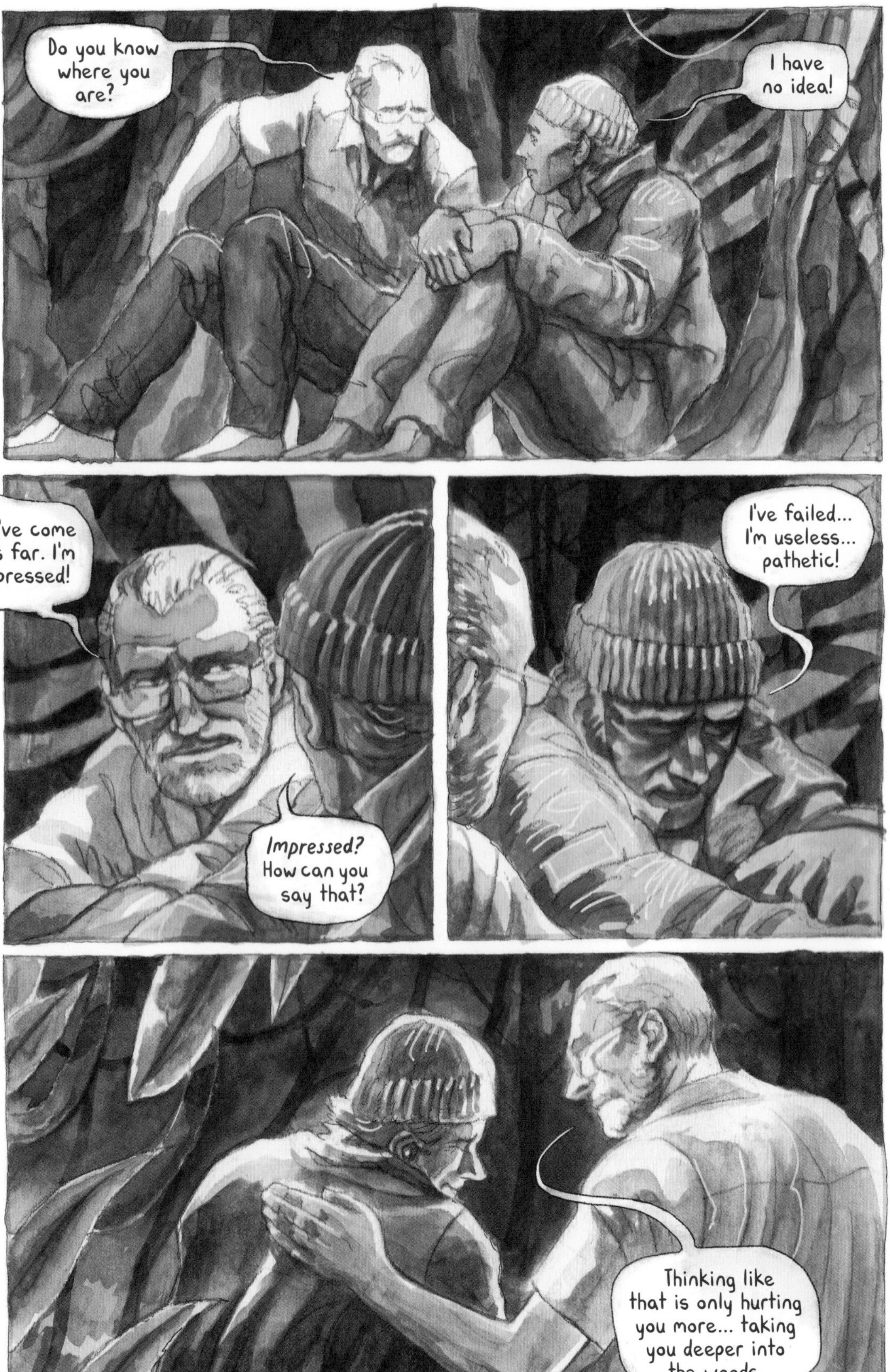
Do you know where you are?
I have no idea!
You've come this far. I'm impressed!
Impressed? How can you say that?
I've failed... I'm useless... pathetic!
Thinking like that is only hurting you more... taking you deeper into the woods.

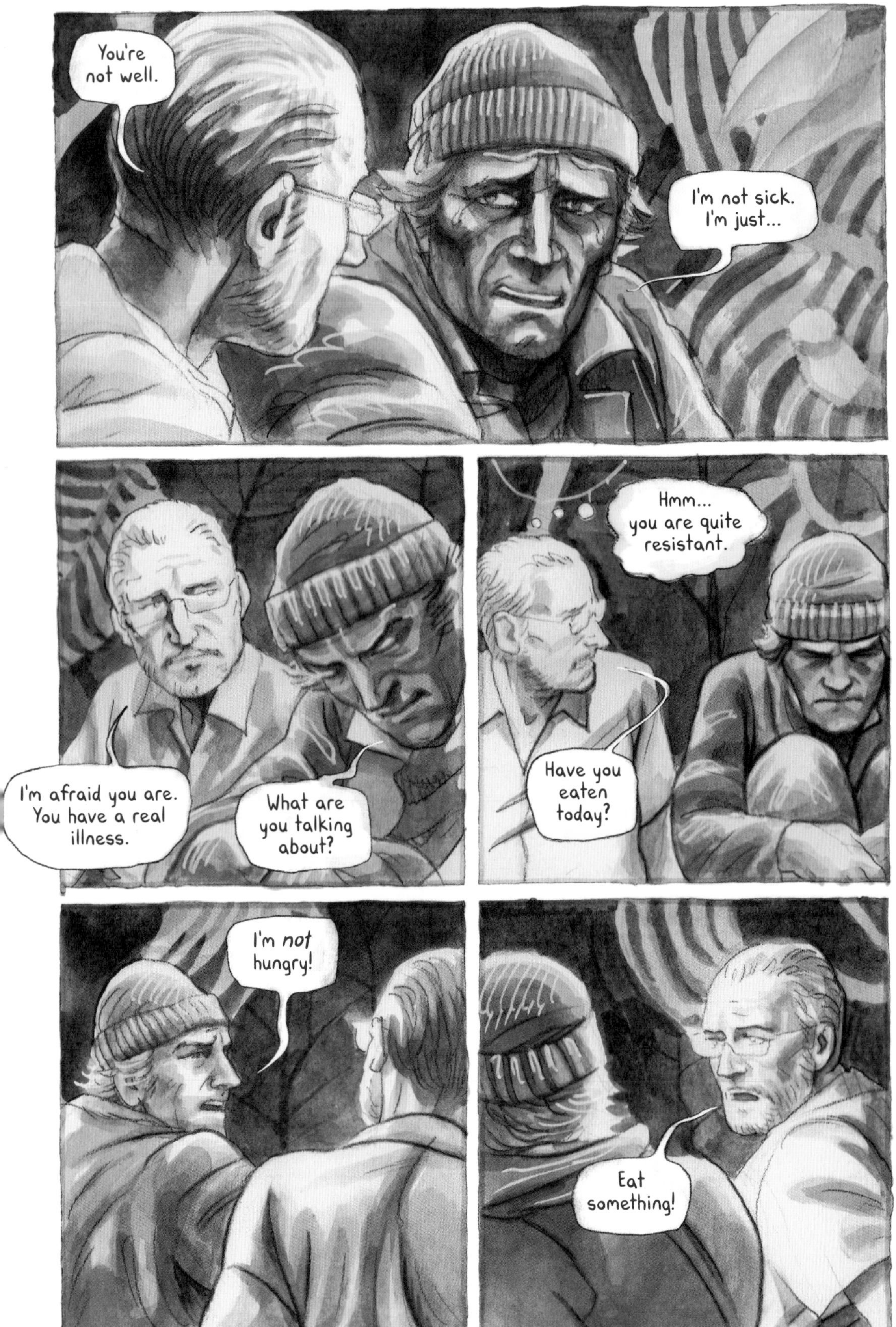
You're not well.
I'm not sick. I'm just...
I'm afraid you are. You have a real illness.
What are you talking about?
Hmm... you are quite resistant.
Have you eaten today?
I'm *not* hungry!
Eat something!

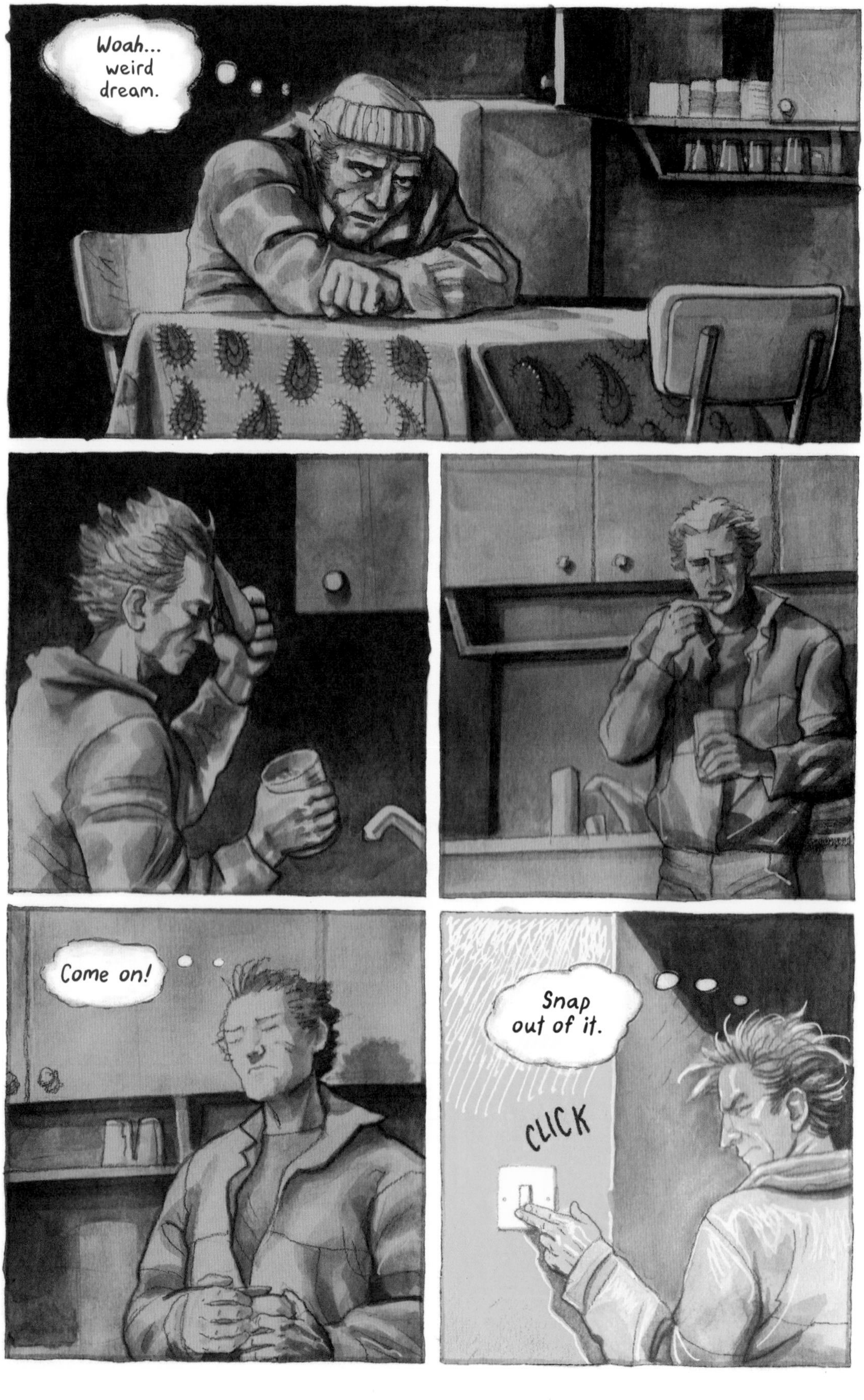
Woah...
weird
dream.
Come on!
Snap
out of it.
CLICK

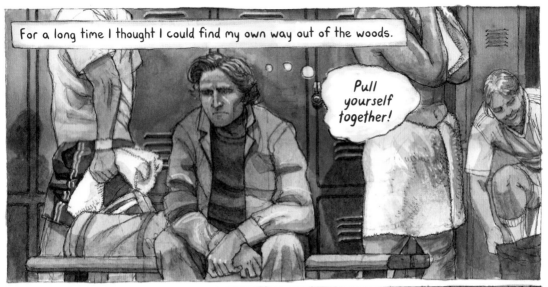

For a long time I thought I could find my own way out of the woods.

Pull yourself together!

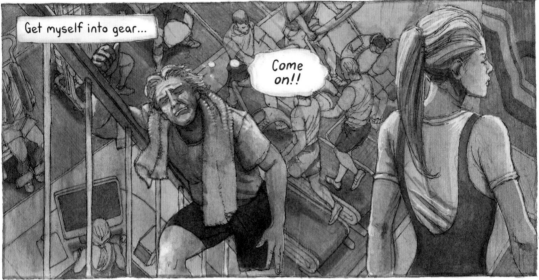

Get myself into gear...

Come on!!

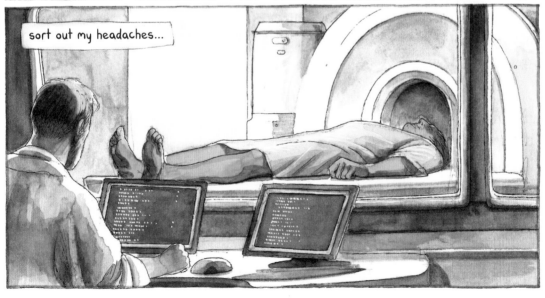

sort out my headaches...

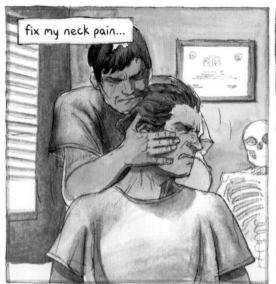

fix my neck pain...
find out why I wasn't sleeping.
I delved into all the possible causes...
I know I can beat this.
or at least the ones I could accept... adrenal fatigue, burnout, chronic fatigue, vitamin deficiency.
Fatigue - Wikipedia, the free encyclopedia
Fatigue (medical) - Wikipedia, the free encyclopedia
What is Fatigue? - Medical News Today
Kullanıcı oyu: 3,9 - 26 oy
Fatigue, Exhaustion and Muscle Weakness: Symptoms ...
I went on retreats and meditated.

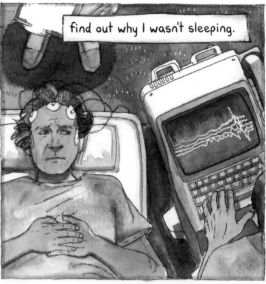

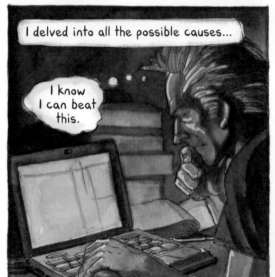

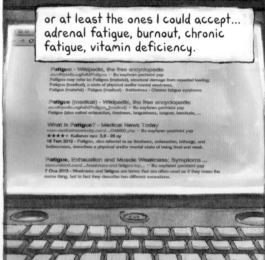

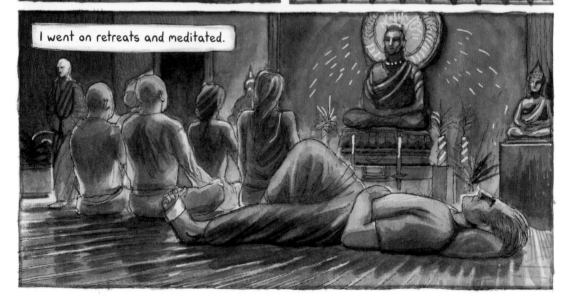

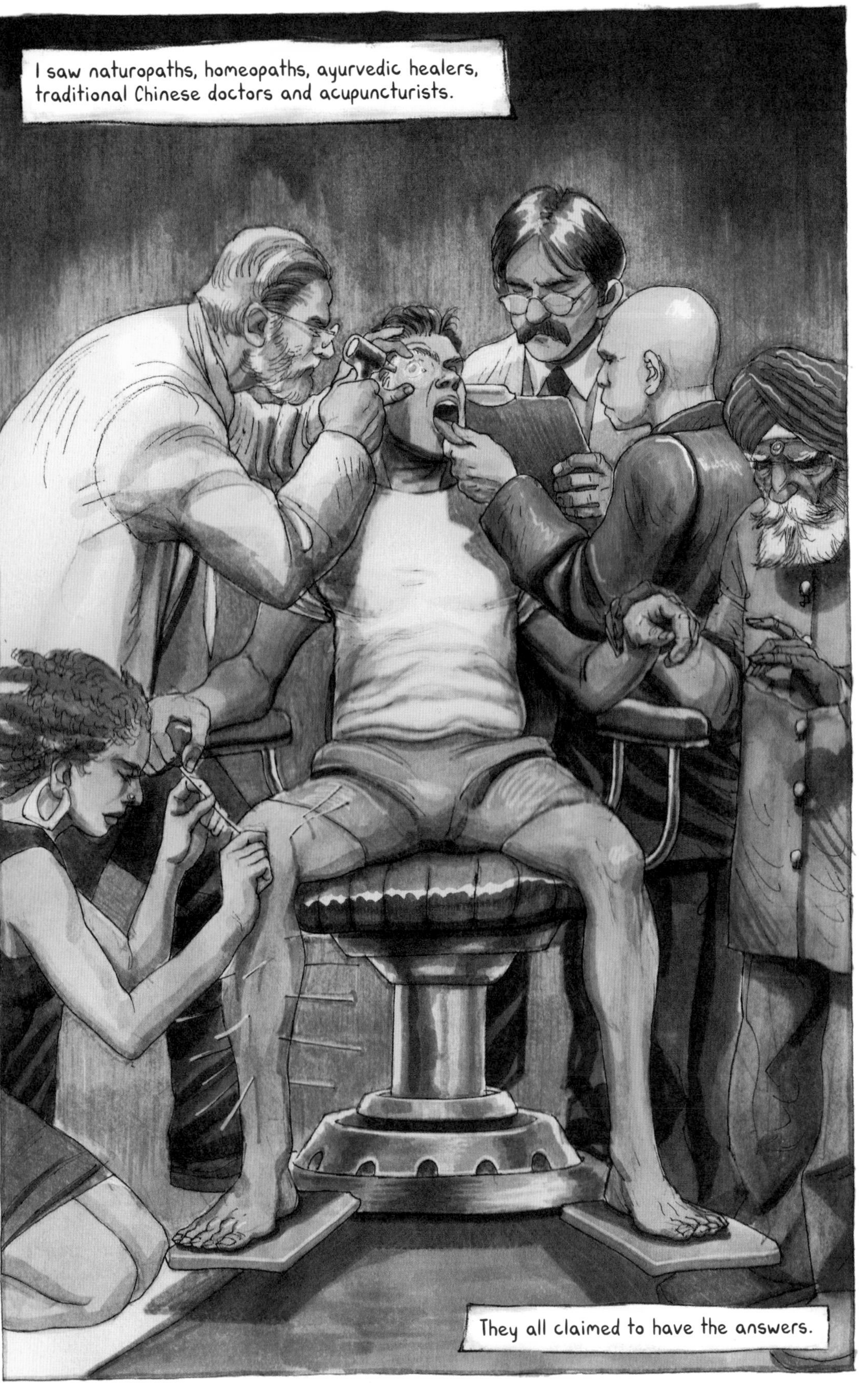
I saw naturopaths, homeopaths, ayurvedic healers, traditional Chinese doctors and acupuncturists.
They all claimed to have the answers.

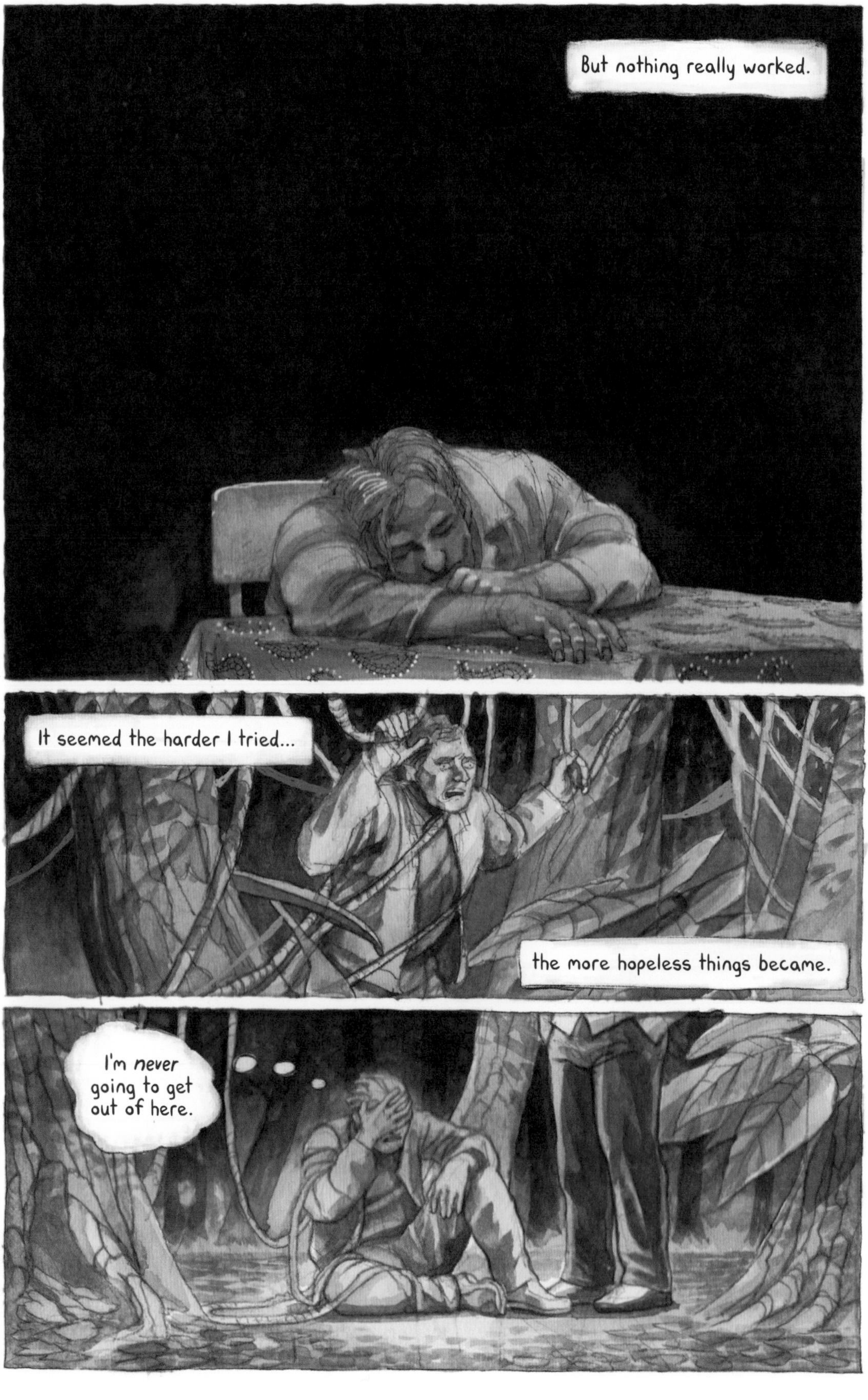
But nothing really worked.
It seemed the harder I tried...
the more hopeless things became.
I'm *never* going to get out of here.

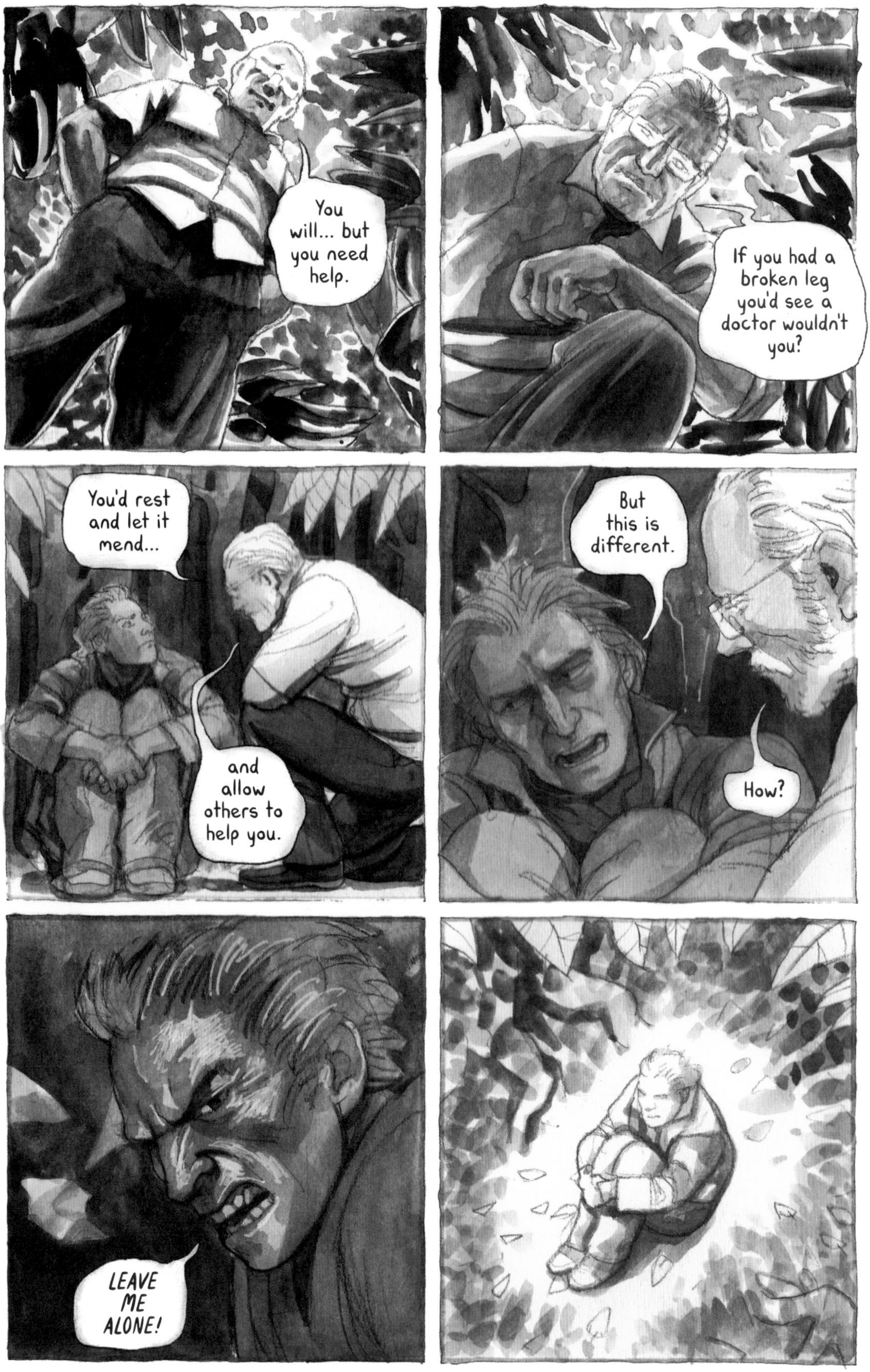
You will... but you need help.
If you had a broken leg you'd see a doctor wouldn't you?
You'd rest and let it mend...
and allow others to help you.
But this is different.
How?
LEAVE ME ALONE!

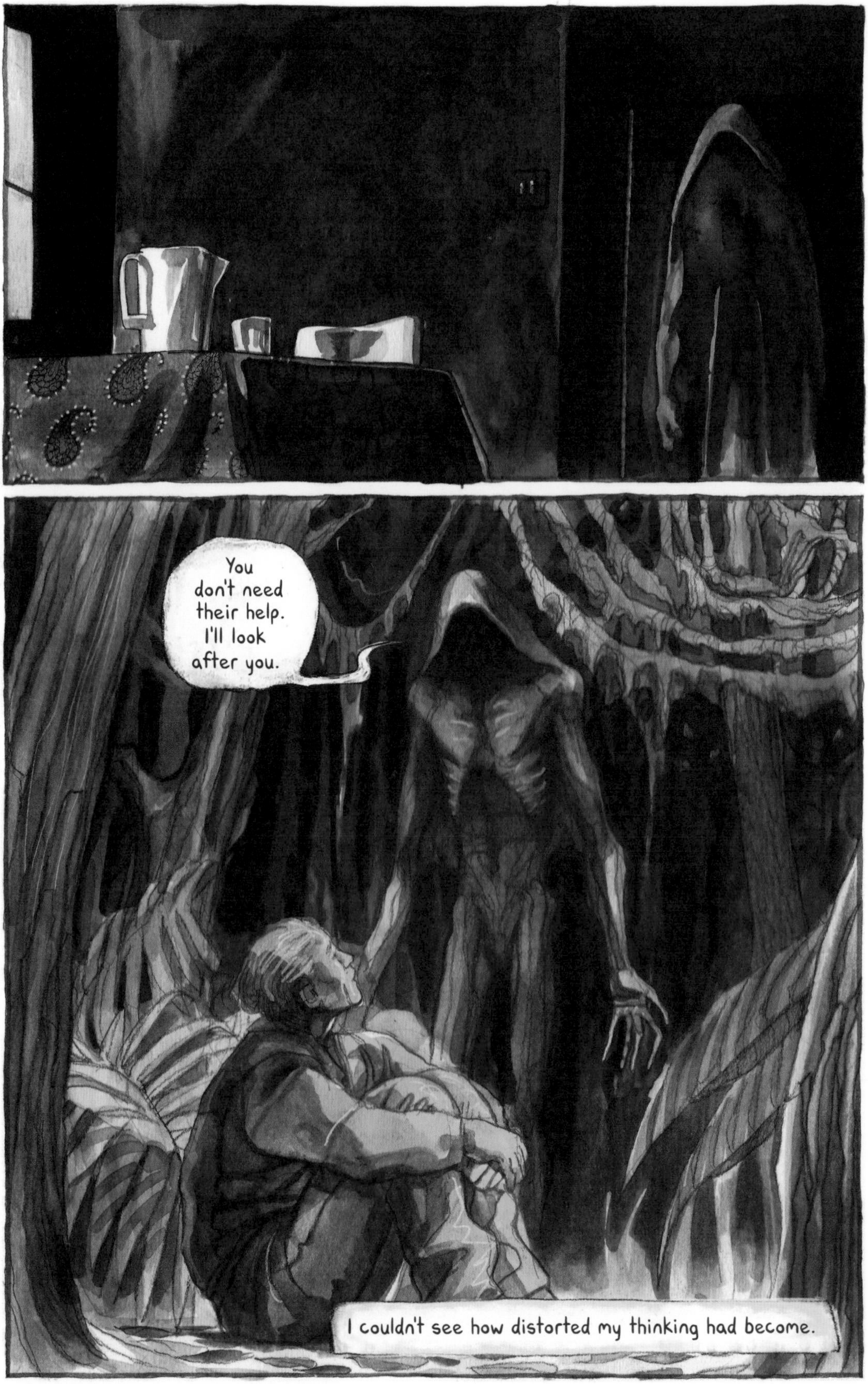
You don't need their help. I'll look after you.
I couldn't see how distorted my thinking had become.

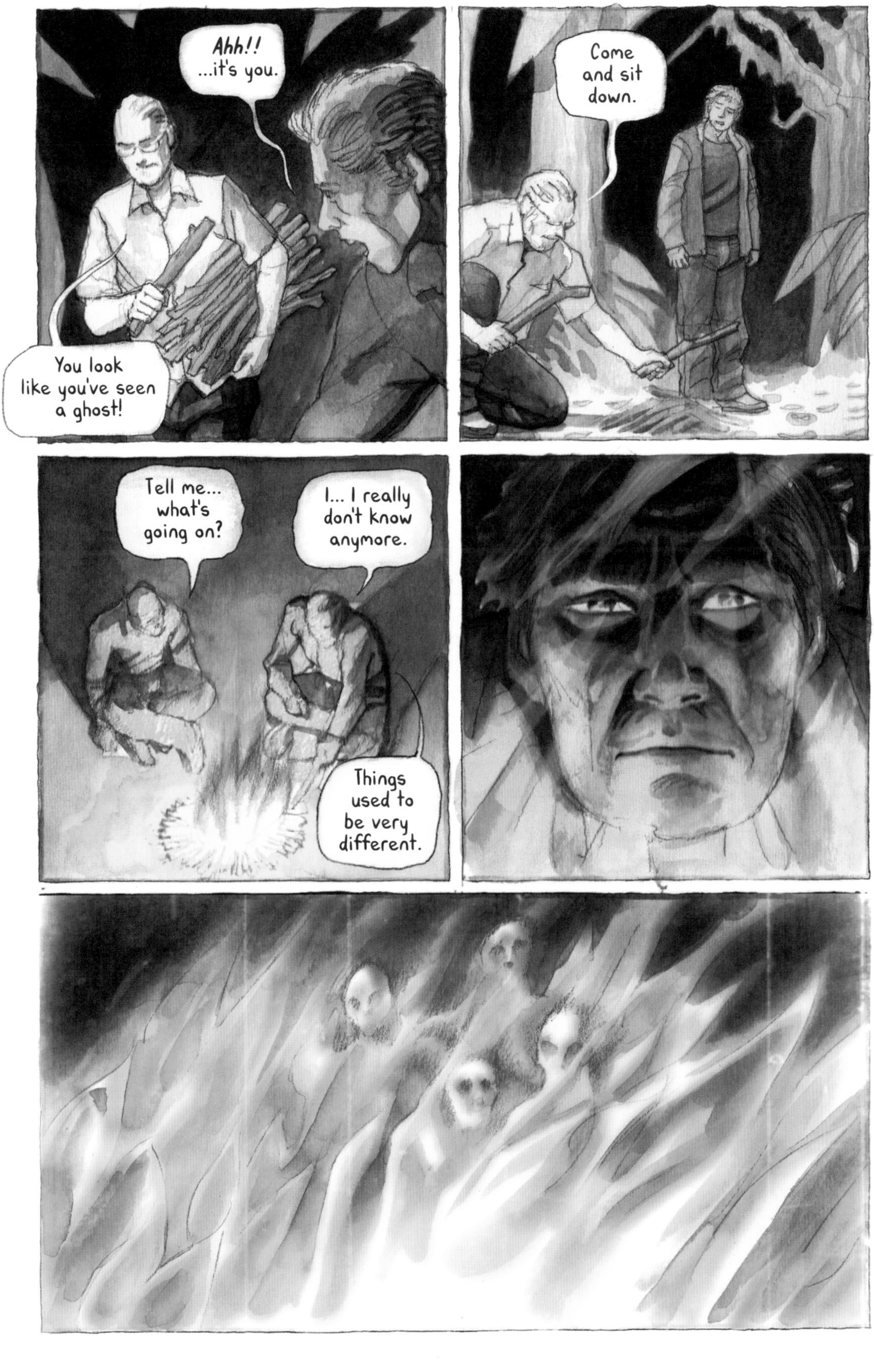
Ahh!! ...it's you.
You look like you've seen a ghost!
Come and sit down.
Tell me... what's going on?
I... I really don't know anymore.
Things used to be very different.

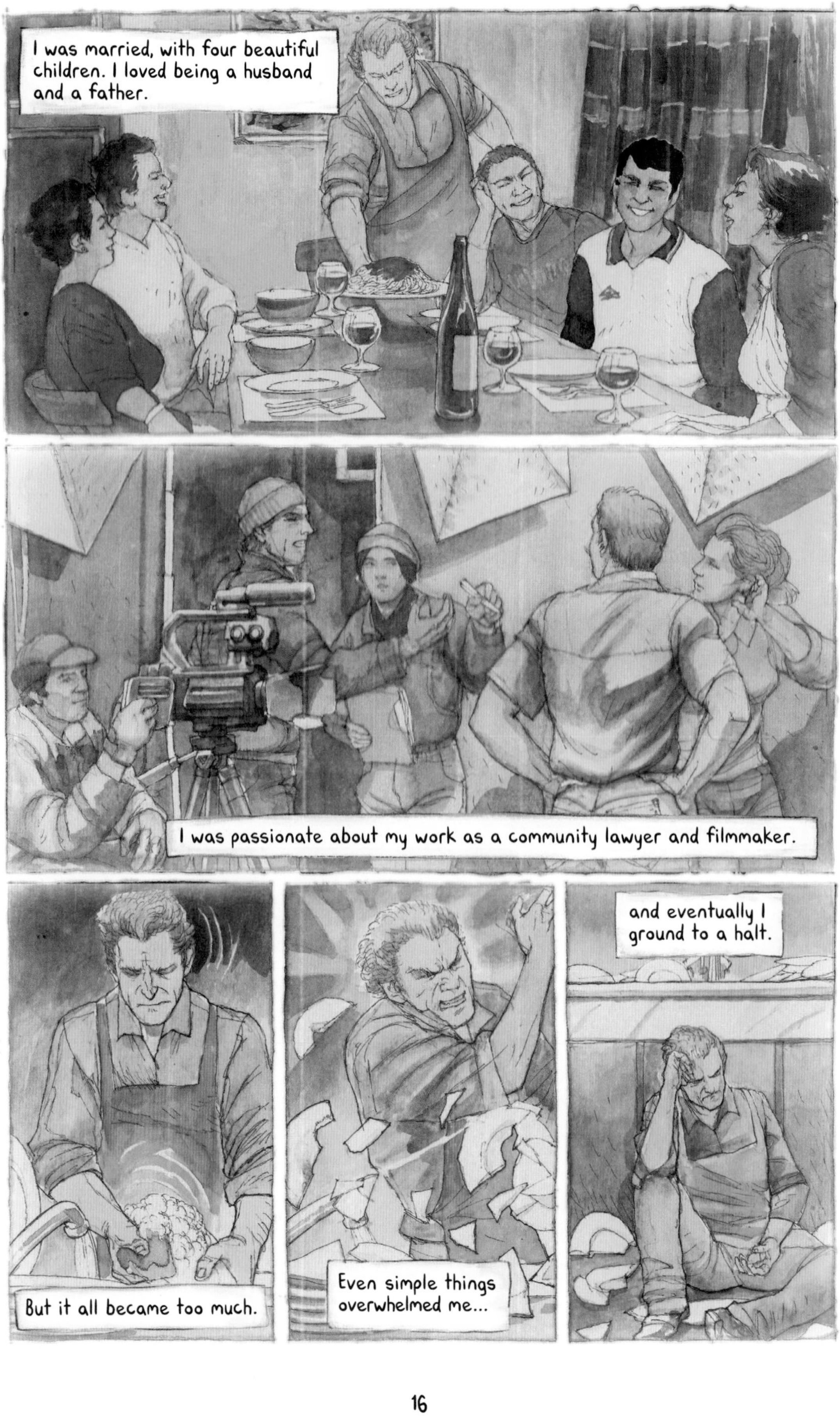
I was married, with four beautiful children. I loved being a husband and a father.
I was passionate about my work as a community lawyer and filmmaker.
But it all became too much.
Even simple things overwhelmed me...
and eventually I ground to a halt.

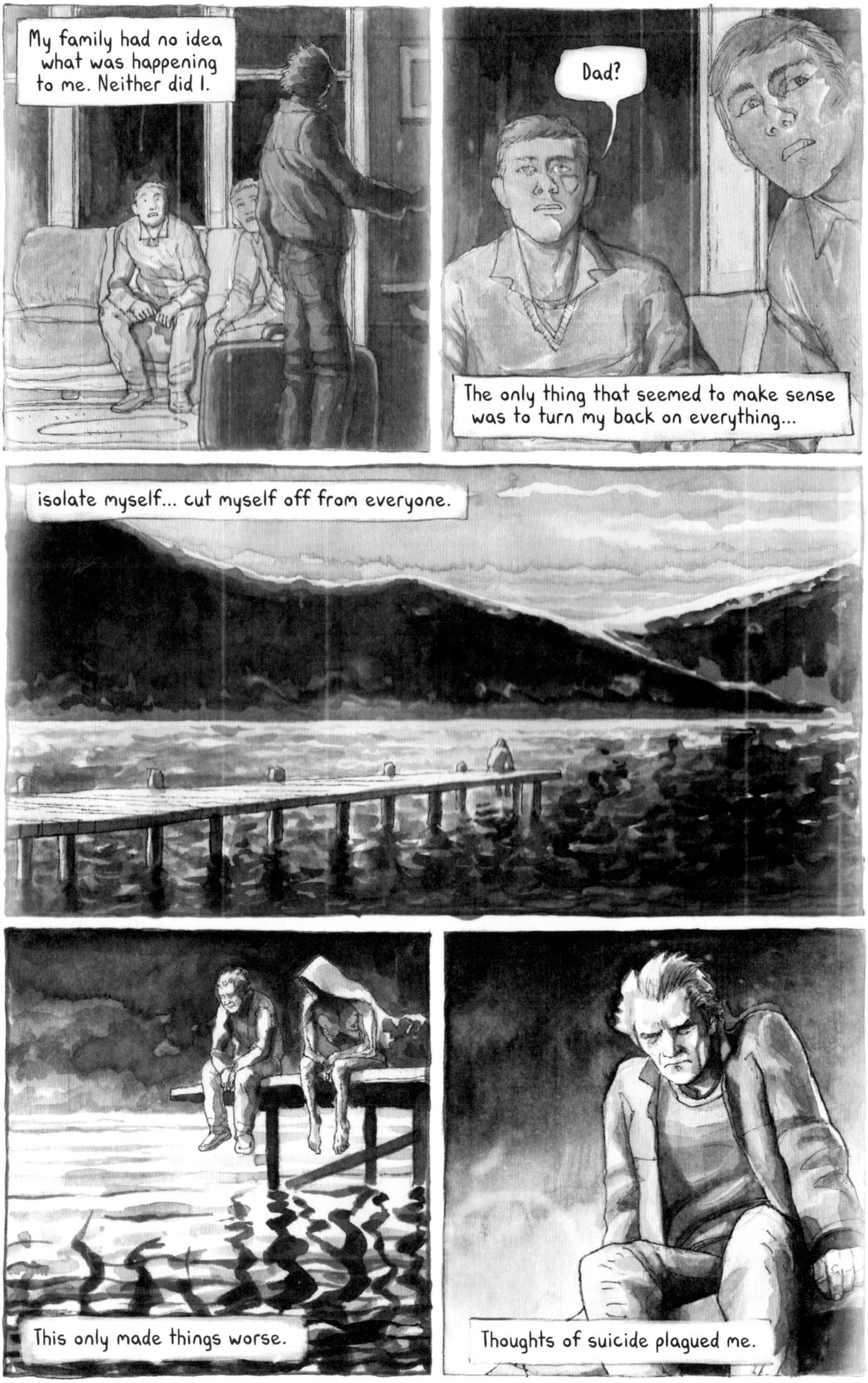
My family had no idea what was happening to me. Neither did I.
Dad?
The only thing that seemed to make sense was to turn my back on everything...
isolate myself... cut myself off from everyone.
This only made things worse.
Thoughts of suicide plagued me.

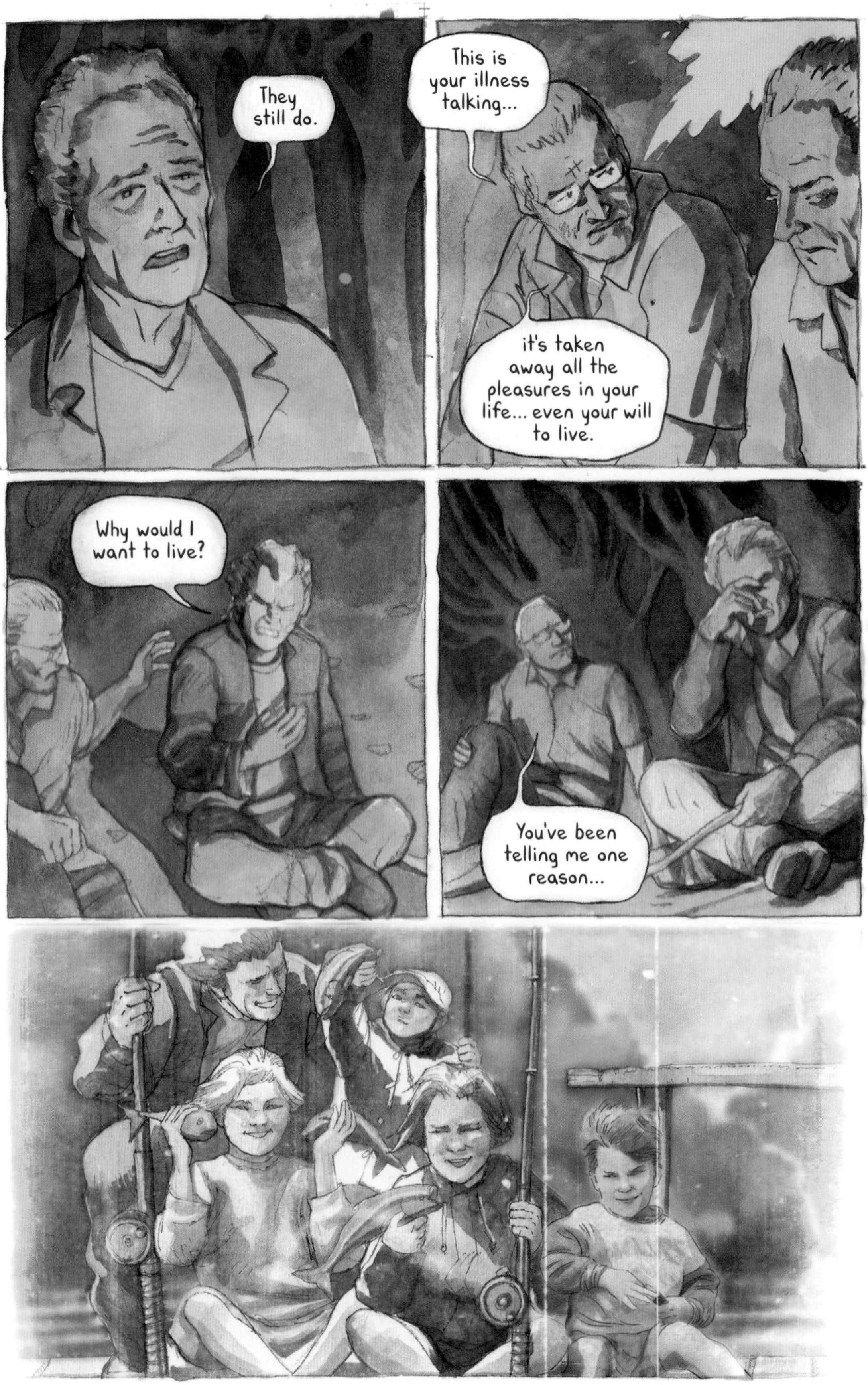
They still do.
This is your illness talking...
it's taken away all the pleasures in your life... even your will to live.
Why would I want to live?
You've been telling me one reason...

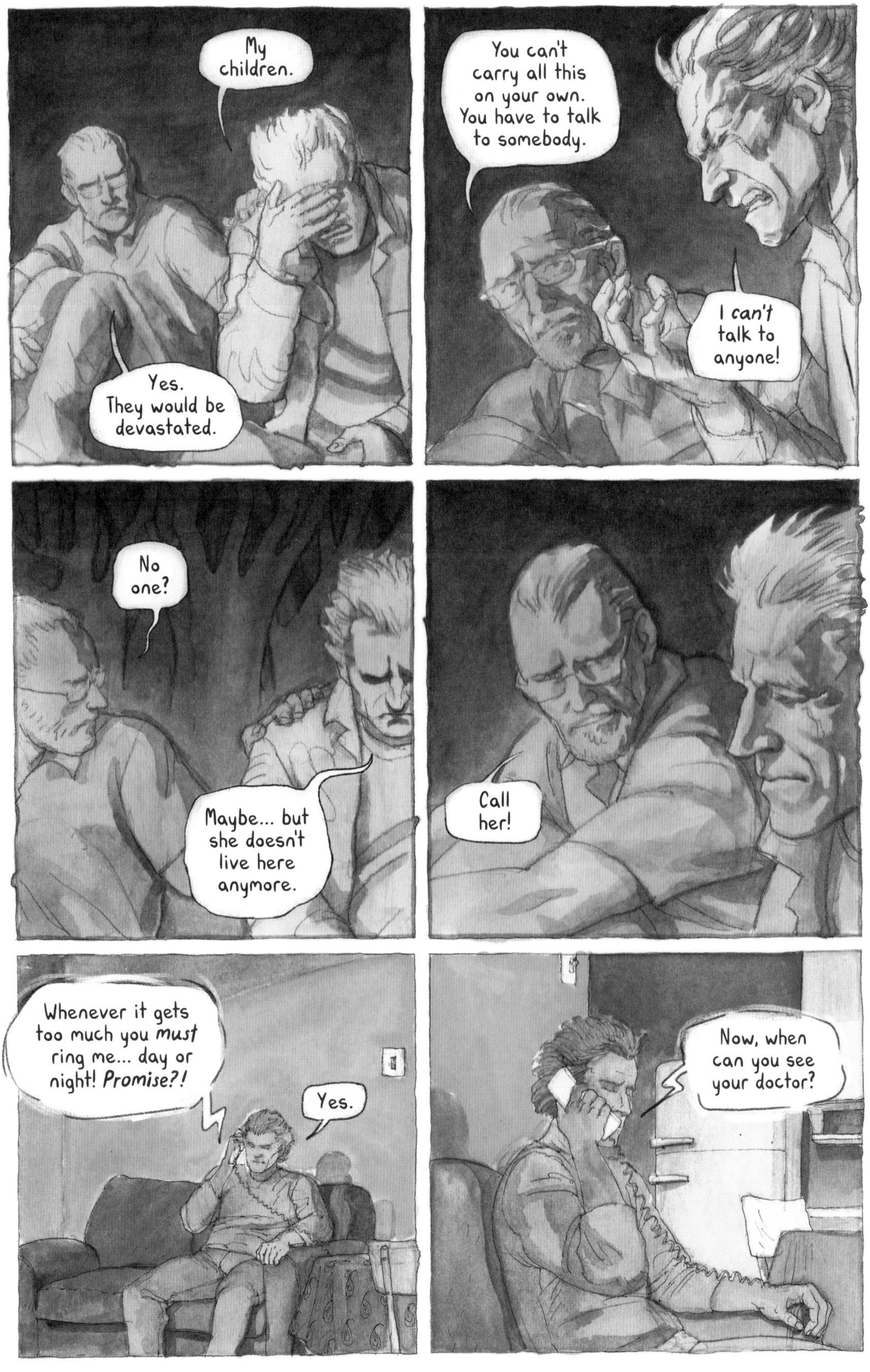
My children.
Yes. They would be devastated.
You can't carry all this on your own. You have to talk to somebody.
I can't talk to anyone!
No one?
Maybe... but she doesn't live here anymore.
Call her!
Whenever it gets too much you *must* ring me... day or night! *Promise?!*
Yes.
Now, when can you see your doctor?

Later that week...
Wellington GPs
Your rash will clear up in a few weeks with this cream. Everything else ok?
Yeah, good thanks.
Ah...
Yes?
Actually... I haven't been feeling so good lately...
Sit down.
What's going on?
I... I don't know. It's so hard to make sense of it.

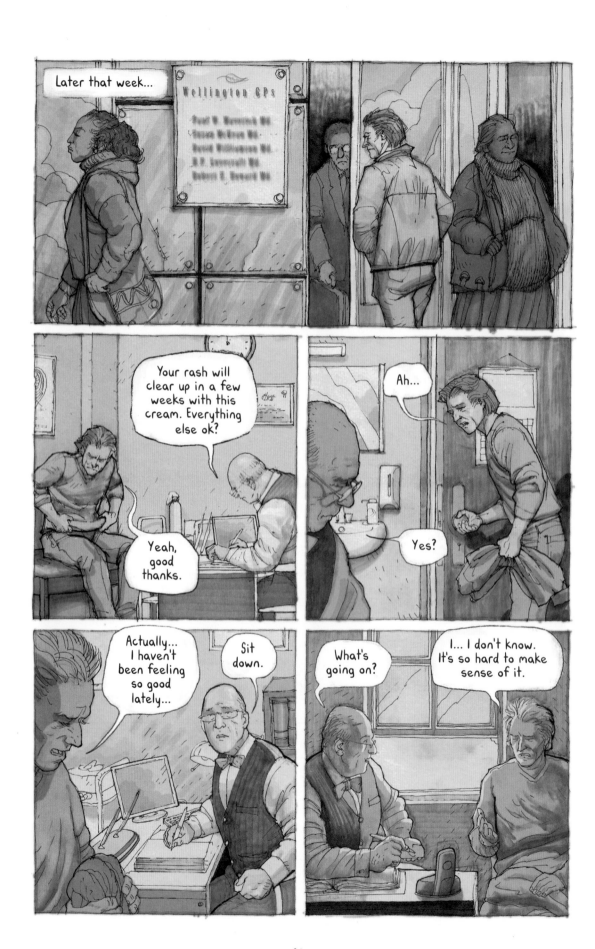

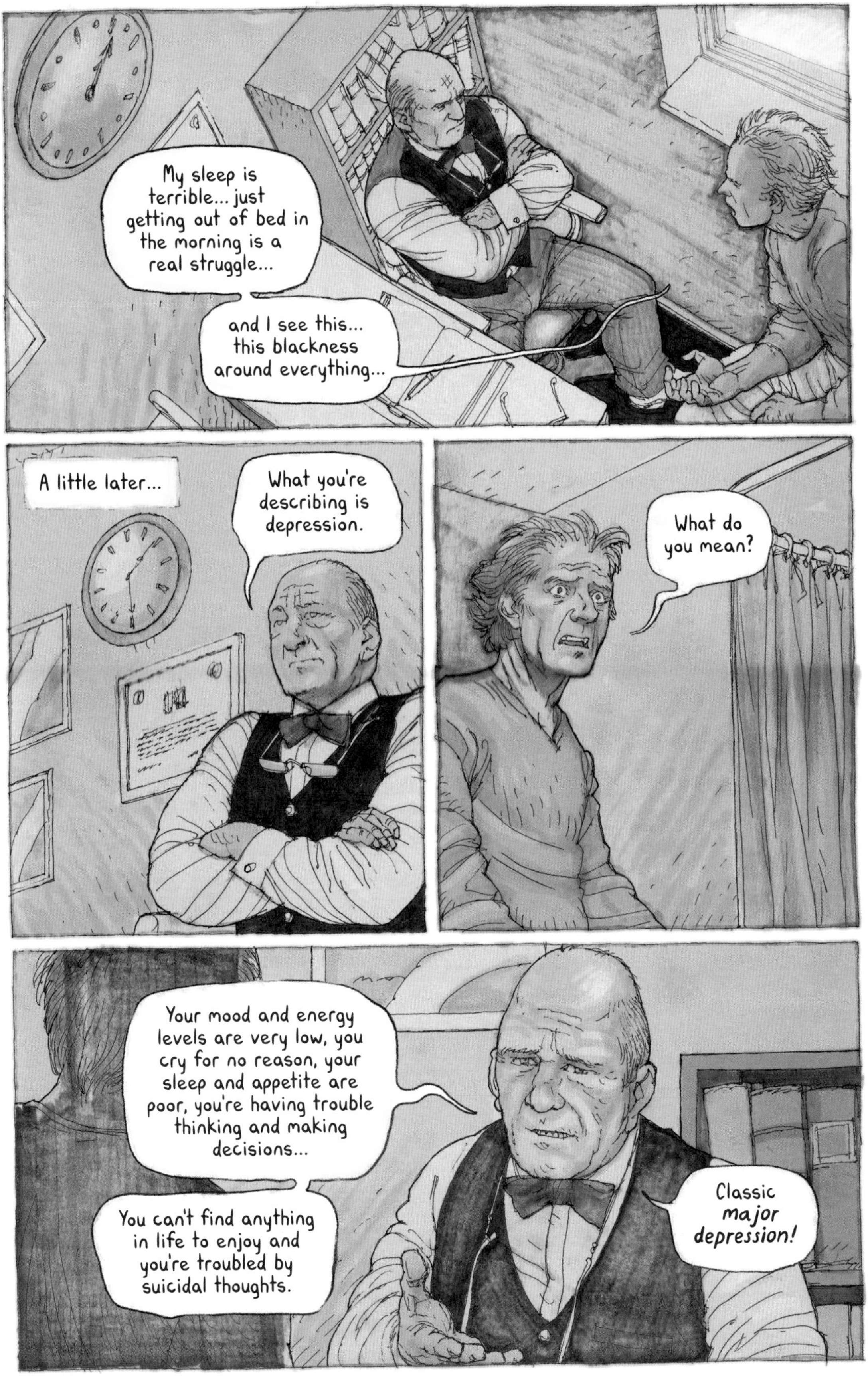
My sleep is terrible... just getting out of bed in the morning is a real struggle...
and I see this... this blackness around everything...
A little later...
What you're describing is depression.
What do you mean?
Your mood and energy levels are very low, you cry for no reason, your sleep and appetite are poor, you're having trouble thinking and making decisions...
You can't find anything in life to enjoy and you're troubled by suicidal thoughts.
Classic *major depression!*

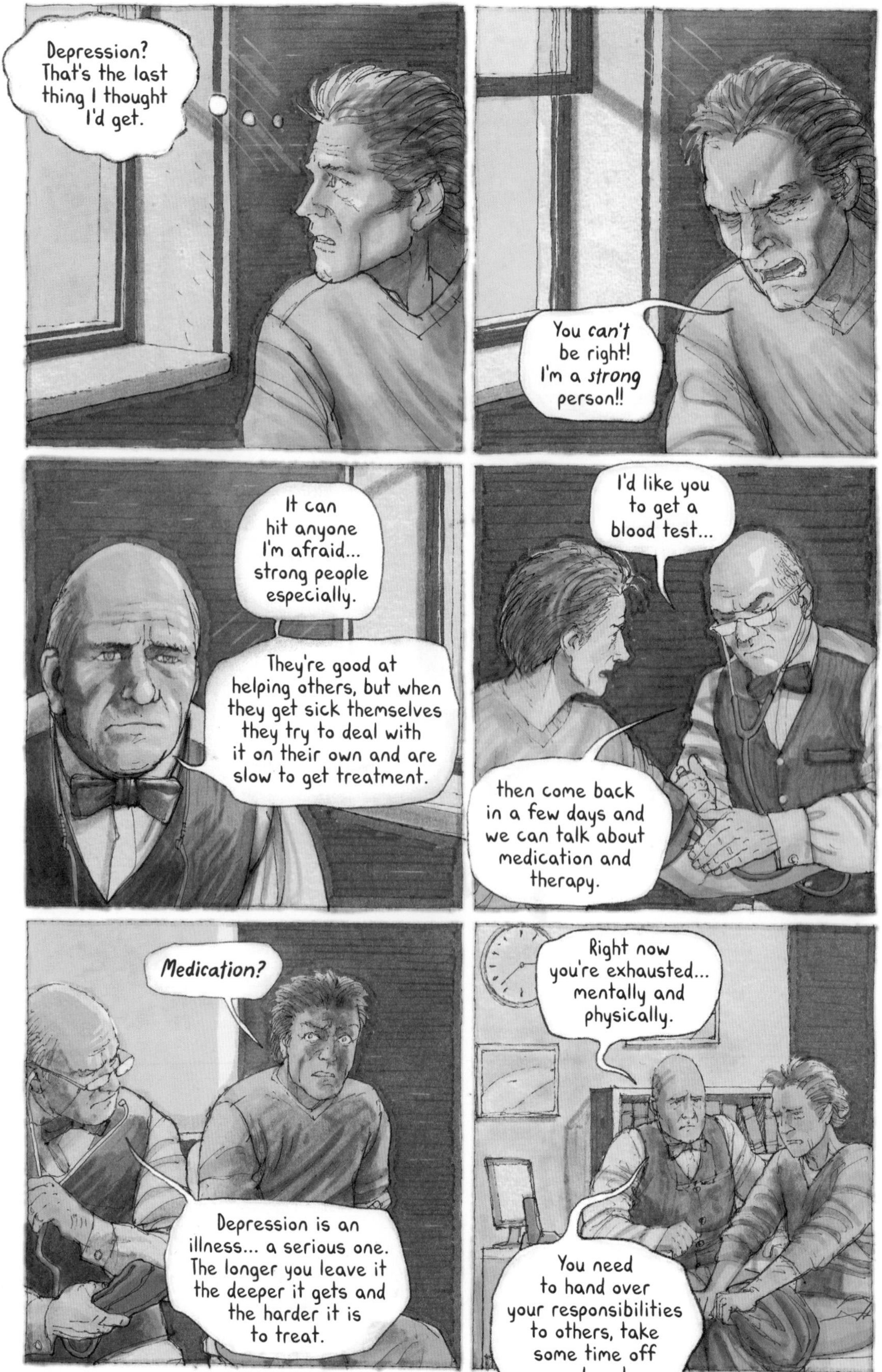
Depression? That's the last thing I thought I'd get.
You can't be right! I'm a strong person!!
It can hit anyone I'm afraid... strong people especially.
They're good at helping others, but when they get sick themselves they try to deal with it on their own and are slow to get treatment.
I'd like you to get a blood test...
then come back in a few days and we can talk about medication and therapy.
Medication?
Depression is an illness... a serious one. The longer you leave it the deeper it gets and the harder it is to treat.
Right now you're exhausted... mentally and physically.
You need to hand over your responsibilities to others, take some time off and rest.

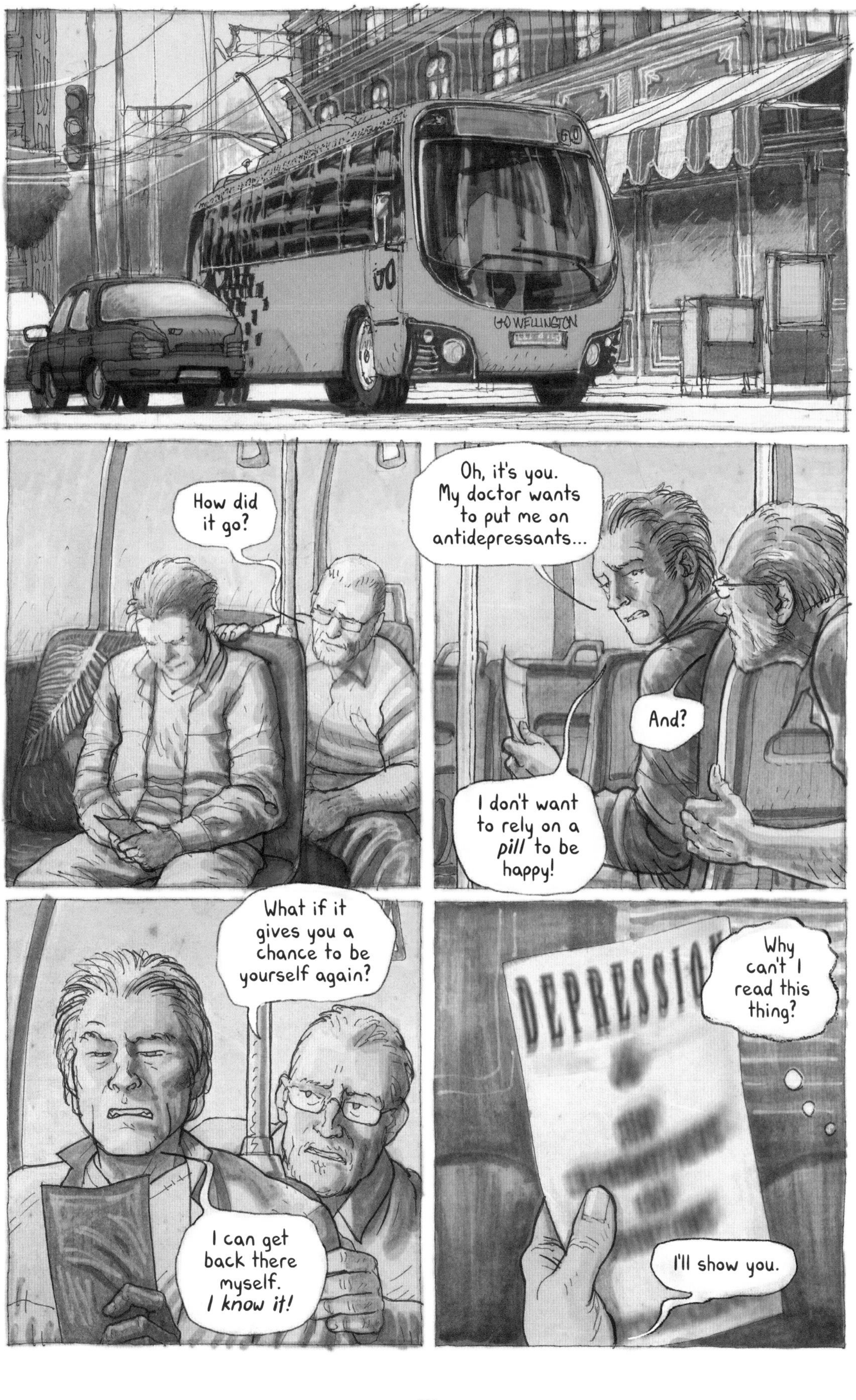
GO WELLINGTON
How did it go?
Oh, it's you. My doctor wants to put me on antidepressants...
And?
I don't want to rely on a *pill* to be happy!
What if it gives you a chance to be yourself again?
I can get back there myself. *I know it!*
DEPRESSIO
Why can't I read this thing?
I'll show you.

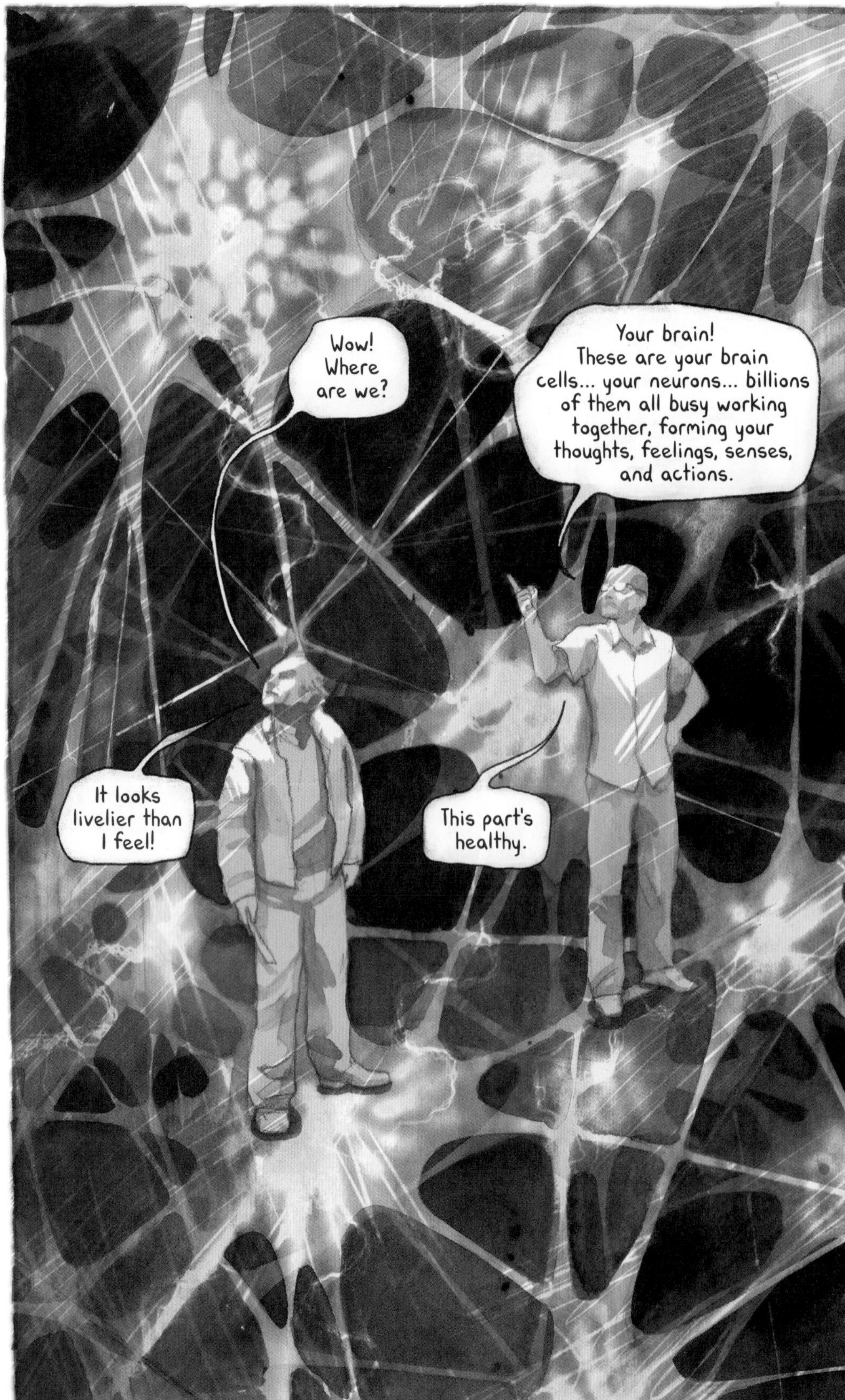
Wow! Where are we?
Your brain! These are your brain cells... your neurons... billions of them all busy working together, forming your thoughts, feelings, senses, and actions.
It looks livelier than I feel!
This part's healthy.

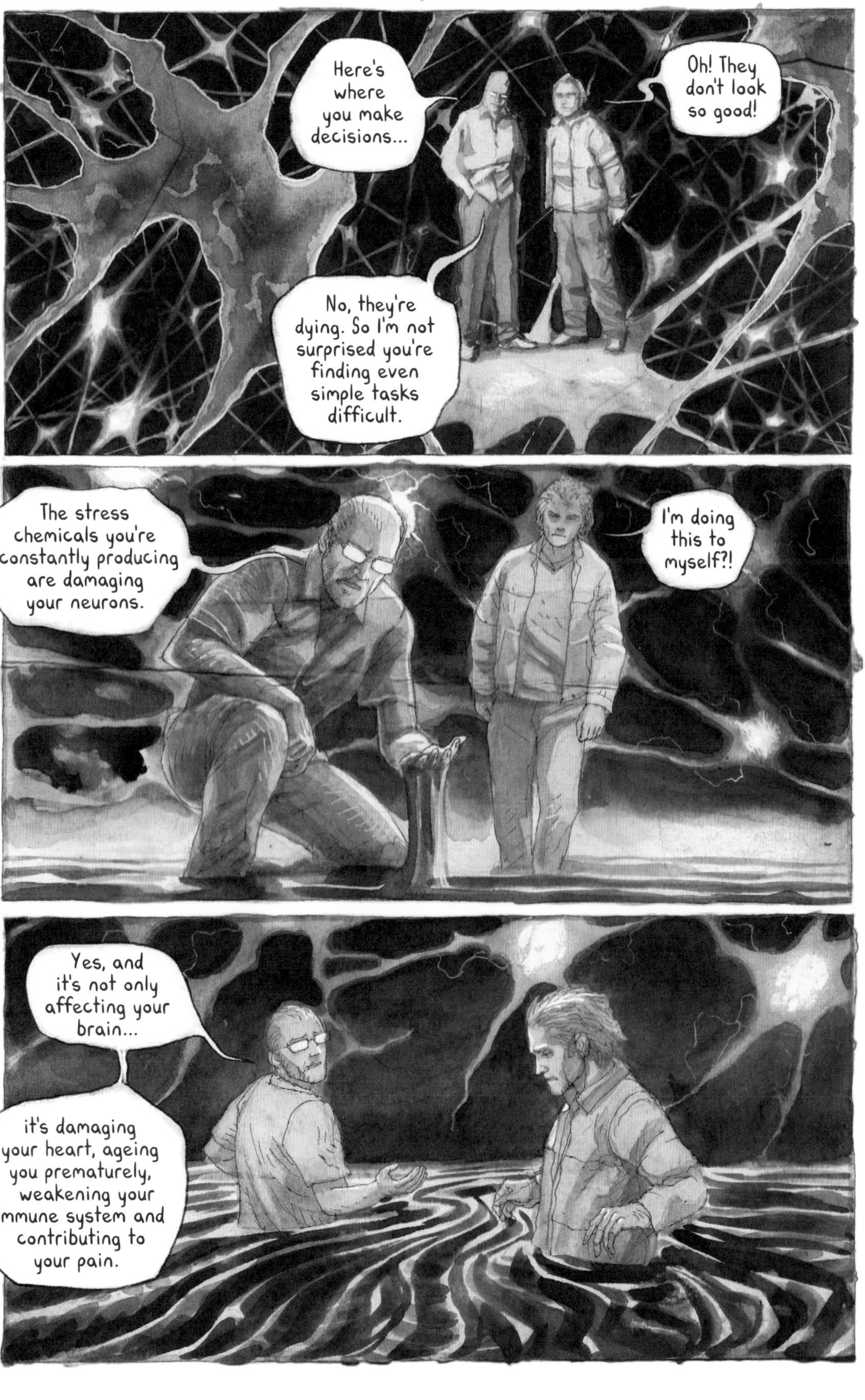
Here's where you make decisions...
Oh! They don't look so good!
No, they're dying. So I'm not surprised you're finding even simple tasks difficult.
The stress chemicals you're constantly producing are damaging your neurons.
I'm doing this to myself?!
Yes, and it's not only affecting your brain...
it's damaging your heart, ageing you prematurely, weakening your immune system and contributing to your pain.

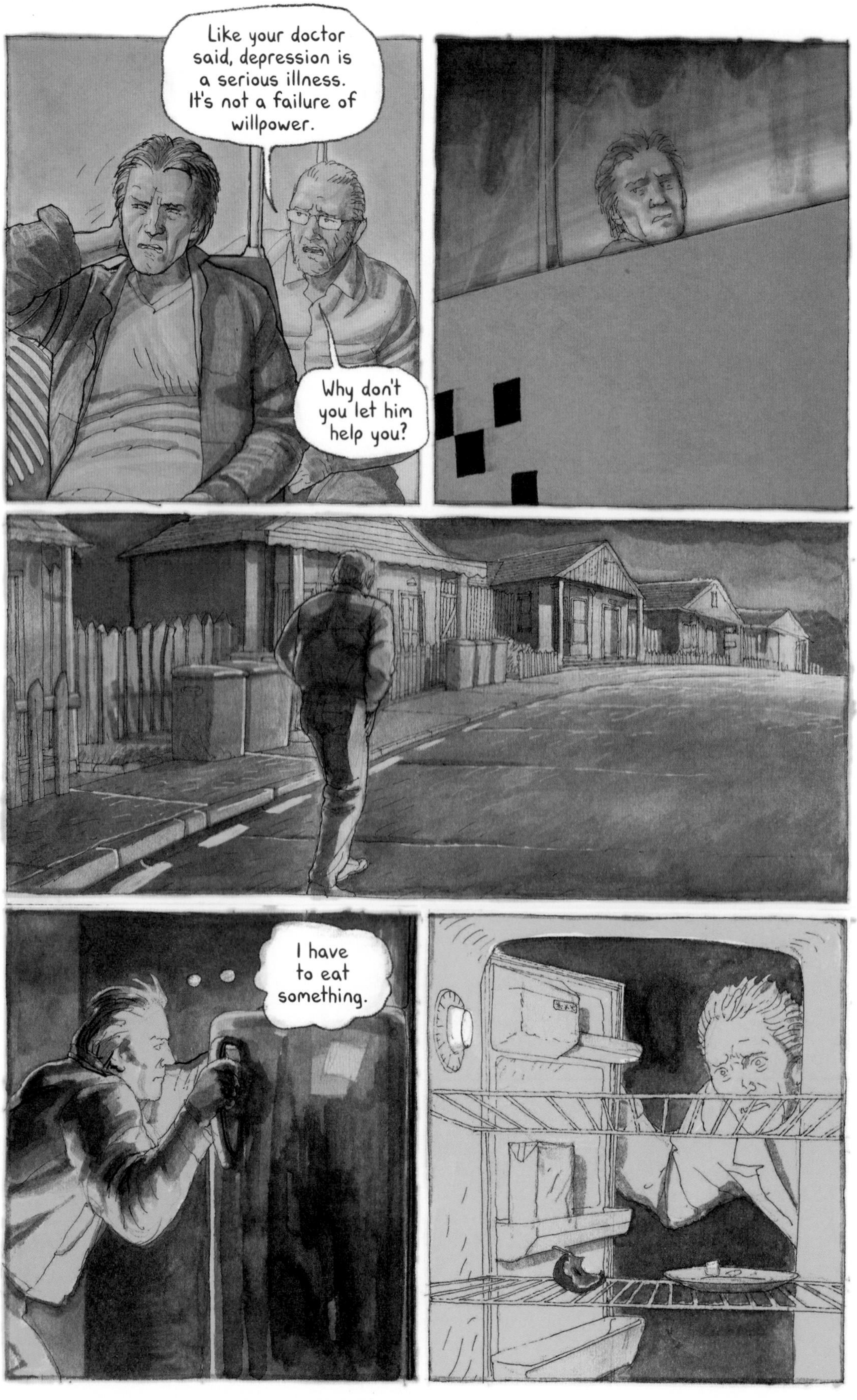
Like your doctor said, depression is a serious illness. It's not a failure of willpower.
Why don't you let him help you?
I have to eat something.

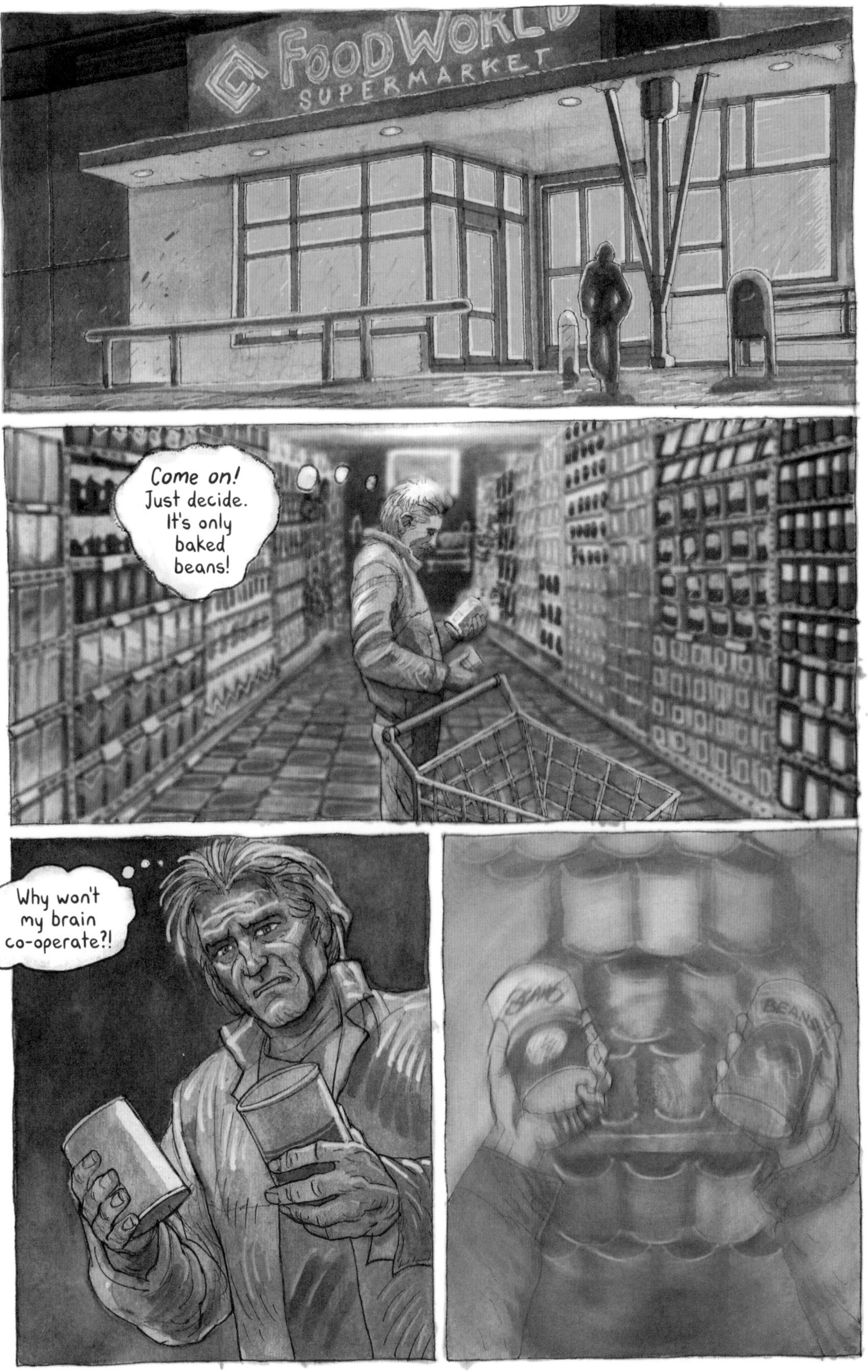
FOOD WORLD
SUPERMARKET
Come on! Just decide. It's only baked beans!
Why won't my brain co-operate?!
BEANS

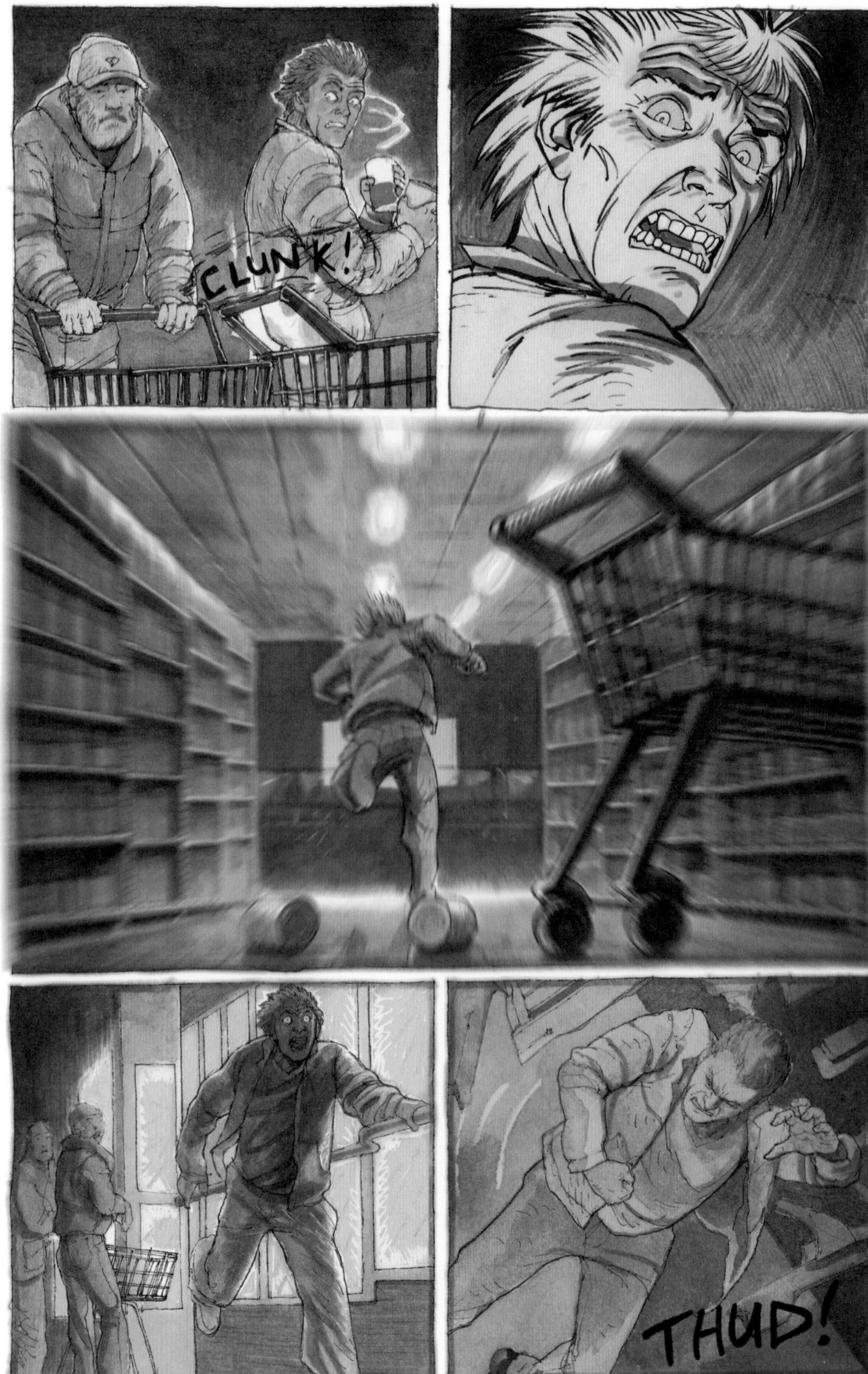
CLUNK!
THUD!

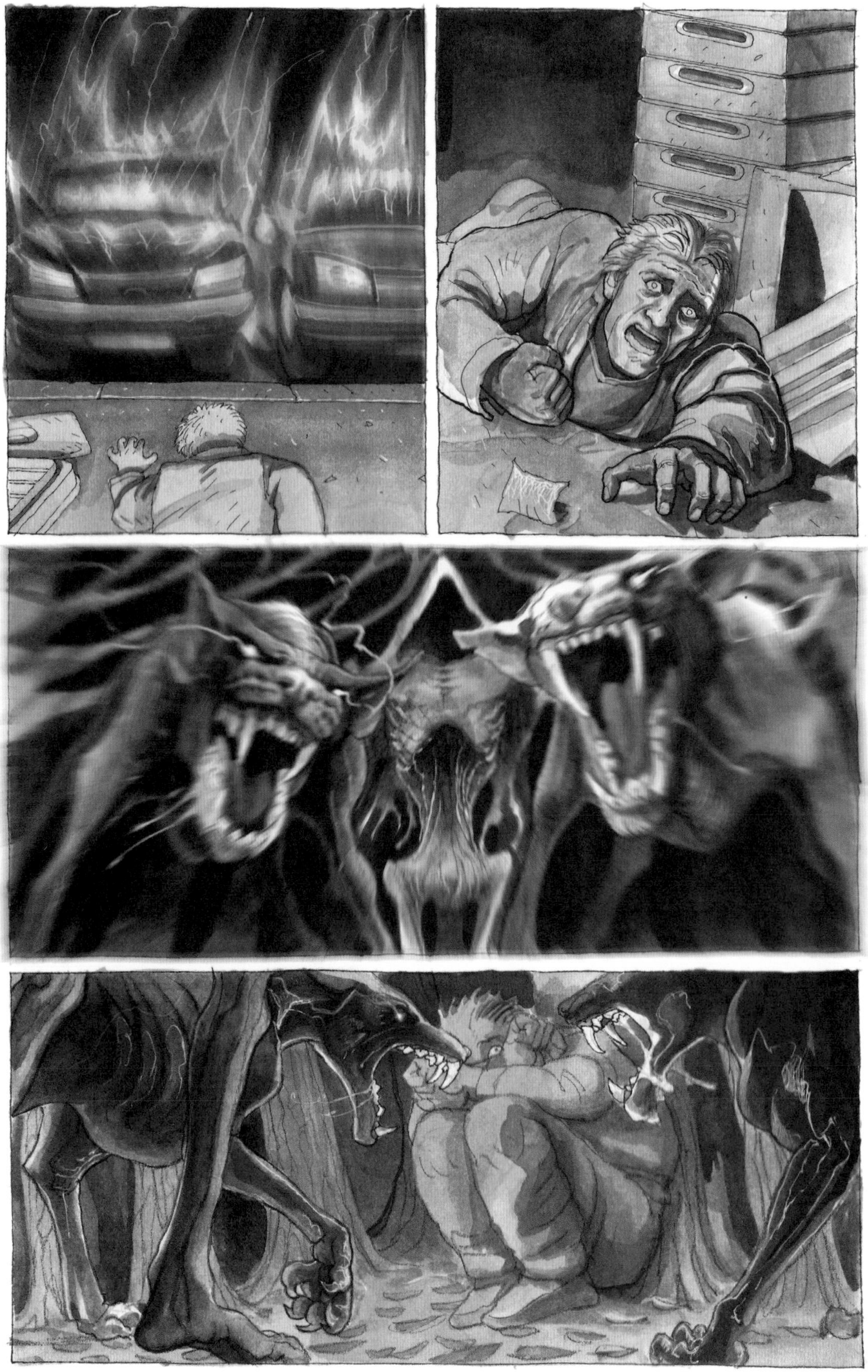

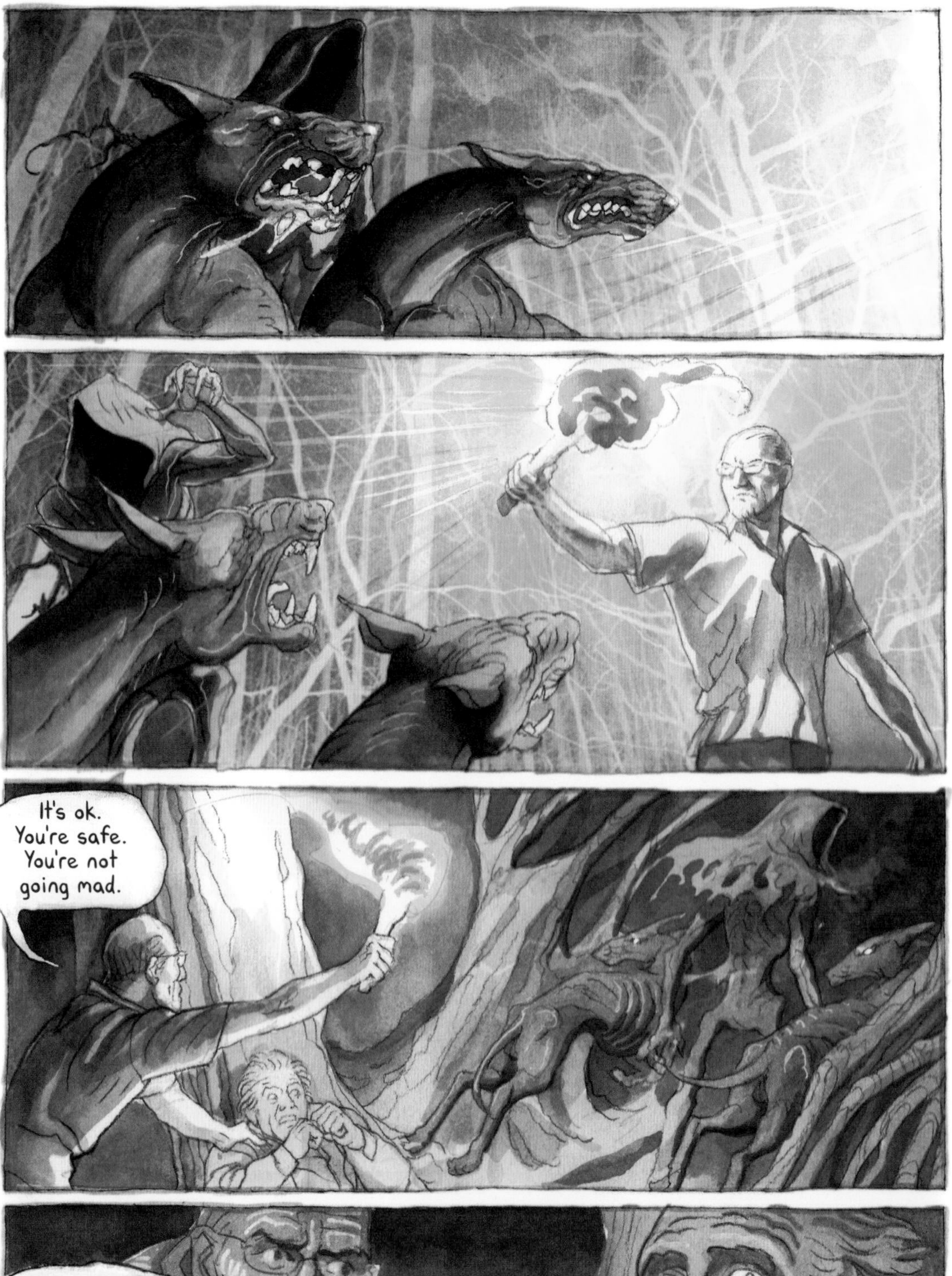
It's ok. You're safe. You're not going mad.
Don't fight it. The feelings will pass very soon. Now *breathe*... slowly and gently.

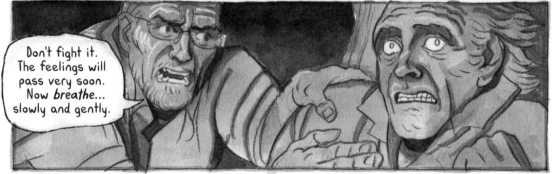

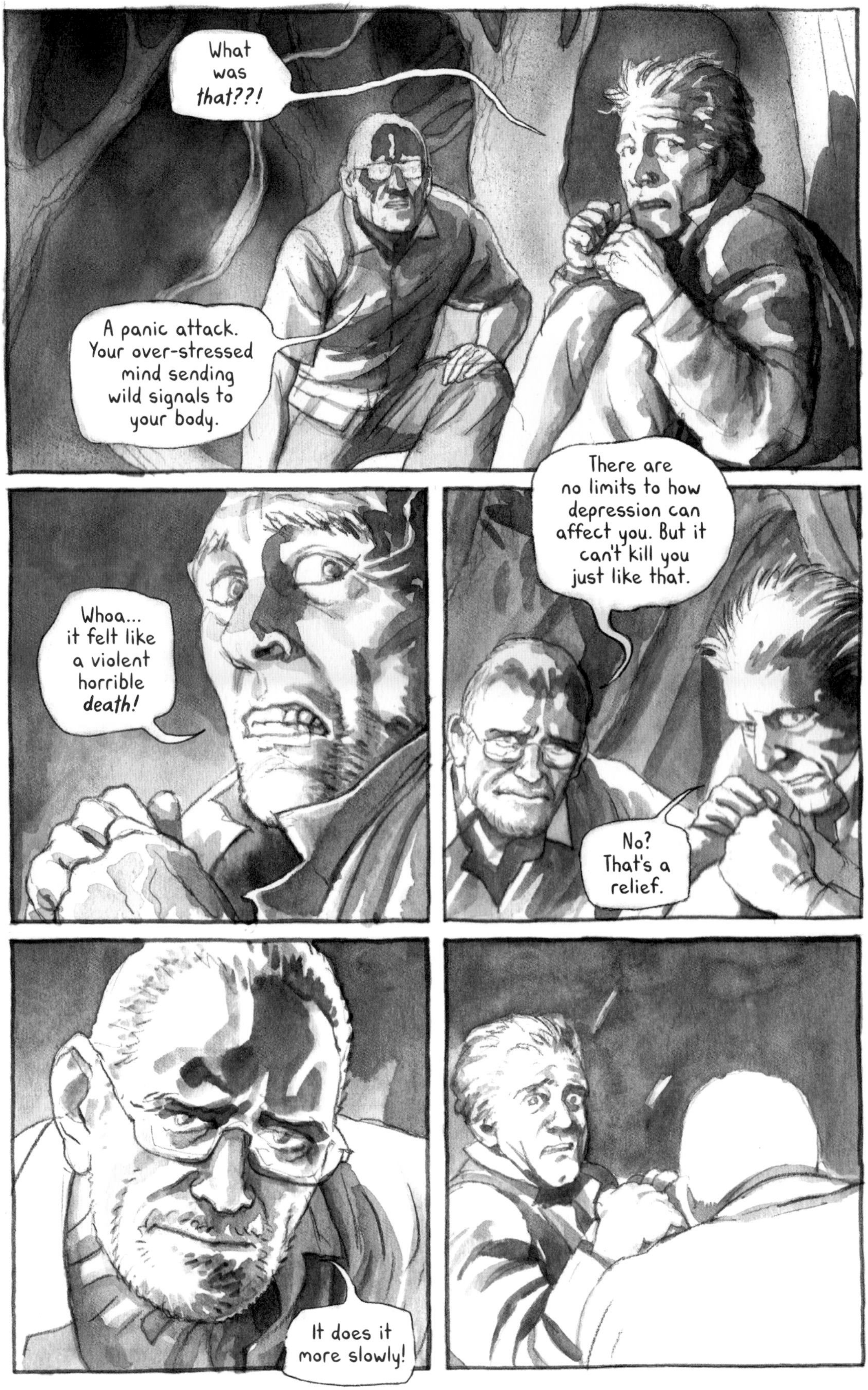
What was *that??!*
A panic attack. Your over-stressed mind sending wild signals to your body.
Whoa... it felt like a violent horrible *death!*
There are no limits to how depression can affect you. But it can't kill you just like that.
No? That's a relief.
It does it more slowly!

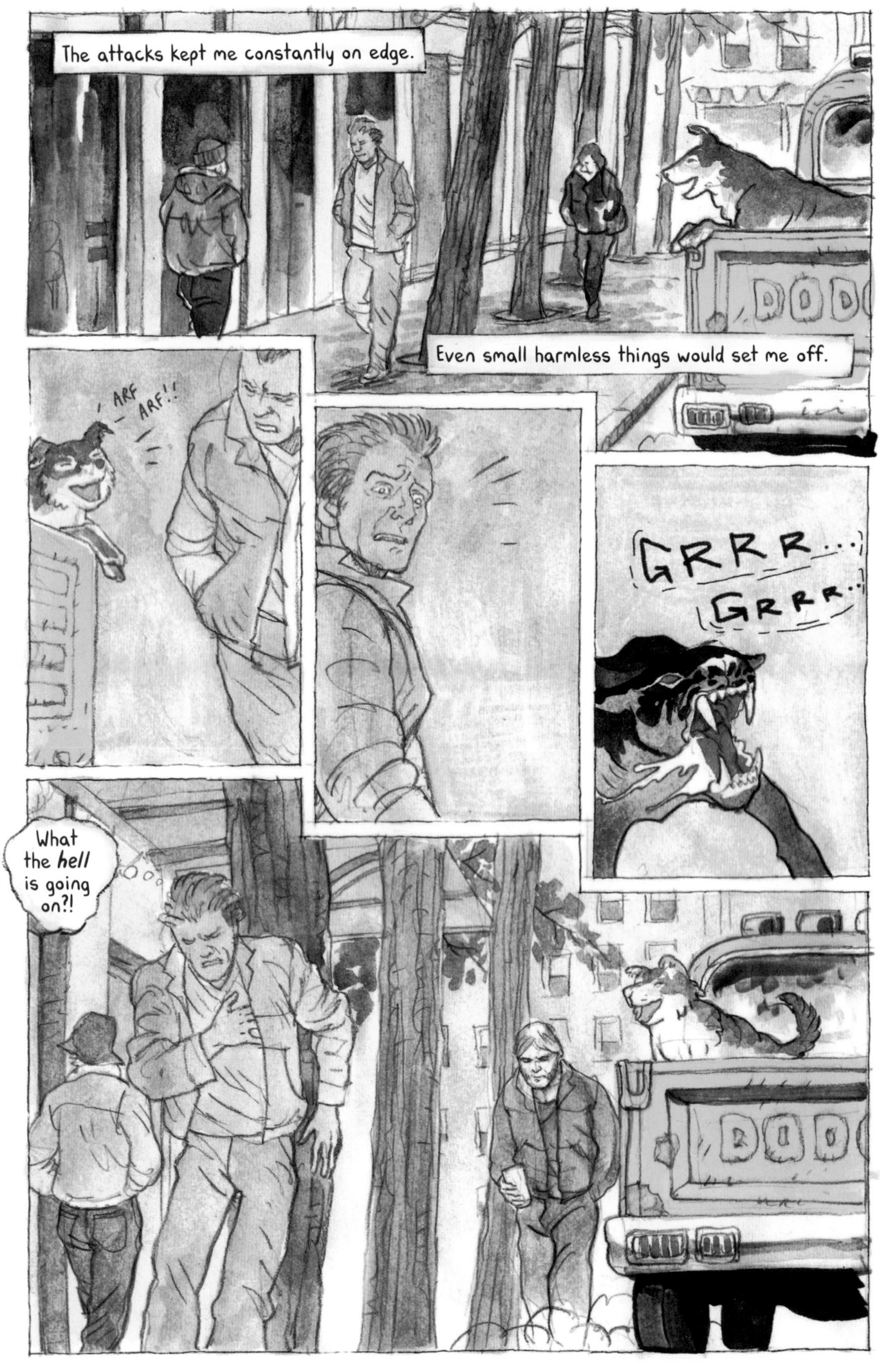
The attacks kept me constantly on edge.
DODG
Even small harmless things would set me off.
ARF ARF!!
GRRR...
GRRR..
What the *hell* is going on?!
DODG

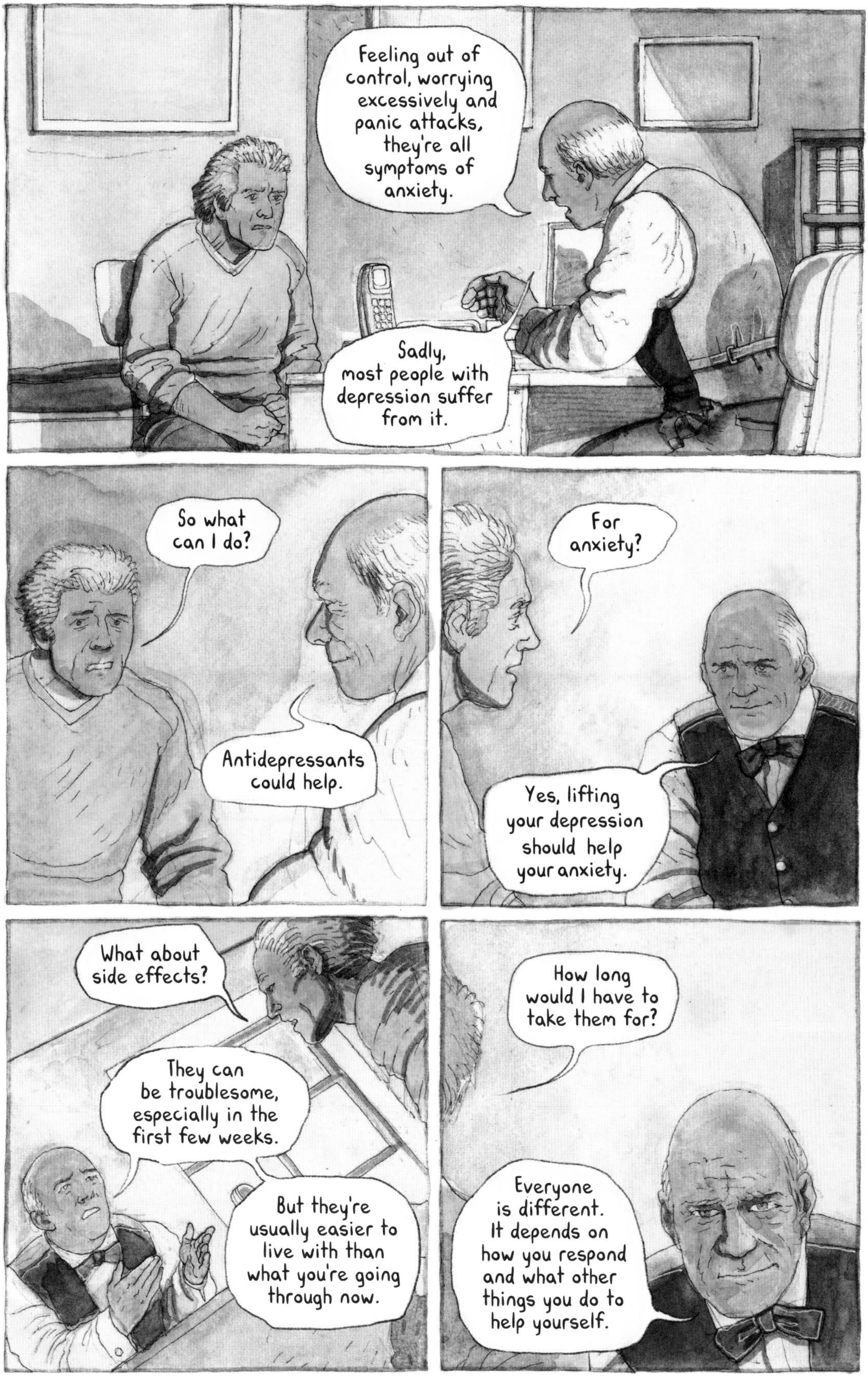
Feeling out of control, worrying excessively and panic attacks, they're all symptoms of anxiety.
Sadly, most people with depression suffer from it.
So what can I do?
Antidepressants could help.
For anxiety?
Yes, lifting your depression should help your anxiety.
What about side effects?
They can be troublesome, especially in the first few weeks.
But they're usually easier to live with than what you're going through now.
How long would I have to take them for?
Everyone is different. It depends on how you respond and what other things you do to help yourself.

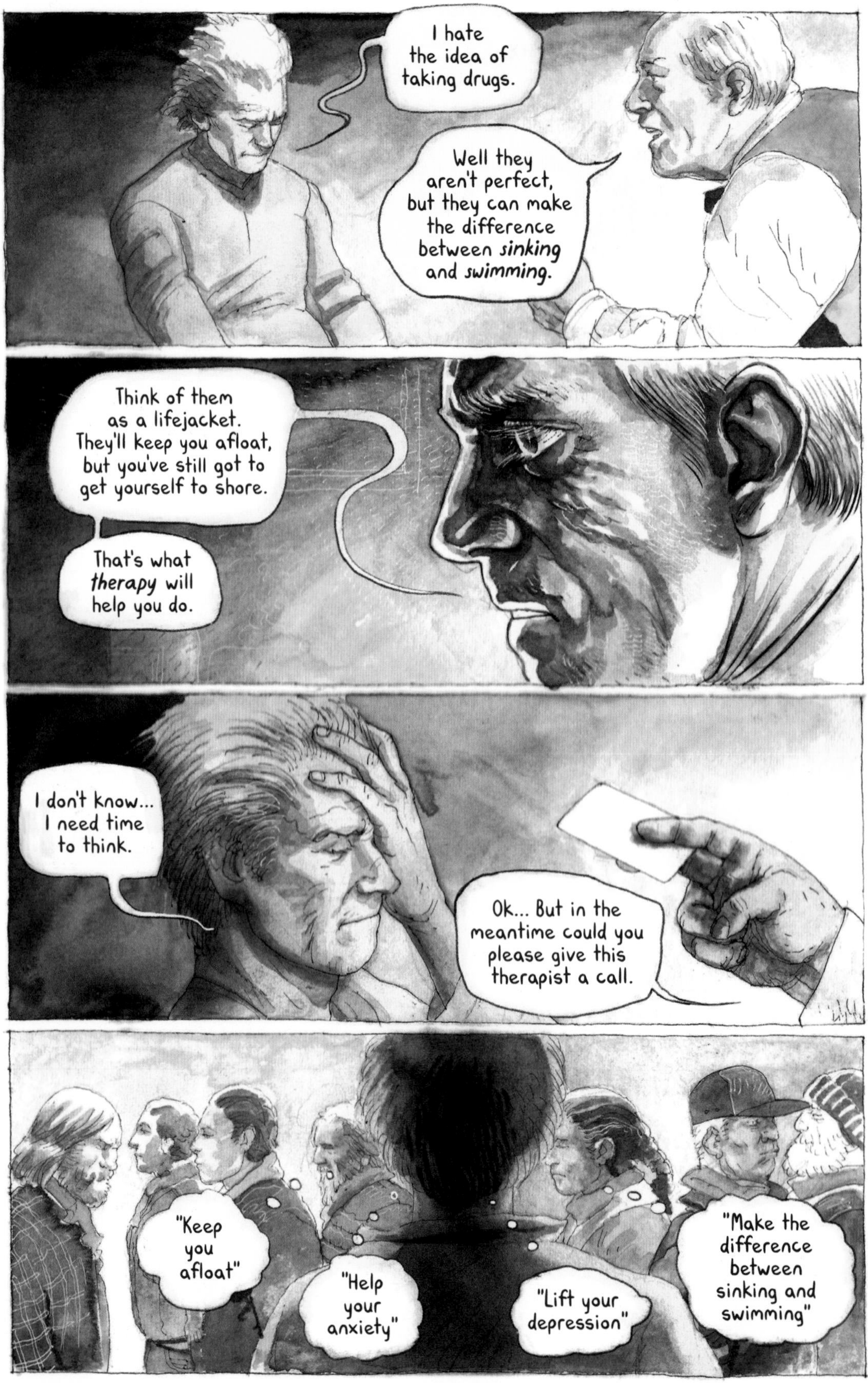
I hate the idea of taking drugs.
Well they aren't perfect, but they can make the difference between *sinking* and *swimming*.
Think of them as a lifejacket. They'll keep you afloat, but you've still got to get yourself to shore.
That's what *therapy* will help you do.
I don't know... I need time to think.
Ok... But in the meantime could you please give this therapist a call.
"Keep you afloat"
"Help your anxiety"
"Lift your depression"
"Make the difference between sinking and swimming"

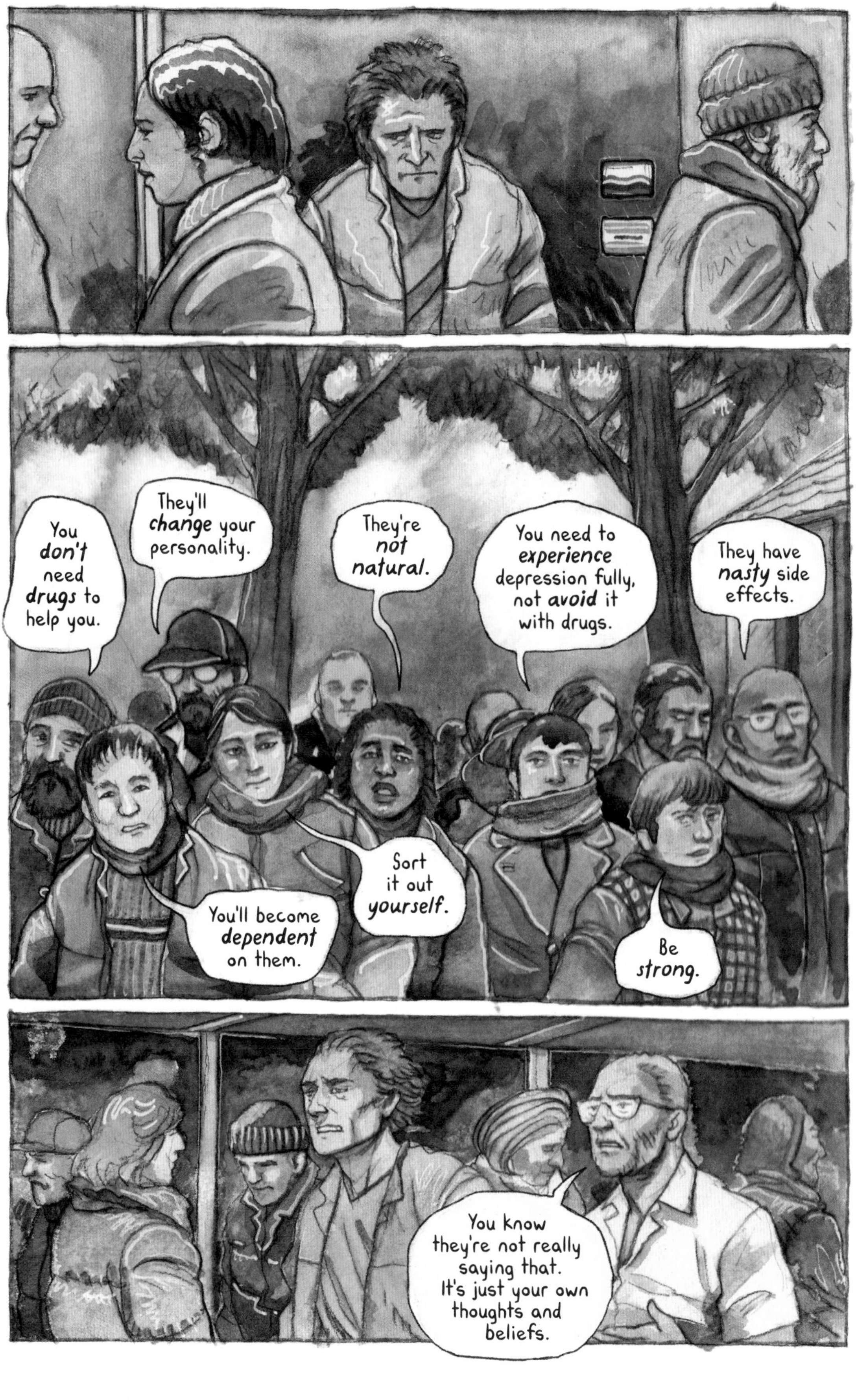
You don't need drugs to help you.
They'll change your personality.
They're not natural.
You need to experience depression fully, not avoid it with drugs.
They have nasty side effects.
You'll become dependent on them.
Sort it out yourself.
Be strong.
You know they're not really saying that. It's just your own thoughts and beliefs.

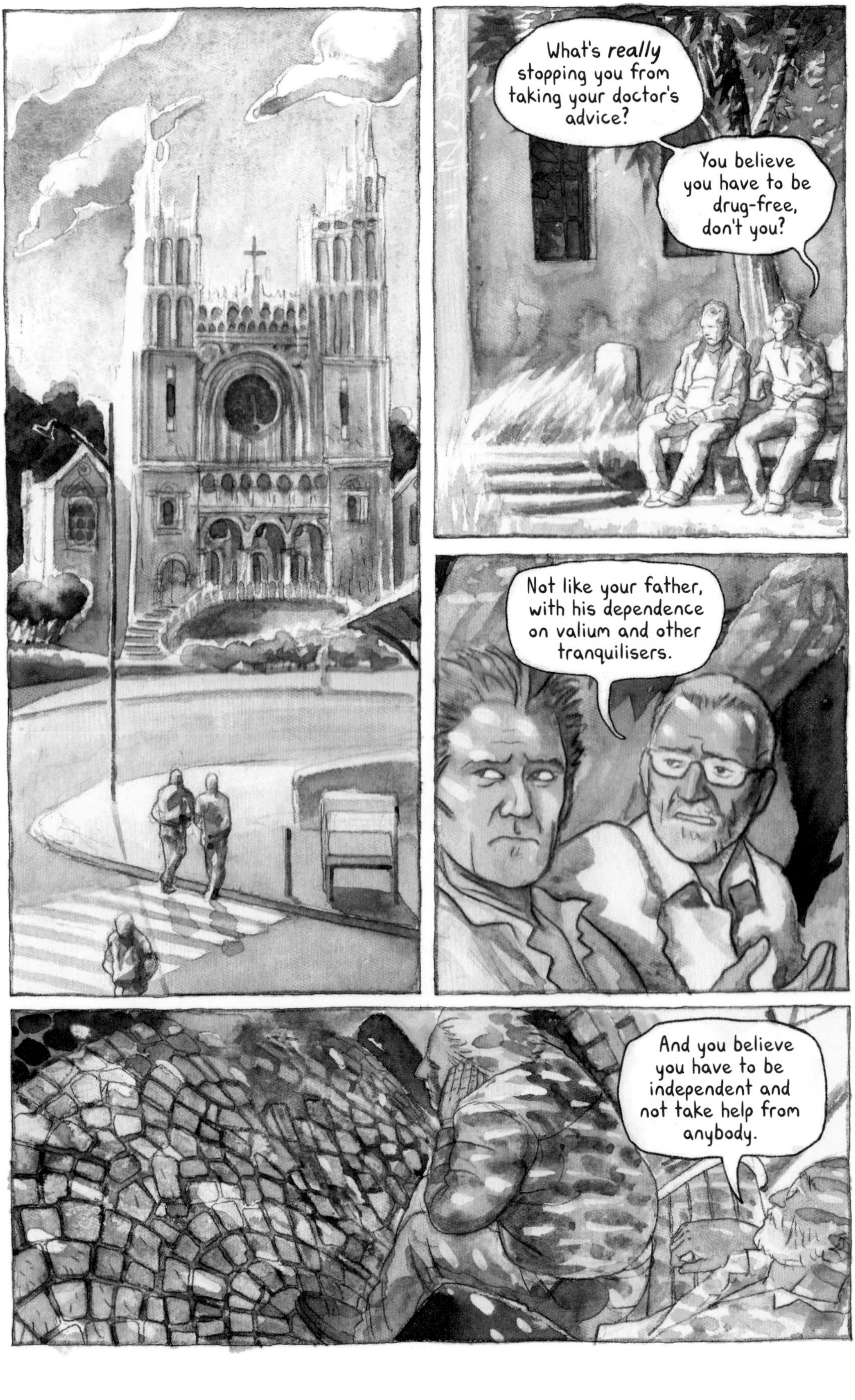
What's *really* stopping you from taking your doctor's advice?
You believe you have to be drug-free, don't you?
Not like your father, with his dependence on valium and other tranquilisers.
And you believe you have to be independent and not take help from anybody.

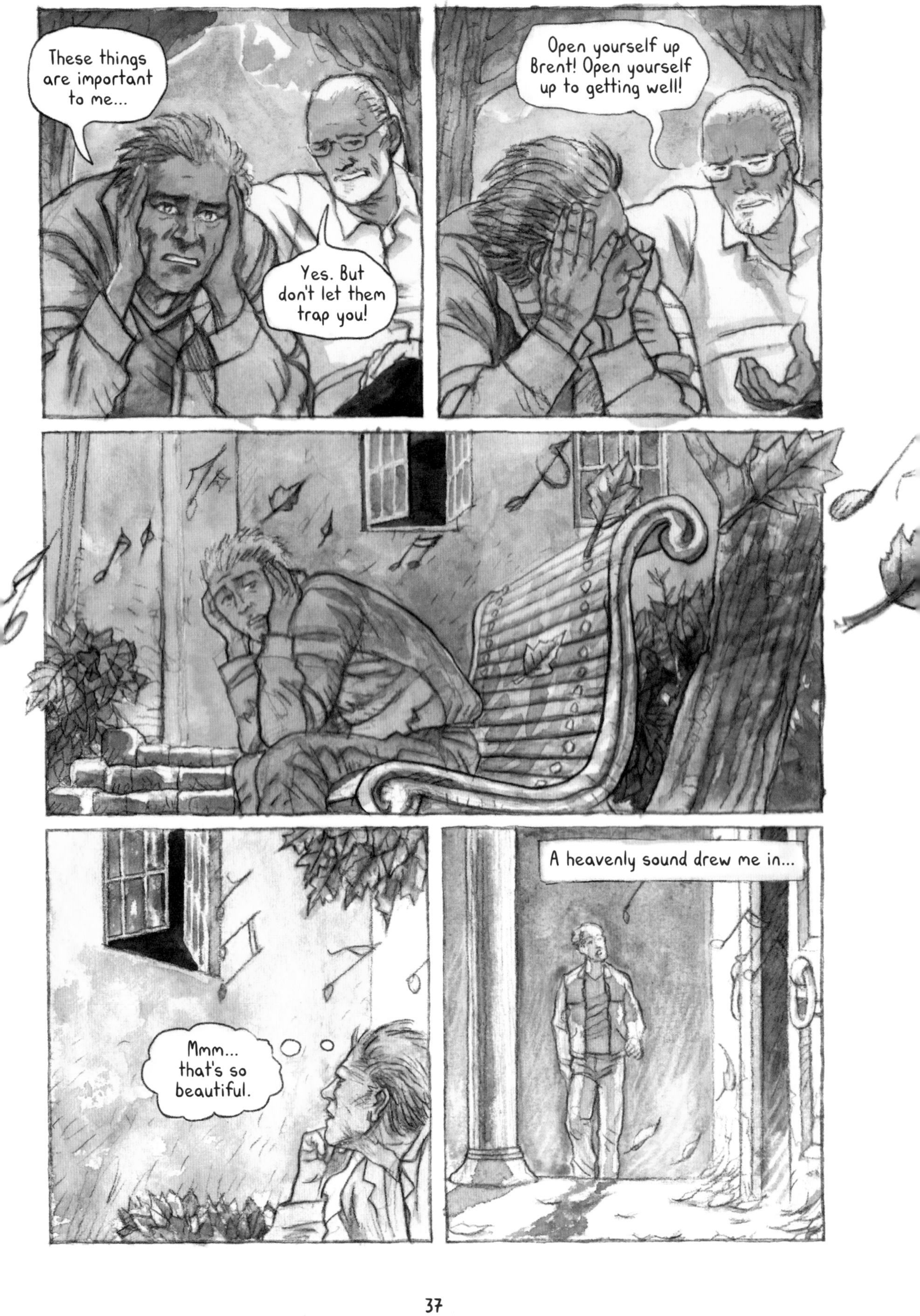
These things are important to me...
Yes. But don't let them trap you!
Open yourself up Brent! Open yourself up to getting well!
Mmm... that's so beautiful.
A heavenly sound drew me in...

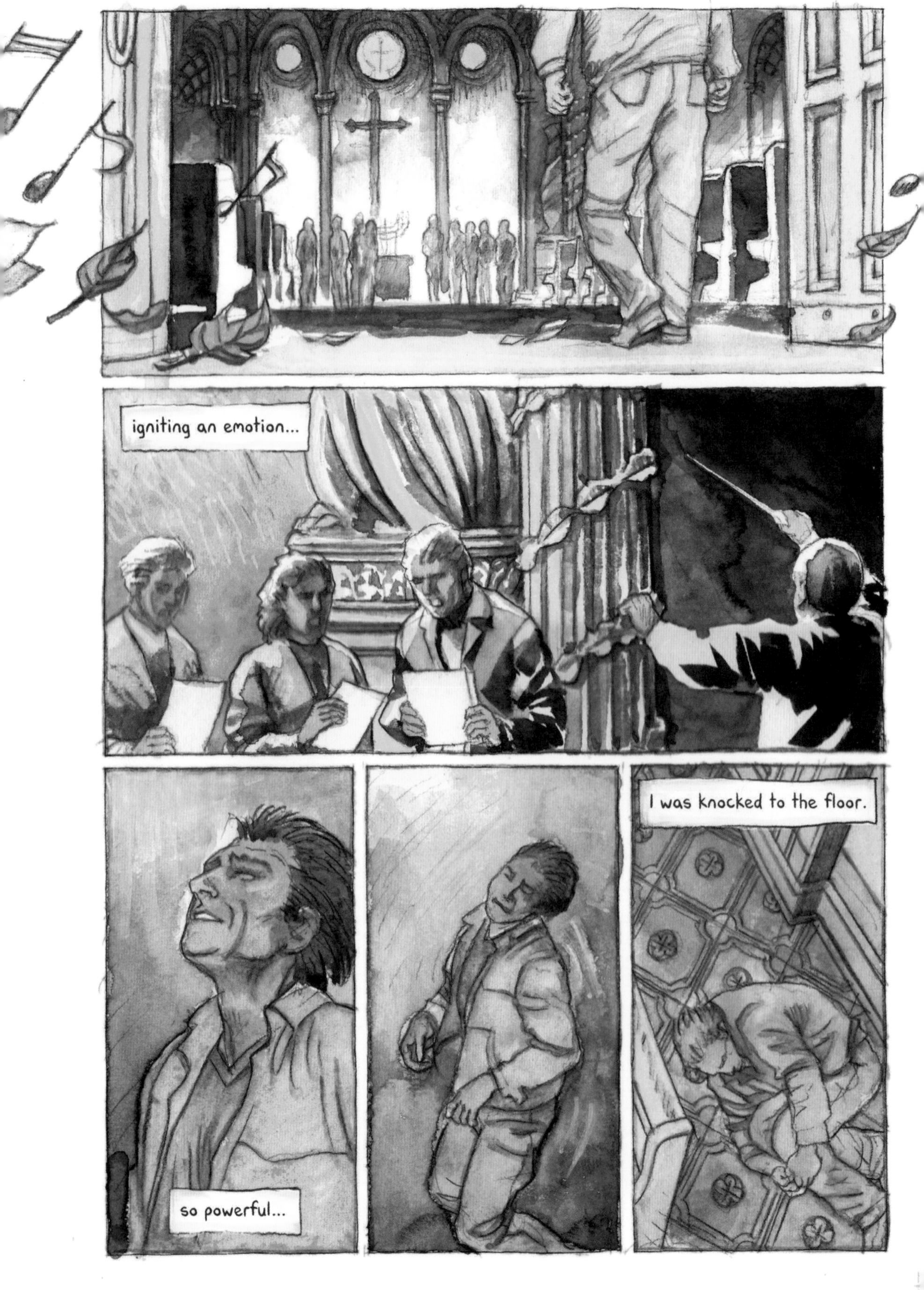
igniting an emotion...
so powerful...
I was knocked to the floor.

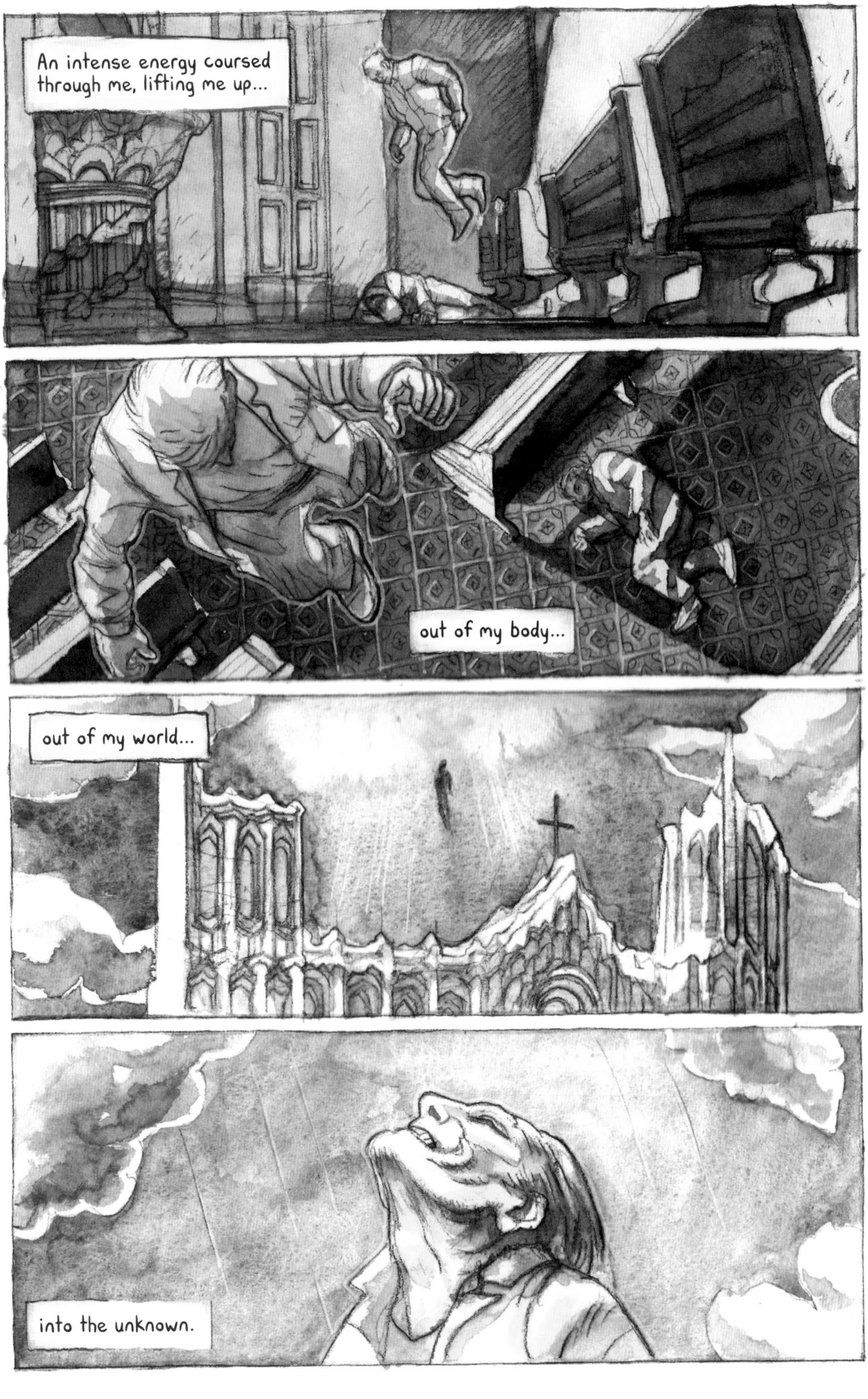
An intense energy coursed through me, lifting me up...
out of my body...
out of my world...
into the unknown.

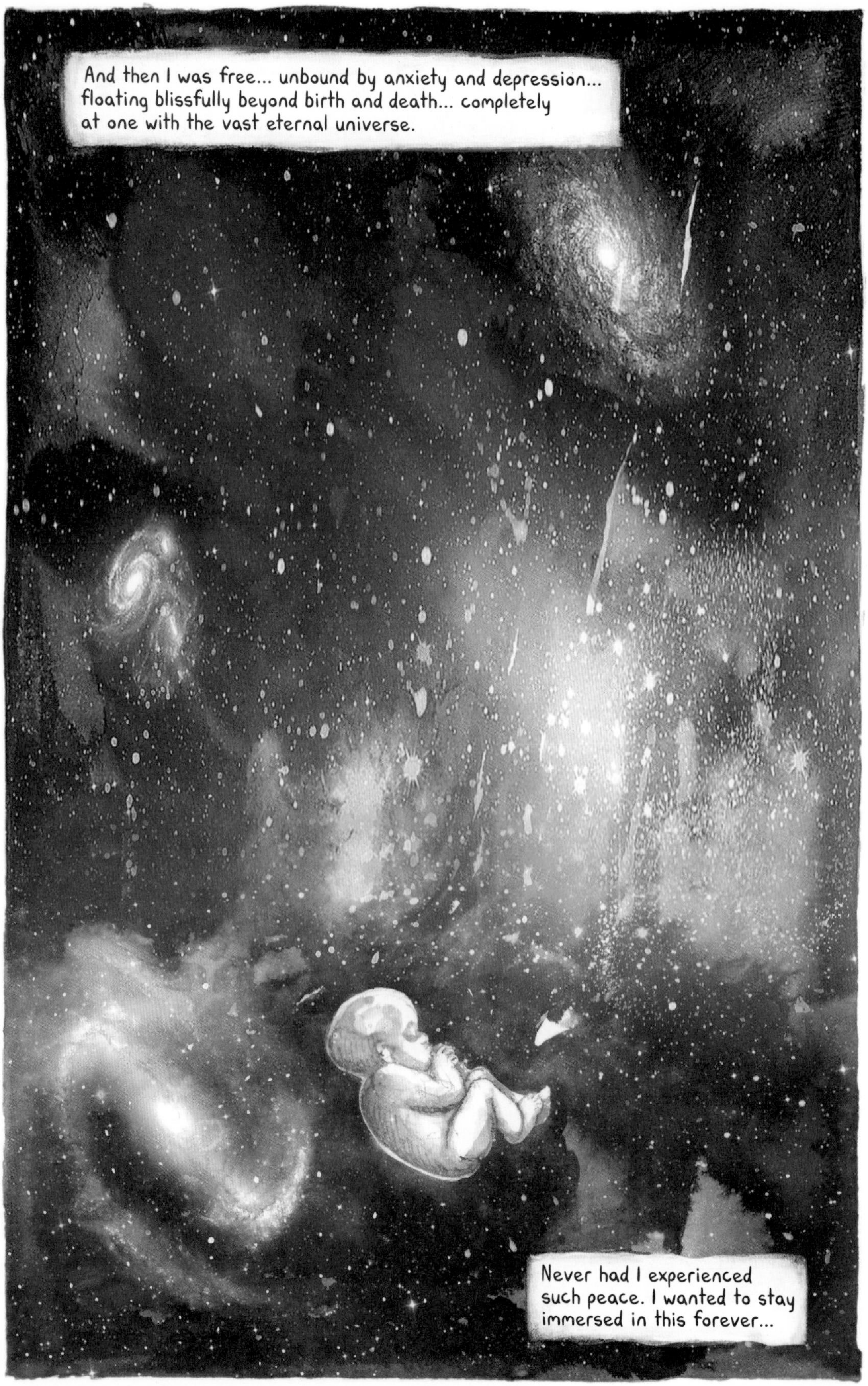
And then I was free... unbound by anxiety and depression... floating blissfully beyond birth and death... completely at one with the vast eternal universe.
Never had I experienced such peace. I wanted to stay immersed in this forever...

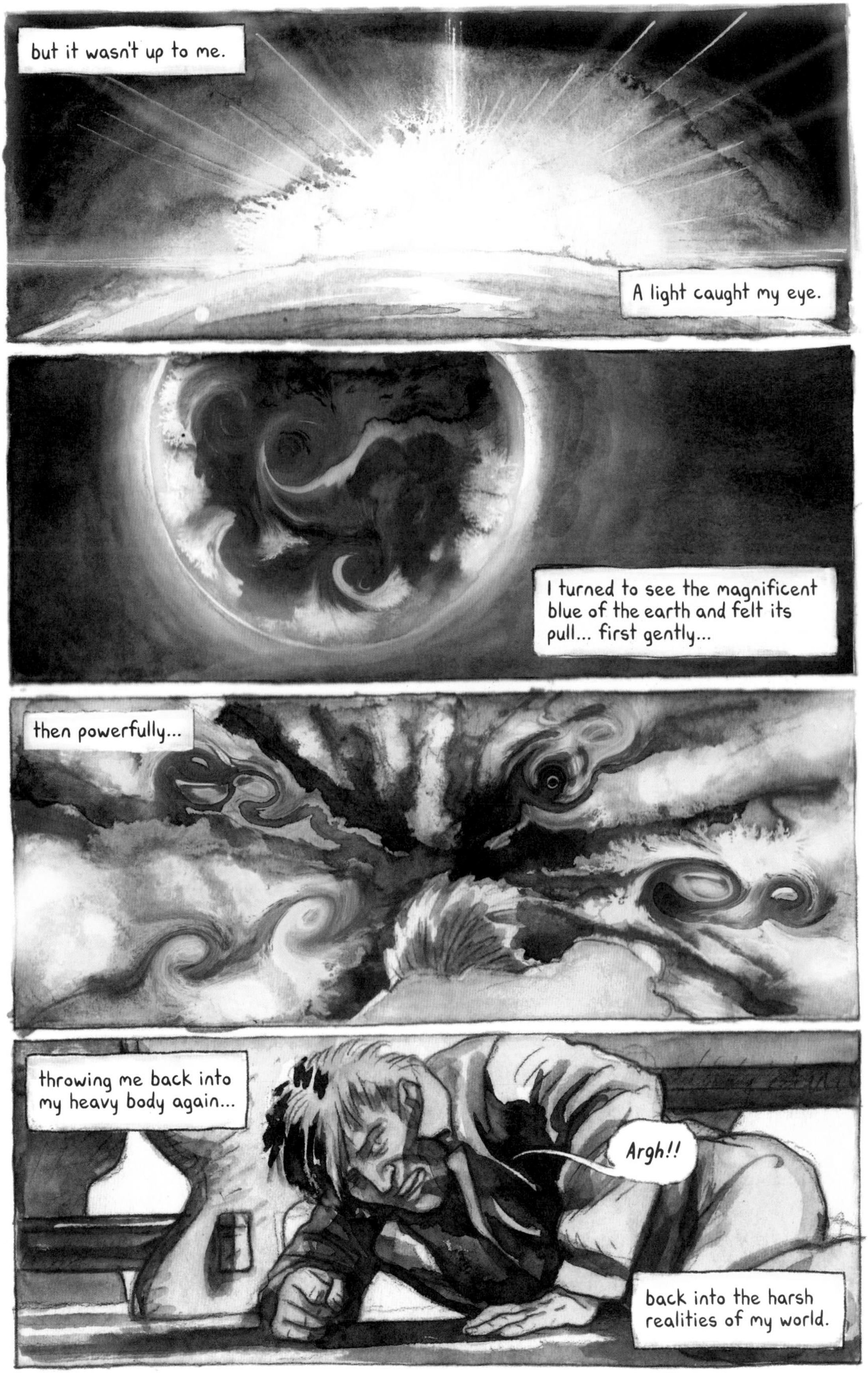
but it wasn't up to me.
A light caught my eye.
I turned to see the magnificent blue of the earth and felt its pull... first gently...
then powerfully...
throwing me back into my heavy body again...
Argh!!
back into the harsh realities of my world.

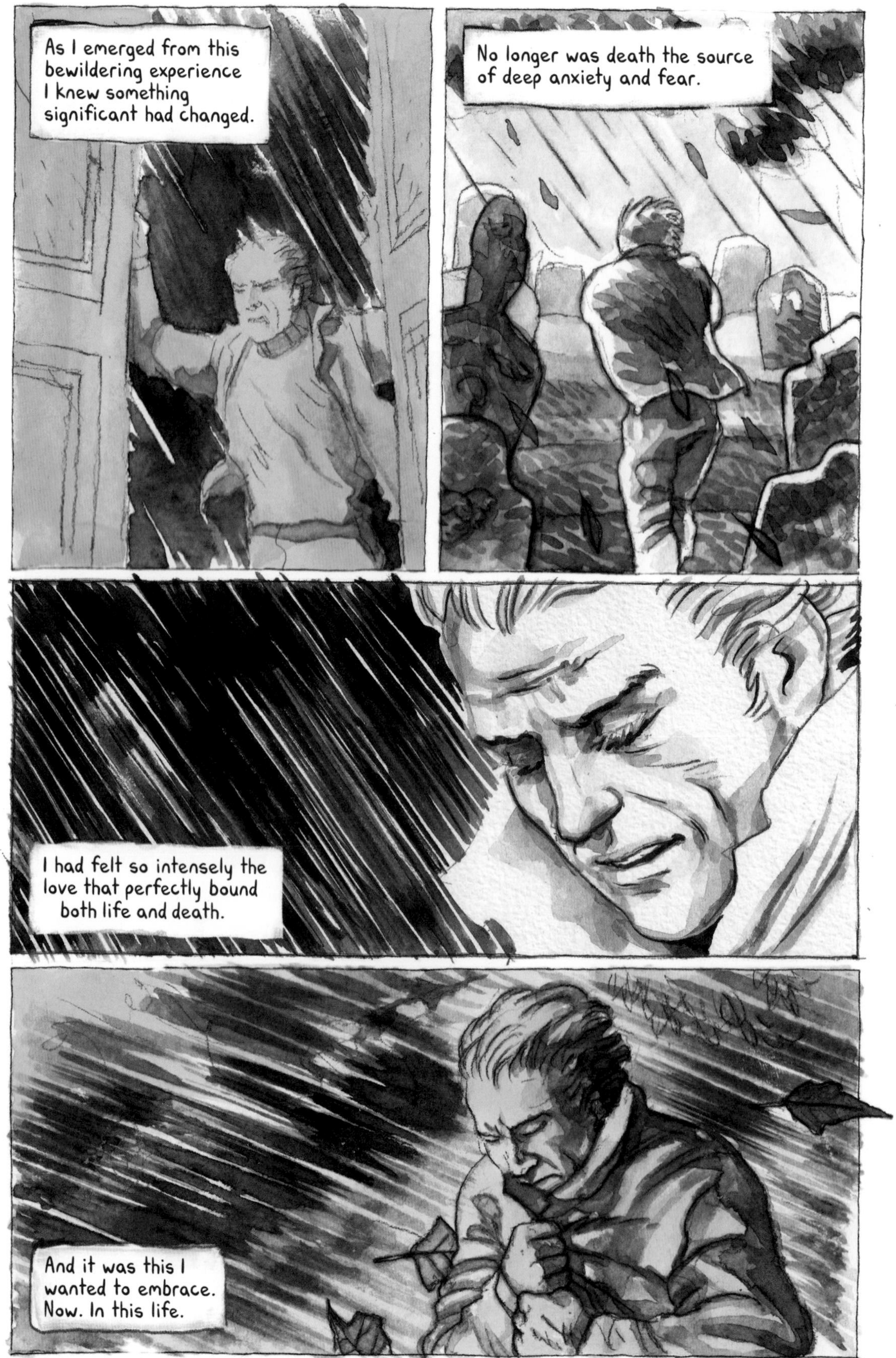
As I emerged from this bewildering experience I knew something significant had changed.
No longer was death the source of deep anxiety and fear.
I had felt so intensely the love that perfectly bound both life and death.
And it was this I wanted to embrace. Now. In this life.

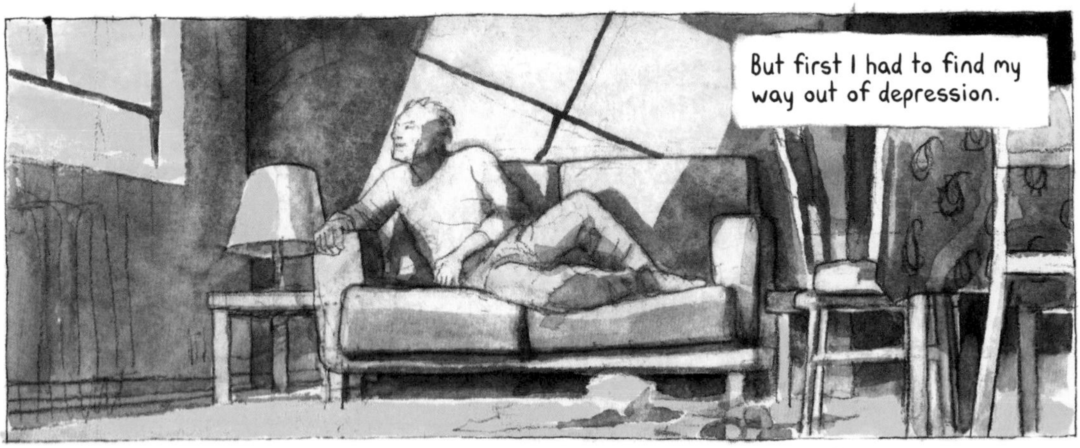
But first I had to find my way out of depression.

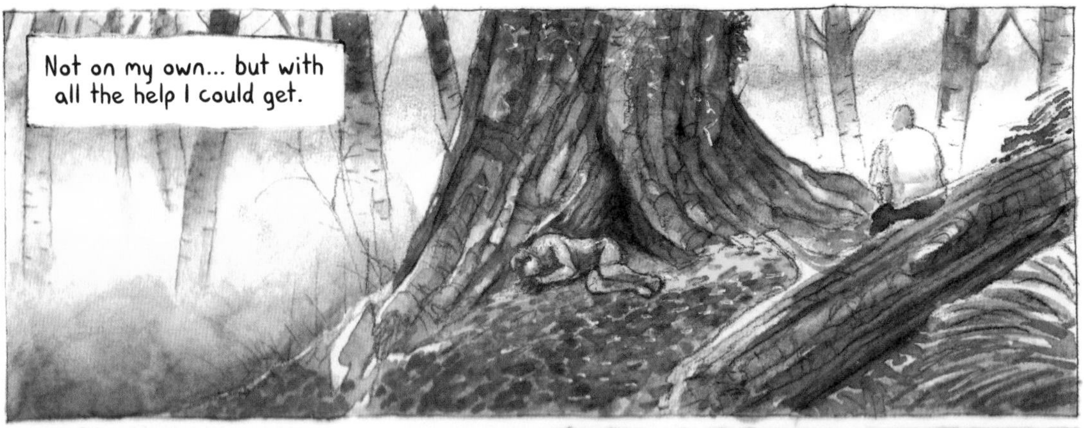
Not on my own... but with all the help I could get.

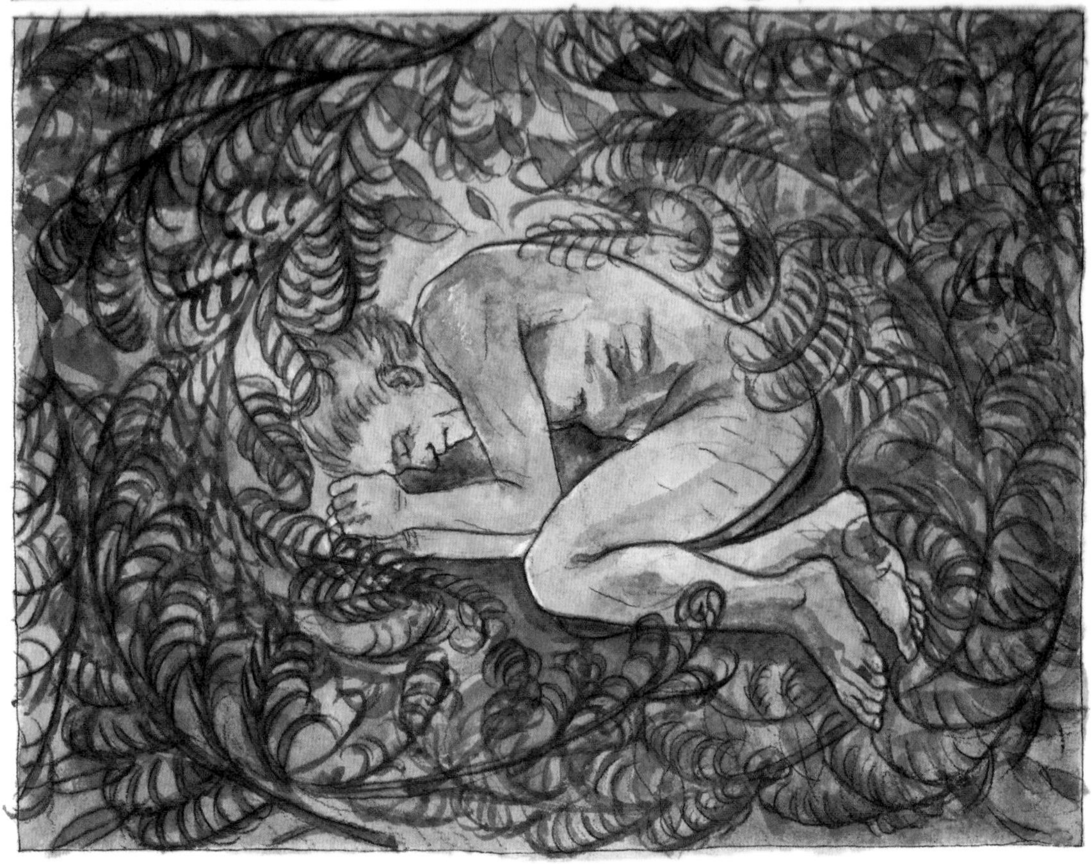

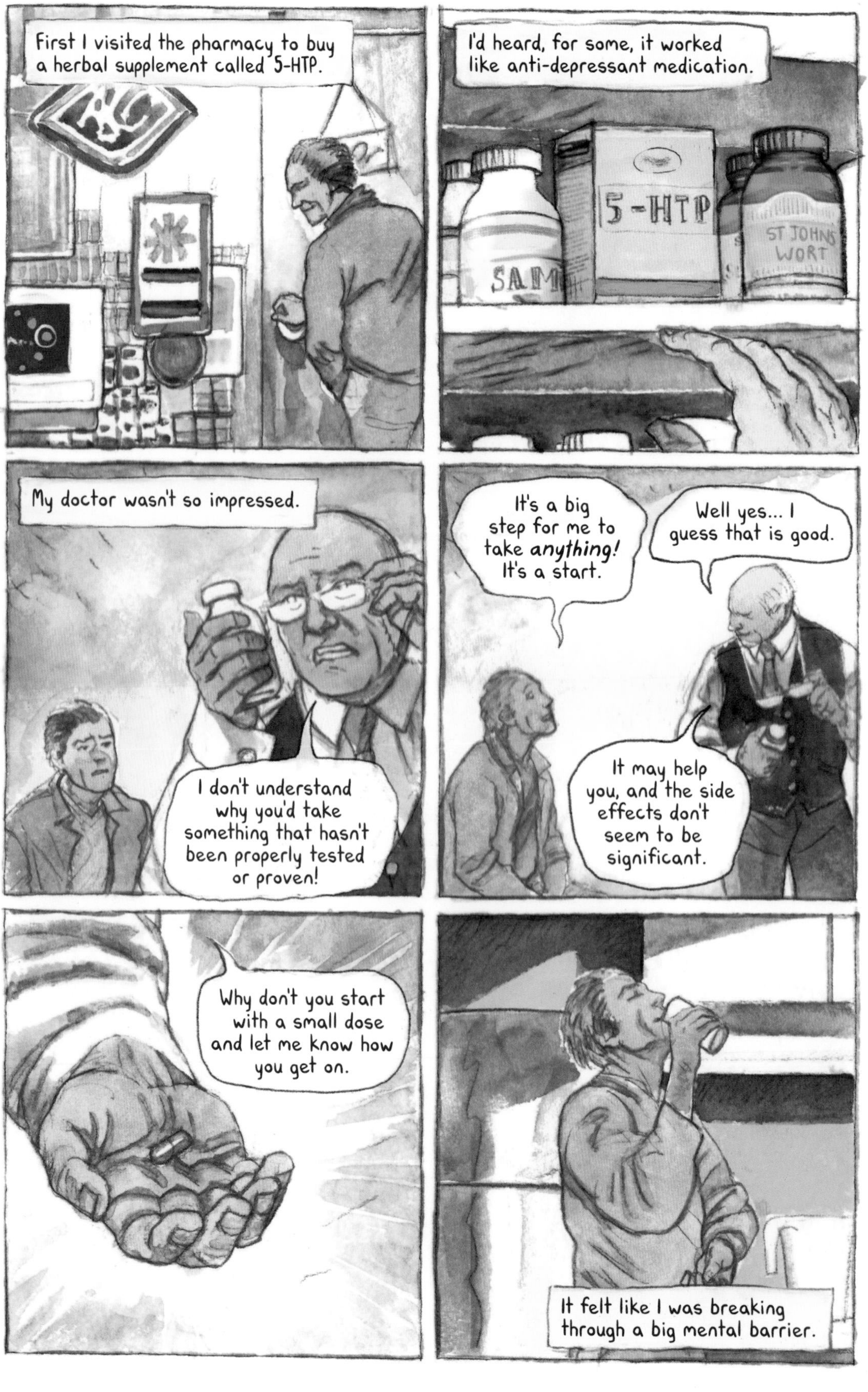
First I visited the pharmacy to buy a herbal supplement called 5-HTP.
I'd heard, for some, it worked like anti-depressant medication.
5-HTP
SAM
ST JOHNS WORT
My doctor wasn't so impressed.
I don't understand why you'd take something that hasn't been properly tested or proven!
It's a big step for me to take *anything!* It's a start.
Well yes... I guess that is good.
It may help you, and the side effects don't seem to be significant.
Why don't you start with a small dose and let me know how you get on.
It felt like I was breaking through a big mental barrier.

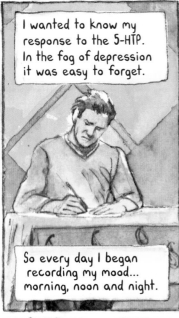

I wanted to know my response to the 5-HTP. In the fog of depression it was easy to forget.
So every day I began recording my mood... morning, noon and night.
-5 was rock bottom, 0 was flat but still functioning, and +5 was feeling really good.
+5
0
-5
Not a place I could imagine at this point.
+5
+4
+3
+2
+1
0
-1
-2
-3
-4
MON
TUES
WED
THURS
FRI
SAT
SUN
Yvonne K. Wraight
Psychological Services
...2pm Friday would be good, thank you.
Two big steps in one day.
Phewww...

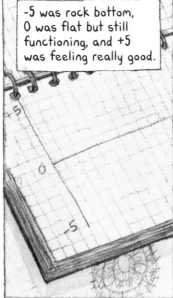

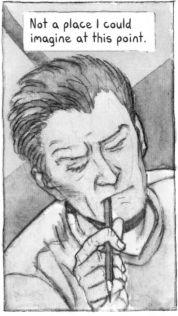

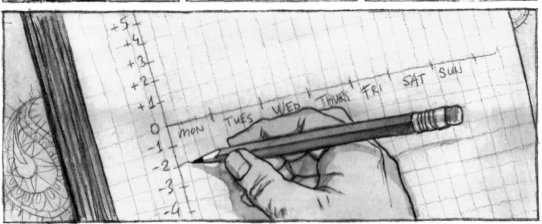

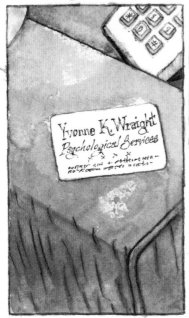

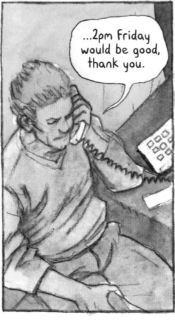

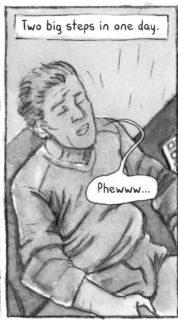

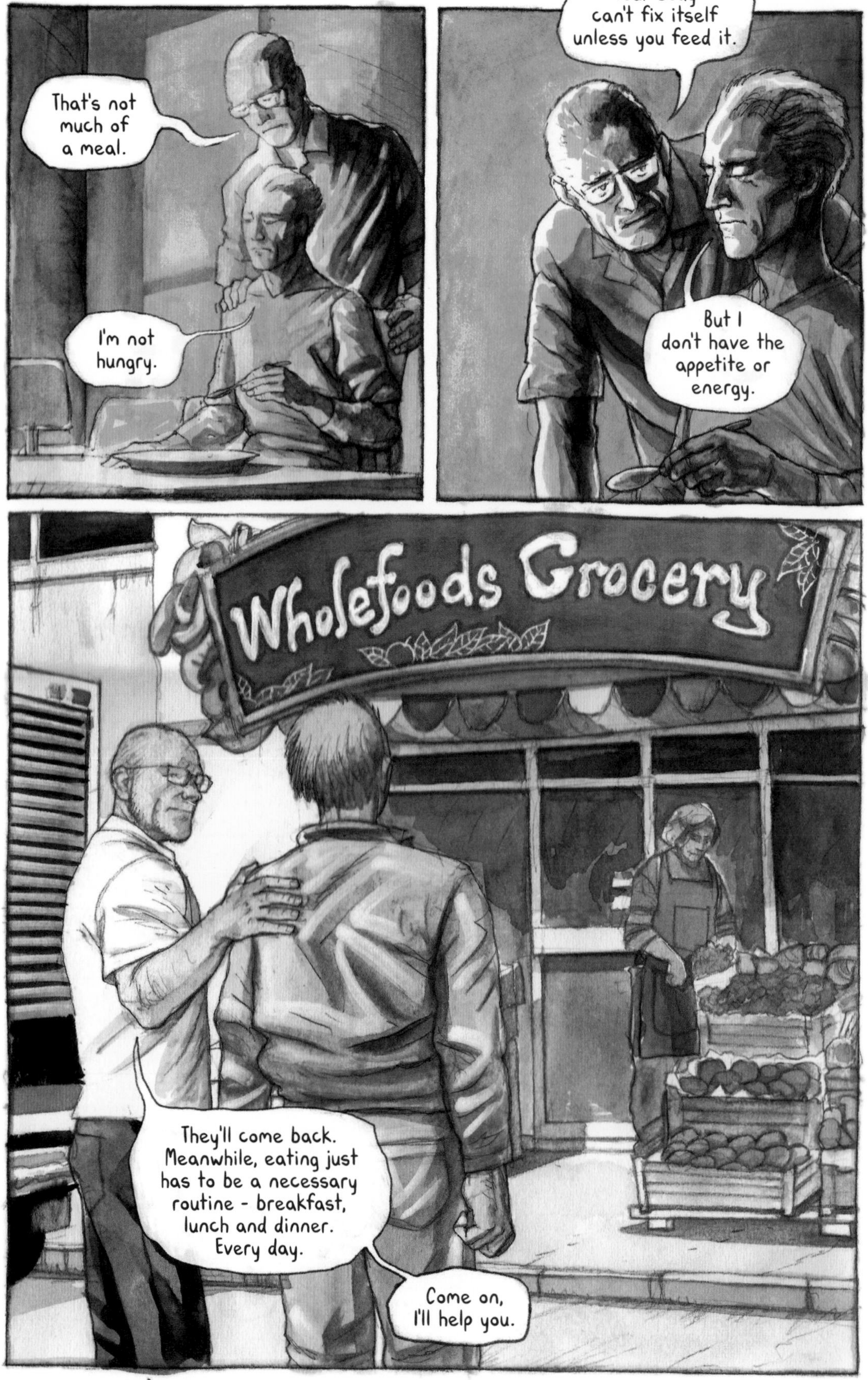
That's not much of a meal.
I'm not hungry.
Your body can't fix itself unless you feed it.
But I don't have the appetite or energy.
Wholefoods Grocery
They'll come back. Meanwhile, eating just has to be a necessary routine - breakfast, lunch and dinner. Every day.
Come on, I'll help you.

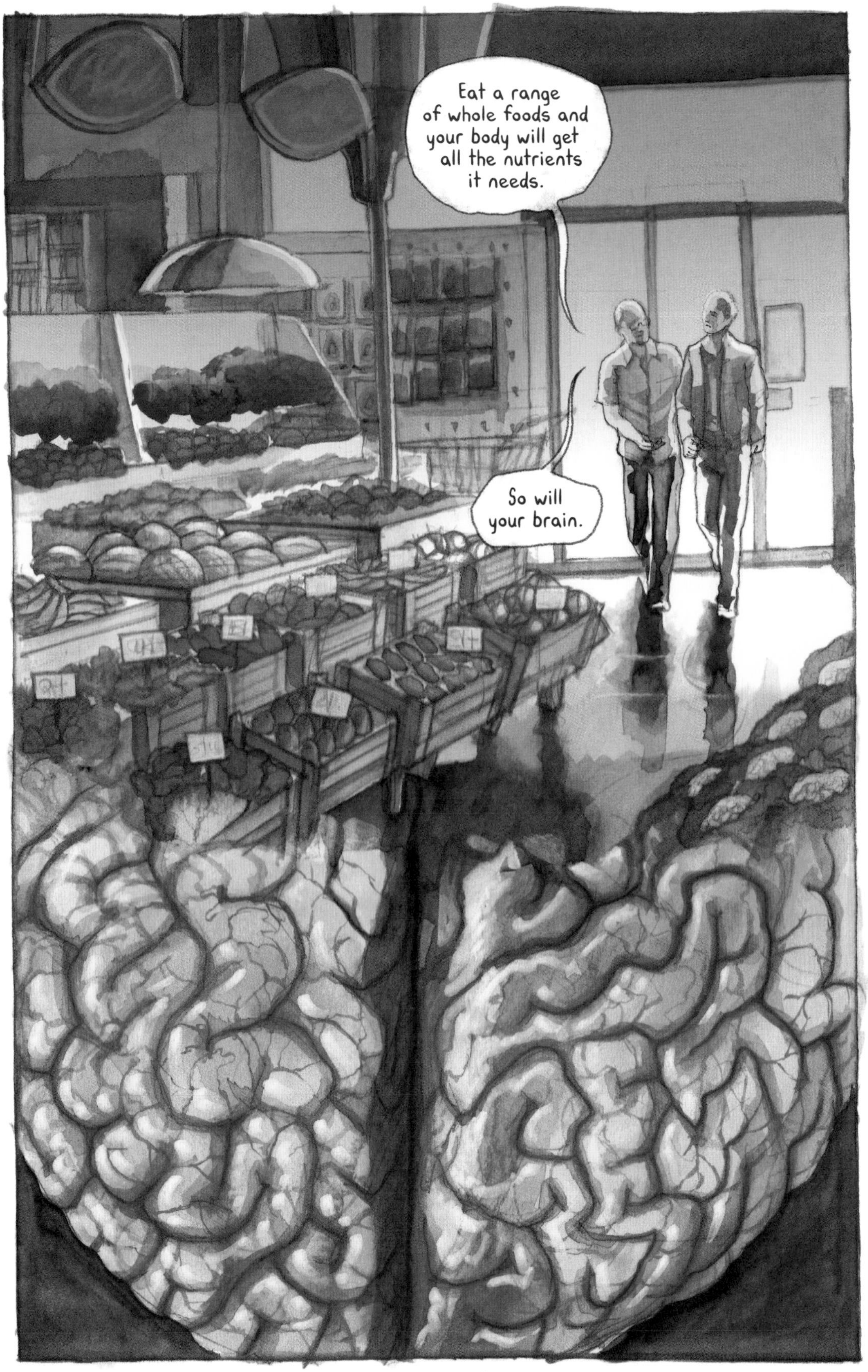
Eat a range of whole foods and your body will get all the nutrients it needs.
So will your brain.

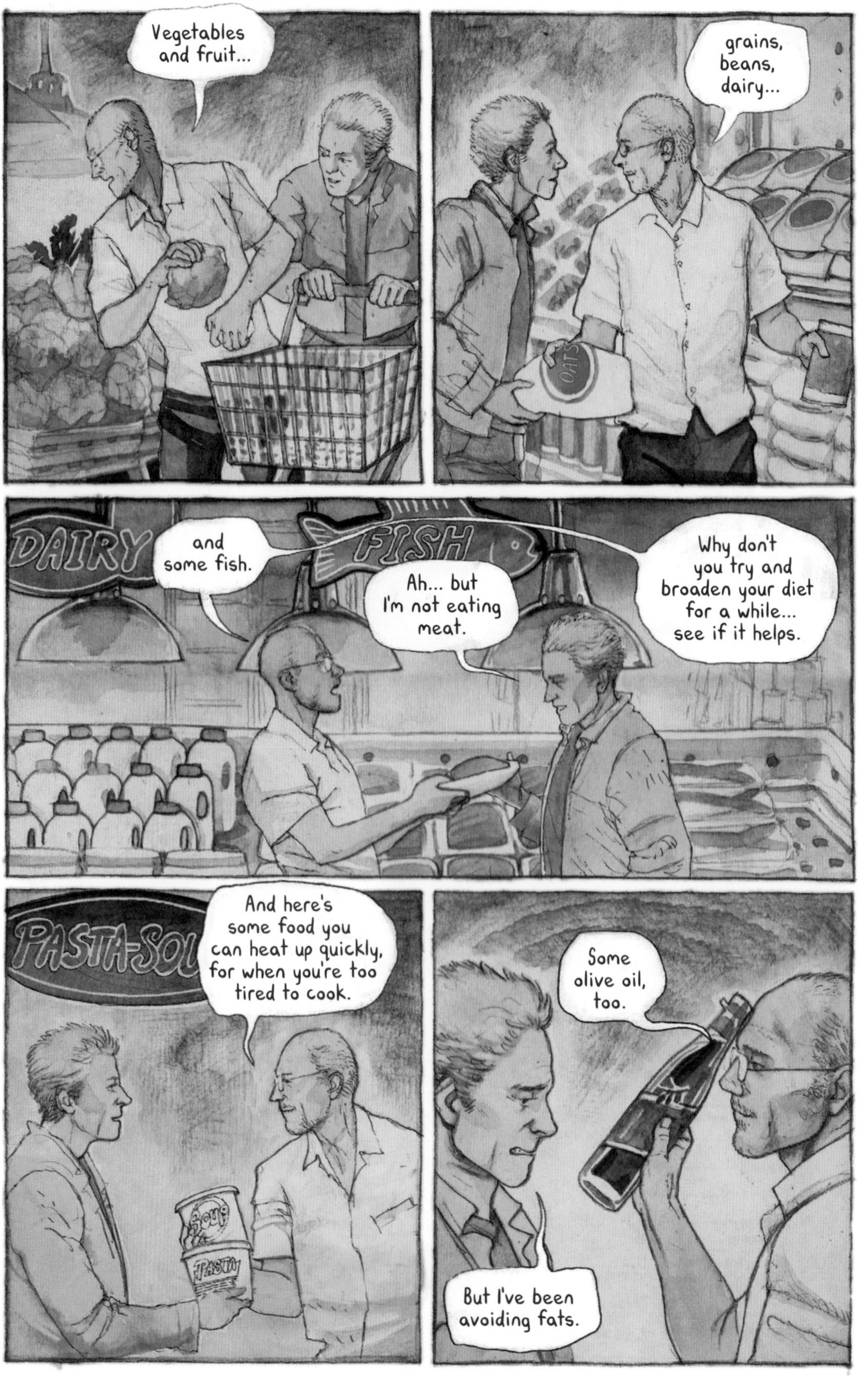
Vegetables and fruit...
grains, beans, dairy...
DAIRY
FISH
and some fish.
Ah... but I'm not eating meat.
Why don't you try and broaden your diet for a while... see if it helps.
PASTA-SOU
And here's some food you can heat up quickly, for when you're too tired to cook.
SOUP
PASTA
Some olive oil, too.
But I've been avoiding fats.

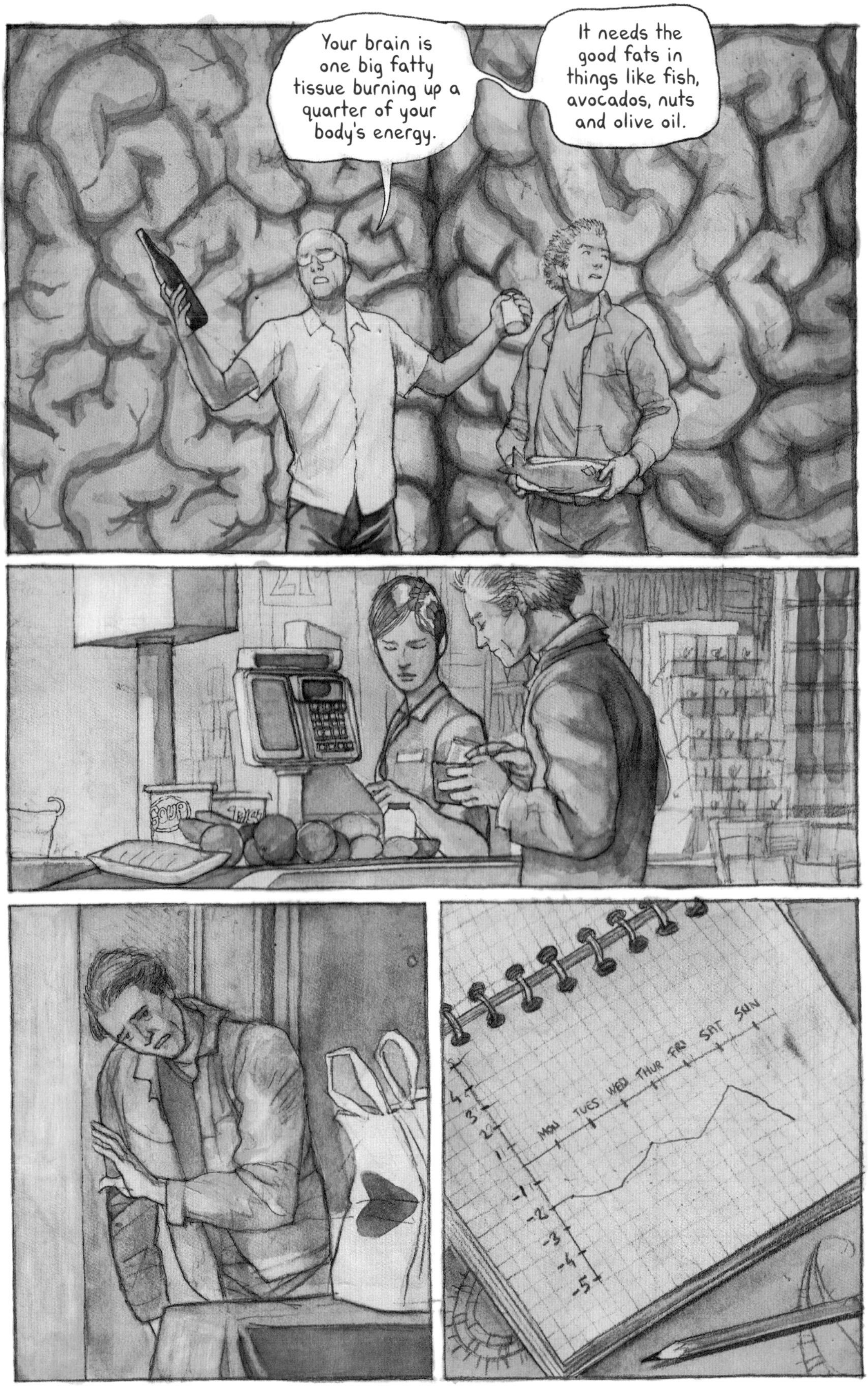
Your brain is one big fatty tissue burning up a quarter of your body's energy.
It needs the good fats in things like fish, avocados, nuts and olive oil.
SOUP
MON TUES WED THUR FRI SAT SUN
4 3 2 1 -1 -2 -3 -4 -5

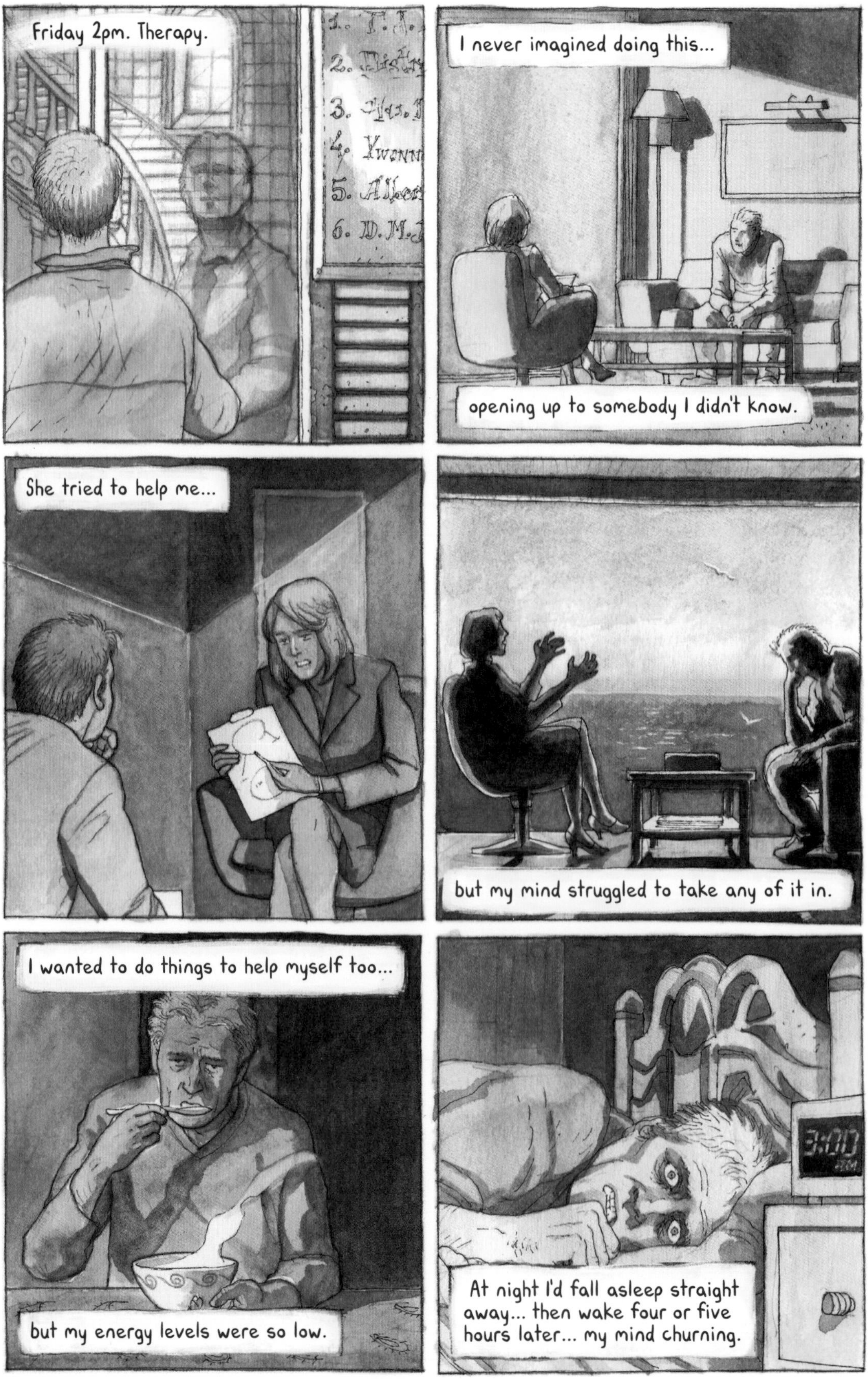
Friday 2pm. Therapy.
I never imagined doing this...
opening up to somebody I didn't know.
She tried to help me...
but my mind struggled to take any of it in.
I wanted to do things to help myself too...
but my energy levels were so low.
At night I'd fall asleep straight away... then wake four or five hours later... my mind churning.

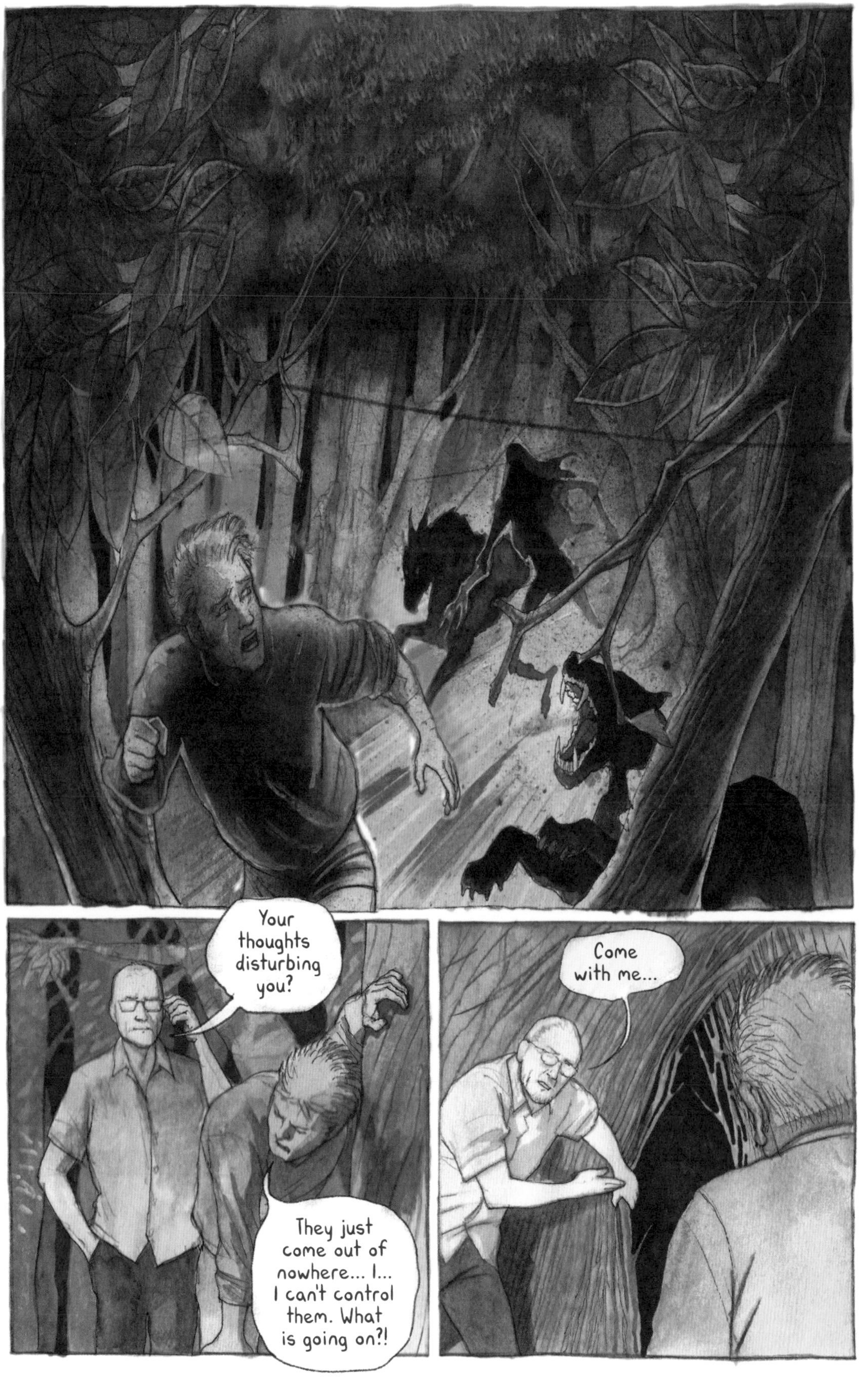
Your thoughts disturbing you?
They just come out of nowhere... I... I can't control them. What is going on?!
Come with me...

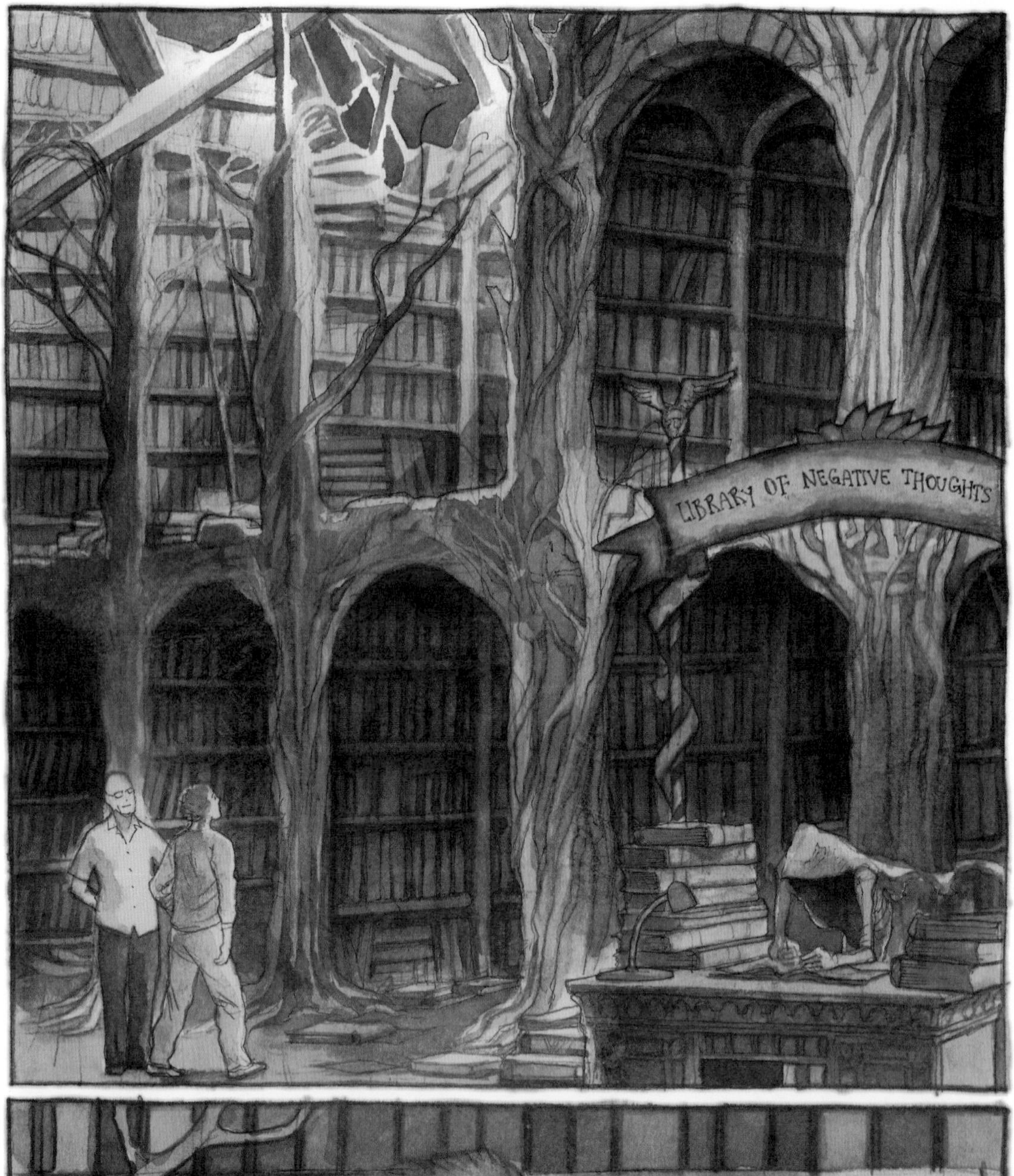
LIBRARY OF NEGATIVE THOUGHTS

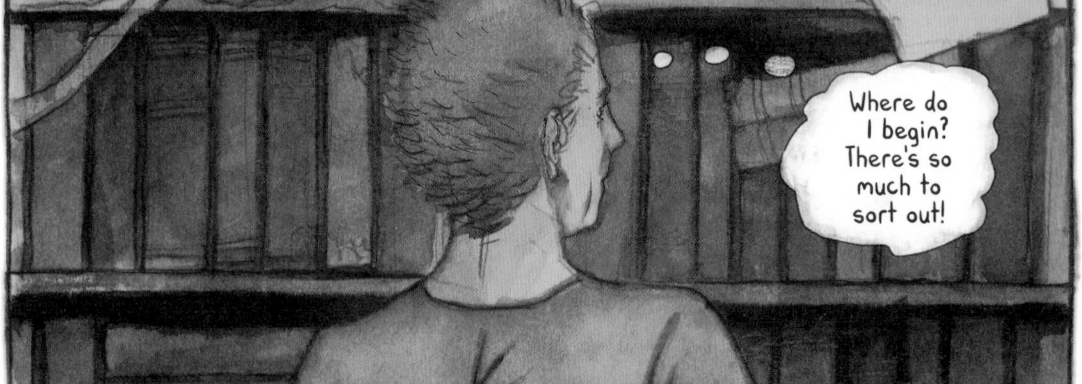
Where do I begin? There's so much to sort out!

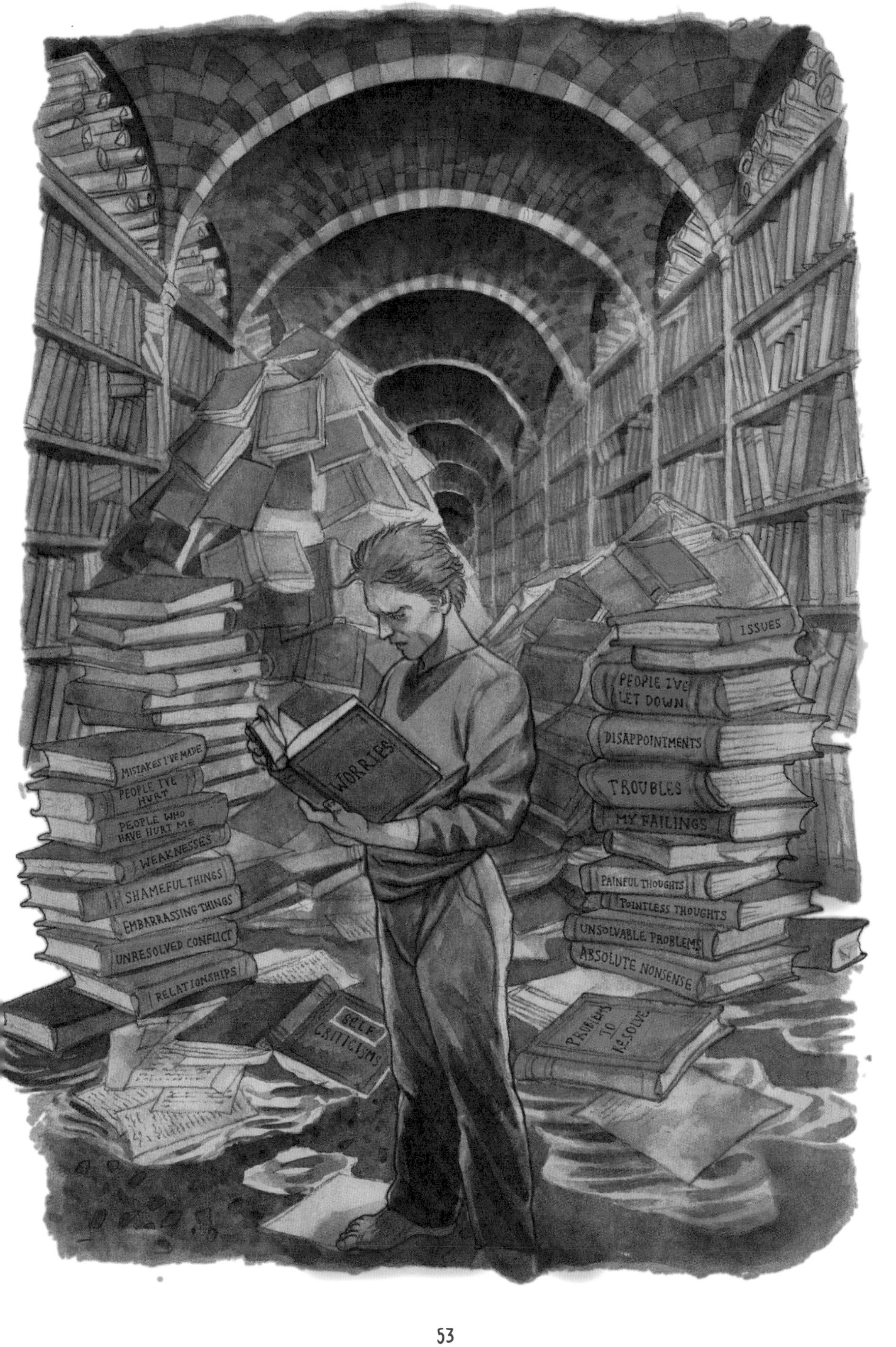
WORRIES
MISTAKES I'VE MADE
PEOPLE I'VE HURT
PEOPLE WHO HAVE HURT ME
WEAKNESSES
SHAMEFUL THINGS
EMBARRASSING THINGS
UNRESOLVED CONFLICT
RELATIONSHIPS
SELF CRITICISMS
ISSUES
PEOPLE I'VE LET DOWN
DISAPPOINTMENTS
TROUBLES
MY FAILINGS
PAINFUL THOUGHTS
POINTLESS THOUGHTS
UNSOLVABLE PROBLEMS
ABSOLUTE NONSENSE
PROBLEMS TO RESOLVE

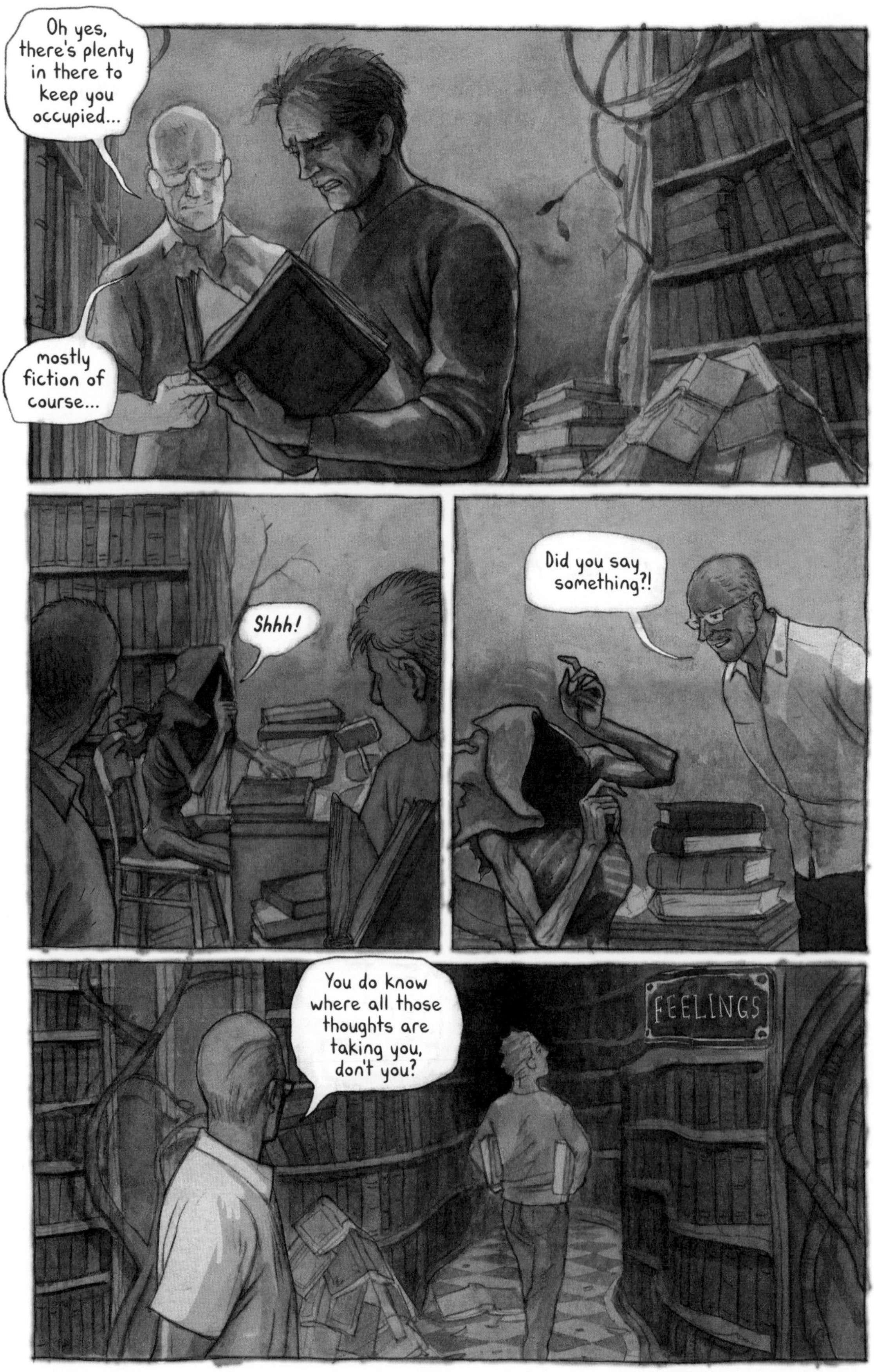
Oh yes, there's plenty in there to keep you occupied...
mostly fiction of course...
Shhh!
Did you say something?!
You do know where all those thoughts are taking you, don't you?
FEELINGS

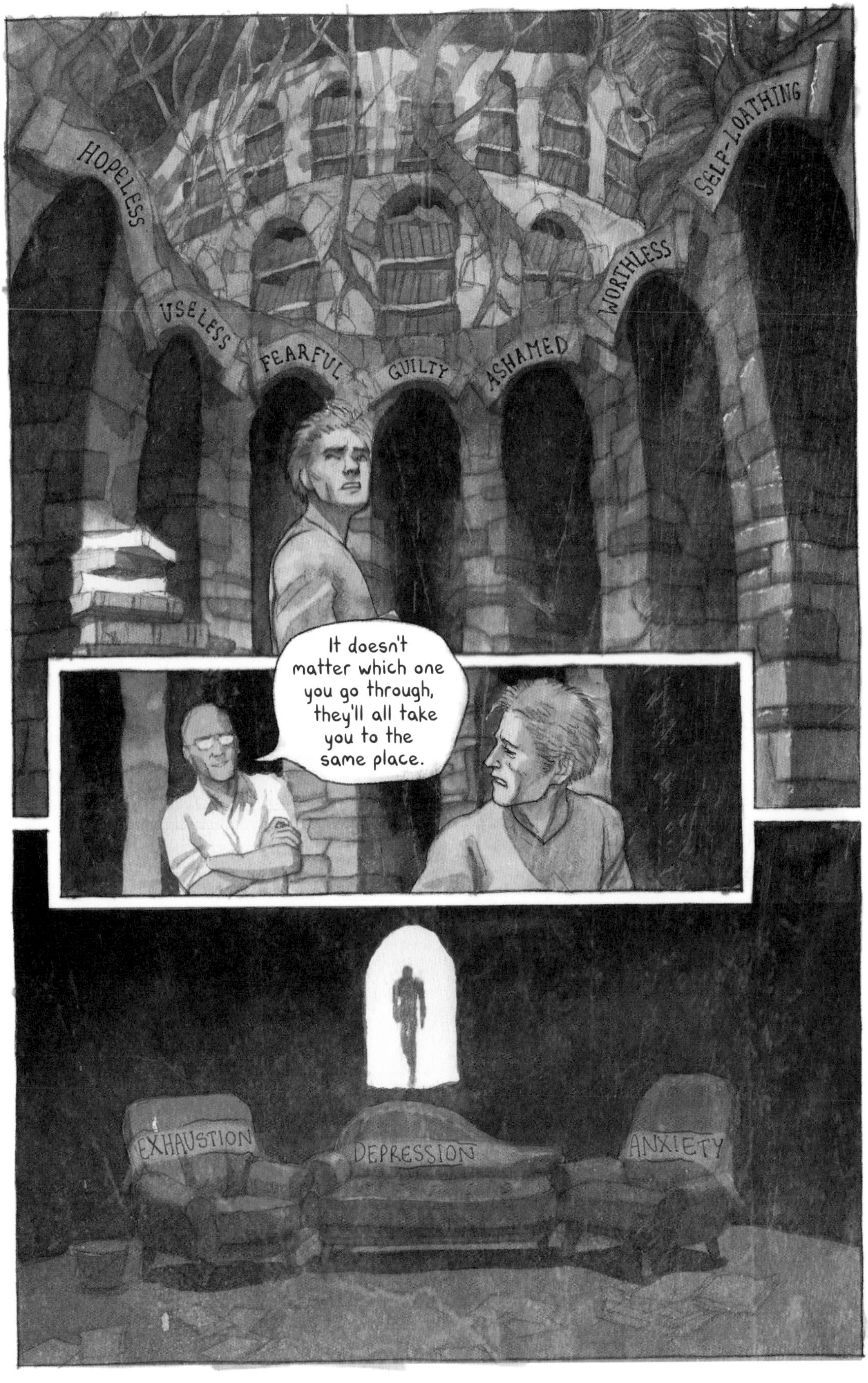
HOPELESS
USELESS
FEARFUL
GUILTY
ASHAMED
WORTHLESS
SELF-LOATHING
It doesn't matter which one you go through, they'll all take you to the same place.
EXHAUSTION
DEPRESSION
ANXIETY

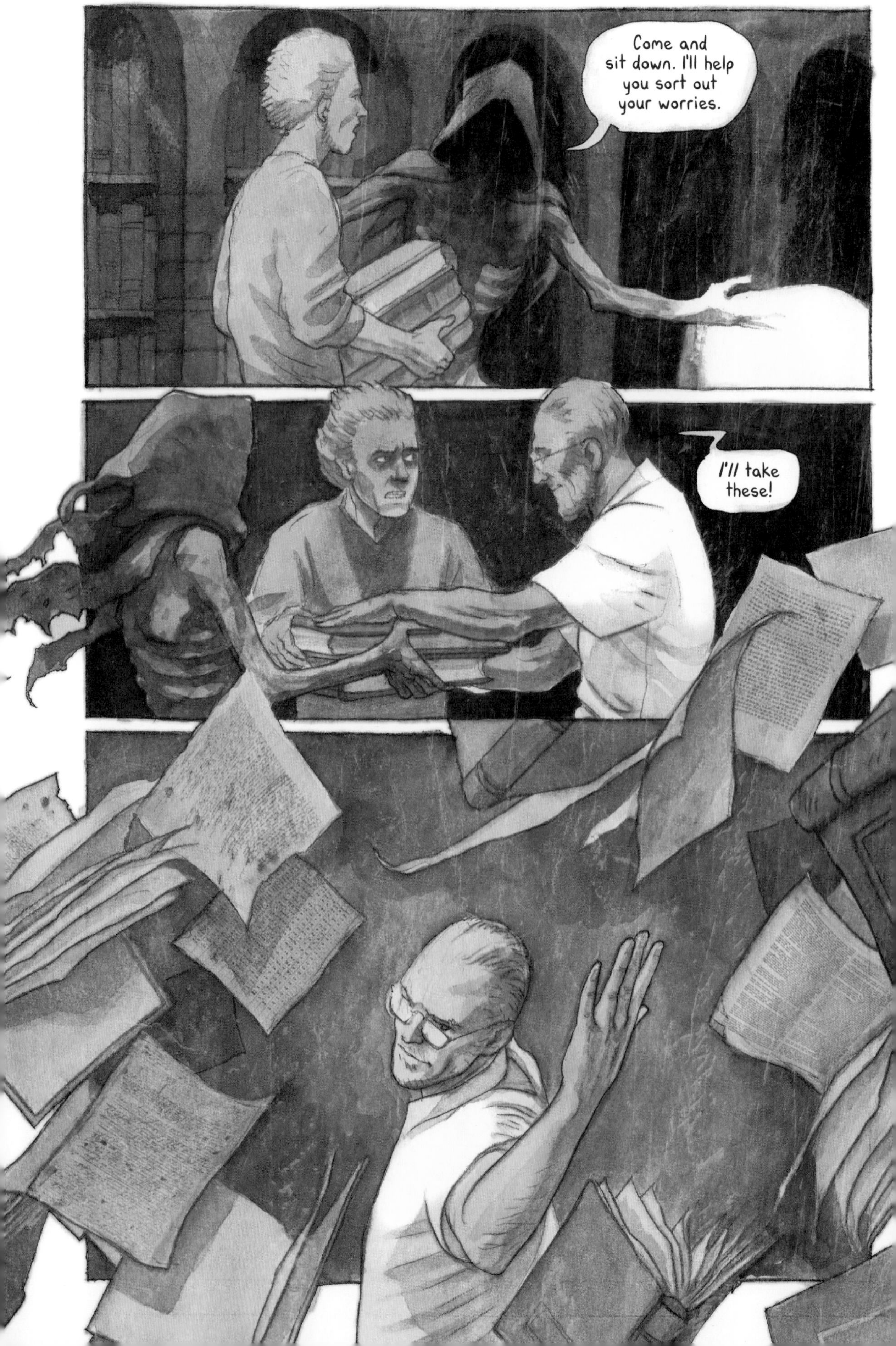
Come and sit down. I'll help you sort out your worries.
I'll take these!

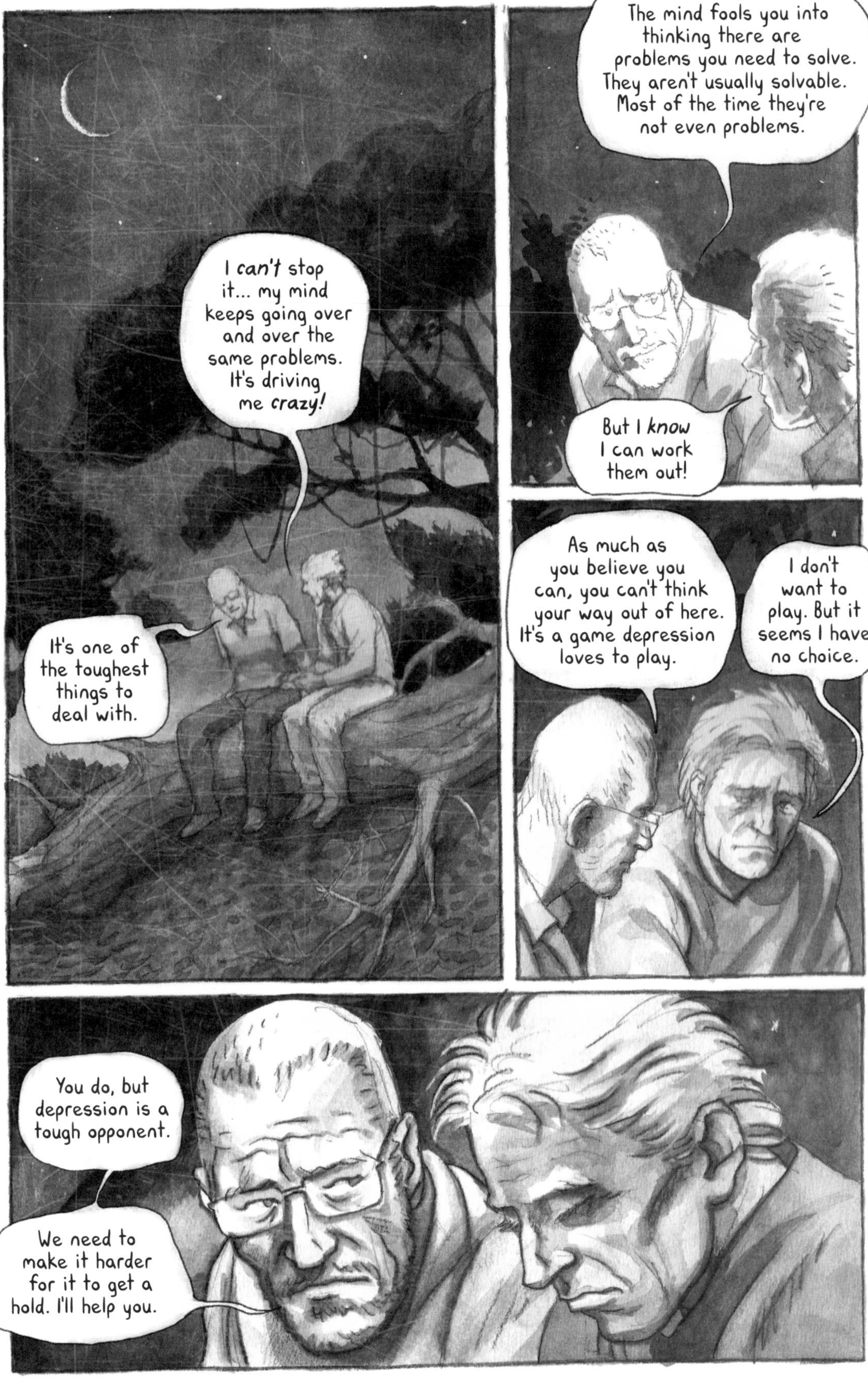
I *can't* stop it... my mind keeps going over and over the same problems. It's driving me *crazy!*
It's one of the toughest things to deal with.
The mind fools you into thinking there are problems you need to solve. They aren't usually solvable. Most of the time they're not even problems.
But I *know* I can work them out!
As much as you believe you can, you can't think your way out of here. It's a game depression loves to play.
I don't want to play. But it seems I have no choice.
You do, but depression is a tough opponent.
We need to make it harder for it to get a hold. I'll help you.

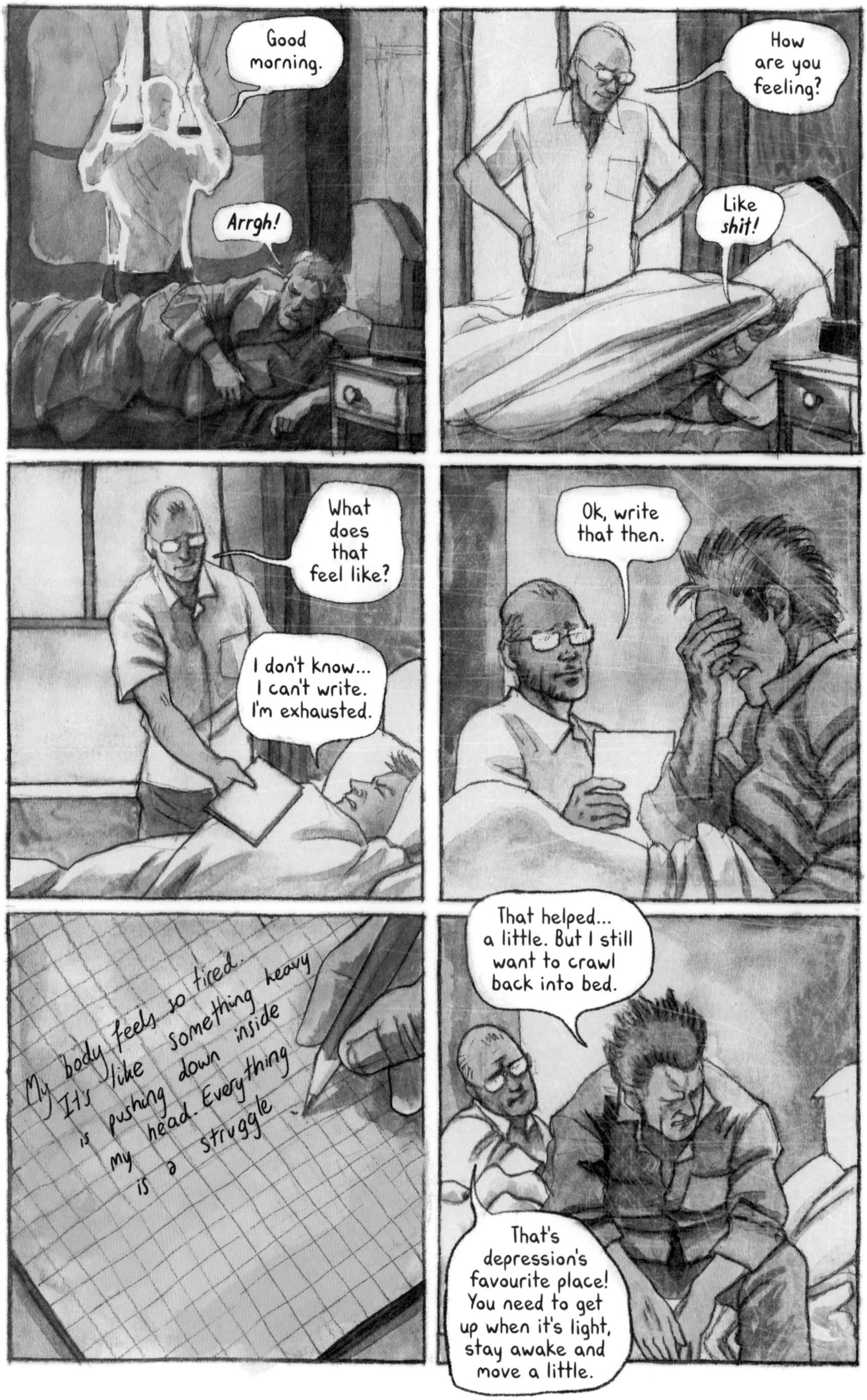
Good morning.
Arrgh!
How are you feeling?
Like shit!
What does that feel like?
I don't know... I can't write. I'm exhausted.
Ok, write that then.
My body feels so tired. It's like something heavy is pushing down inside my head. Everything is a struggle
That helped... a little. But I still want to crawl back into bed.
That's depression's favourite place! You need to get up when it's light, stay awake and move a little.

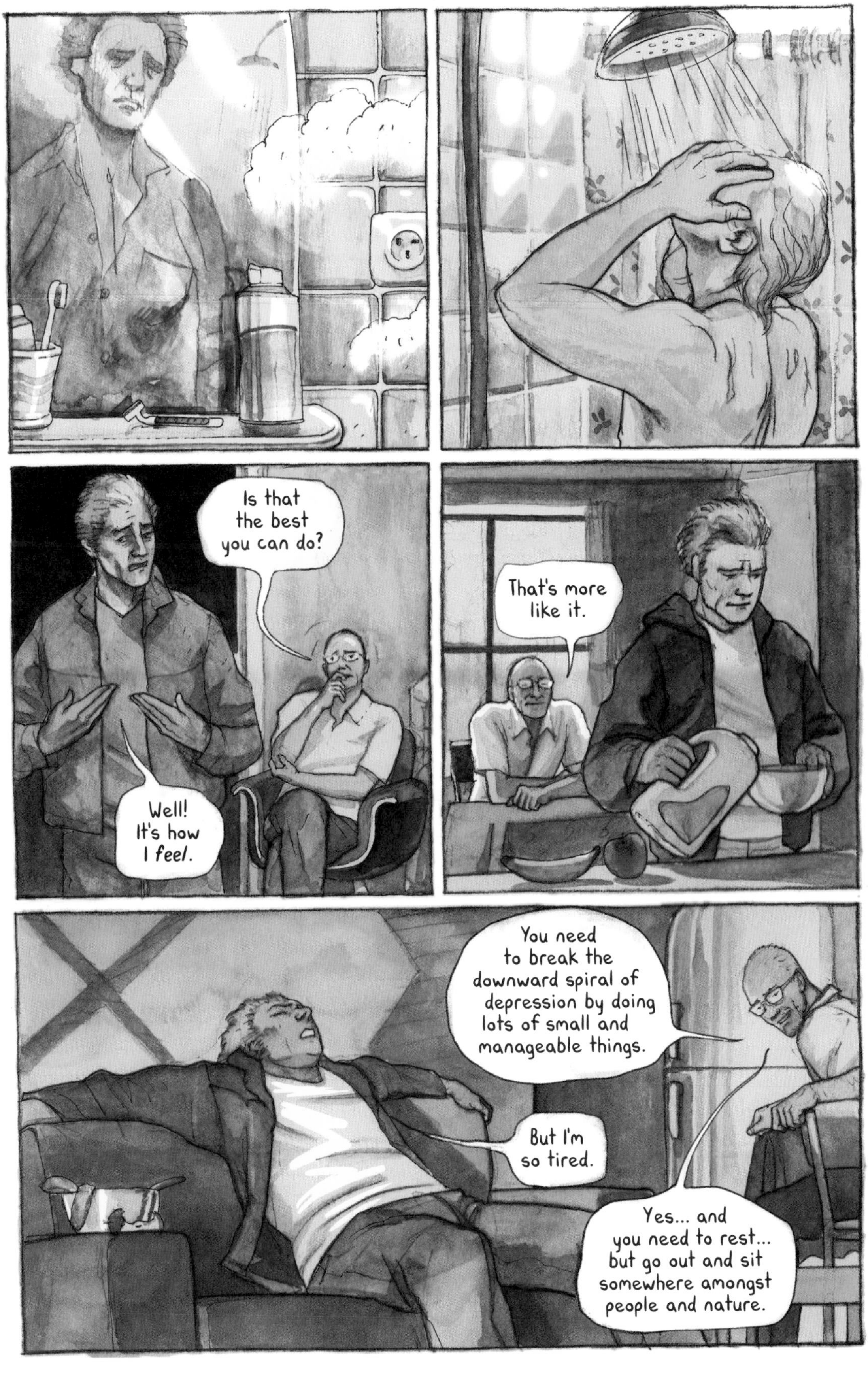
Is that the best you can do?
Well! It's how I *feel*.
That's more like it.
You need to break the downward spiral of depression by doing lots of small and manageable things.
But I'm so tired.
Yes... and you need to rest... but go out and sit somewhere amongst people and nature.

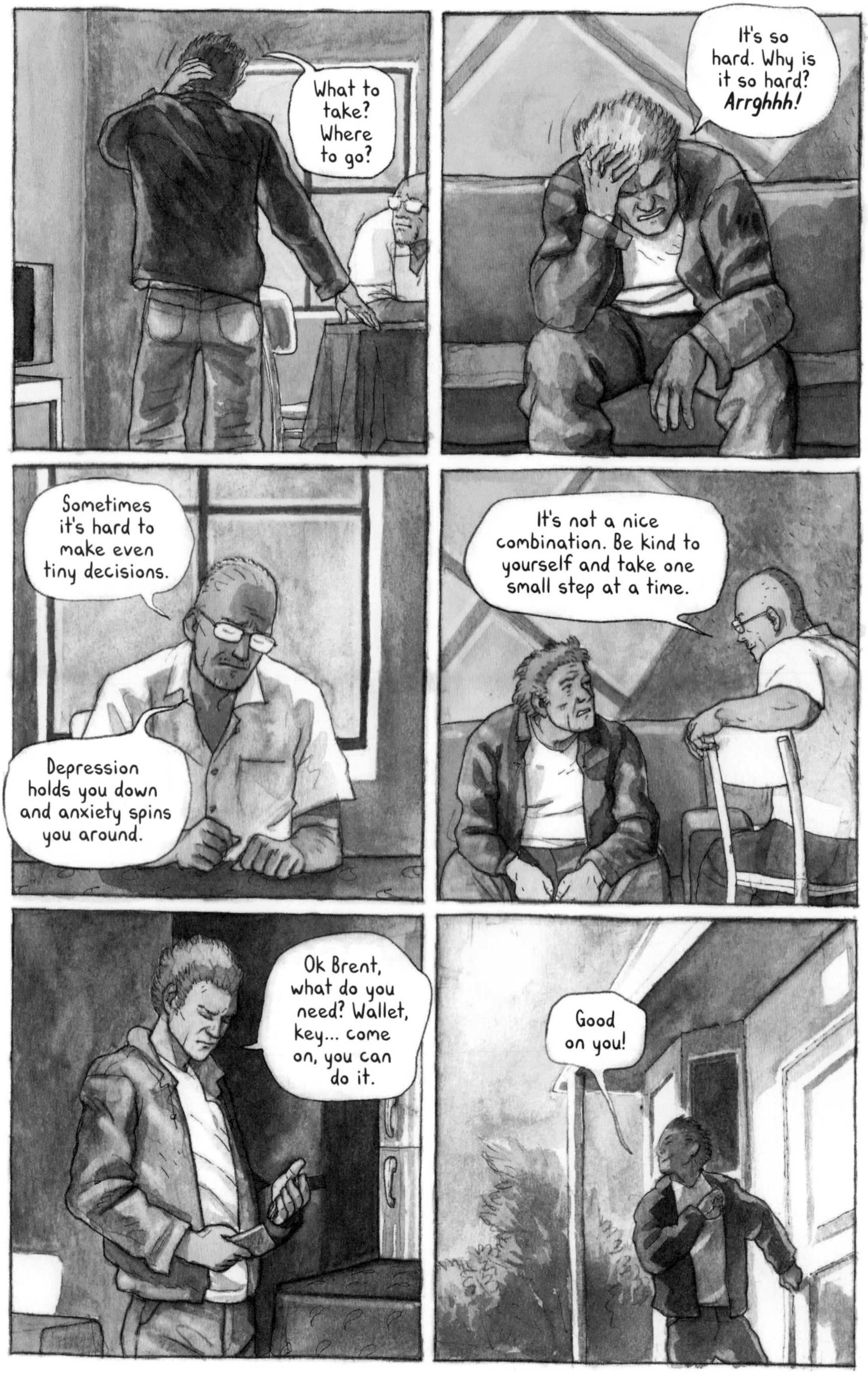
What to take? Where to go?
It's so hard. Why is it so hard? Arrghhh!
Sometimes it's hard to make even tiny decisions.
Depression holds you down and anxiety spins you around.
It's not a nice combination. Be kind to yourself and take one small step at a time.
Ok Brent, what do you need? Wallet, key... come on, you can do it.
Good on you!

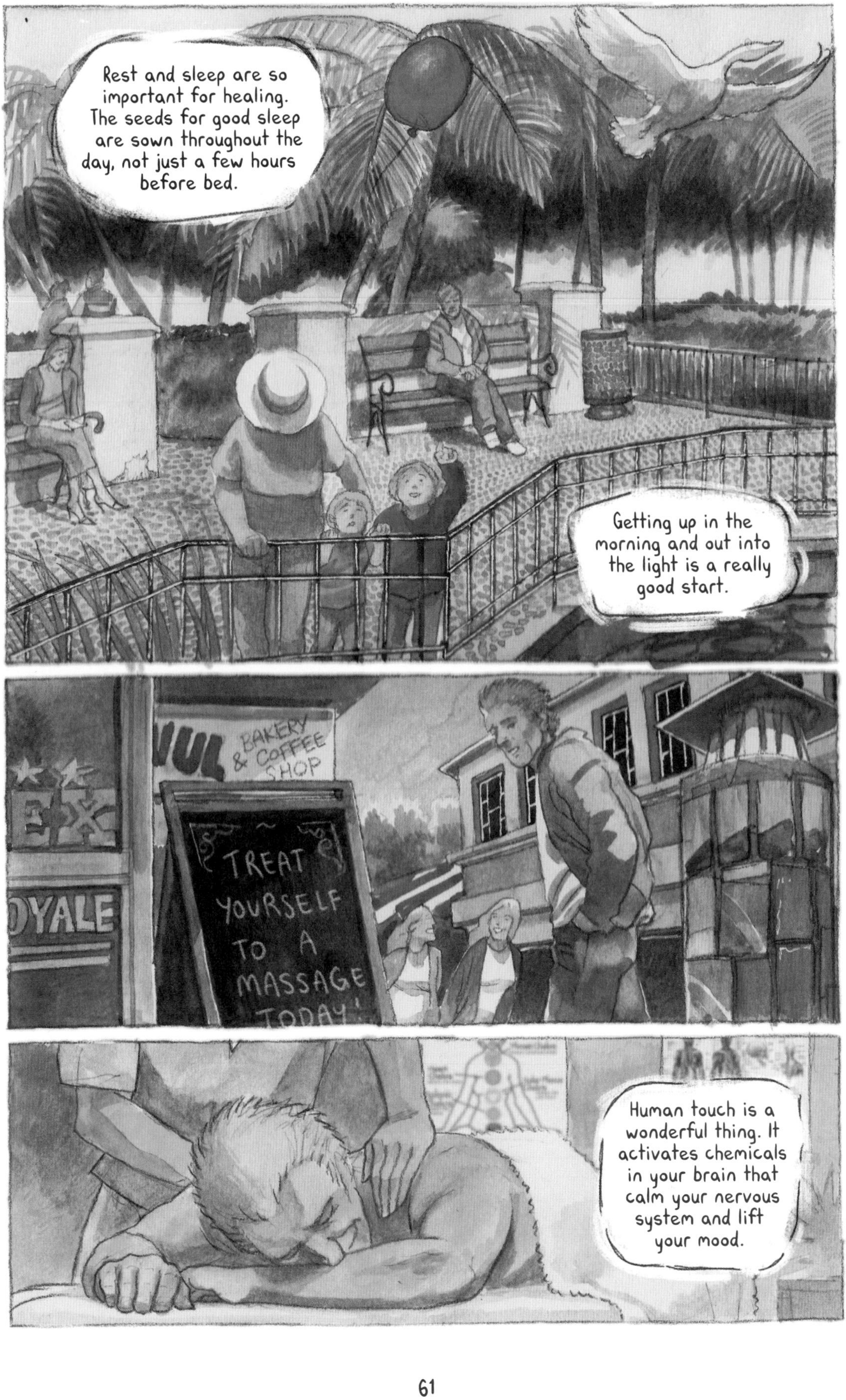
Rest and sleep are so important for healing. The seeds for good sleep are sown throughout the day, not just a few hours before bed.
Getting up in the morning and out into the light is a really good start.
BAKERY & COFFEE SHOP
TREAT YOURSELF TO A MASSAGE TODAY!
Human touch is a wonderful thing. It activates chemicals in your brain that calm your nervous system and lift your mood.

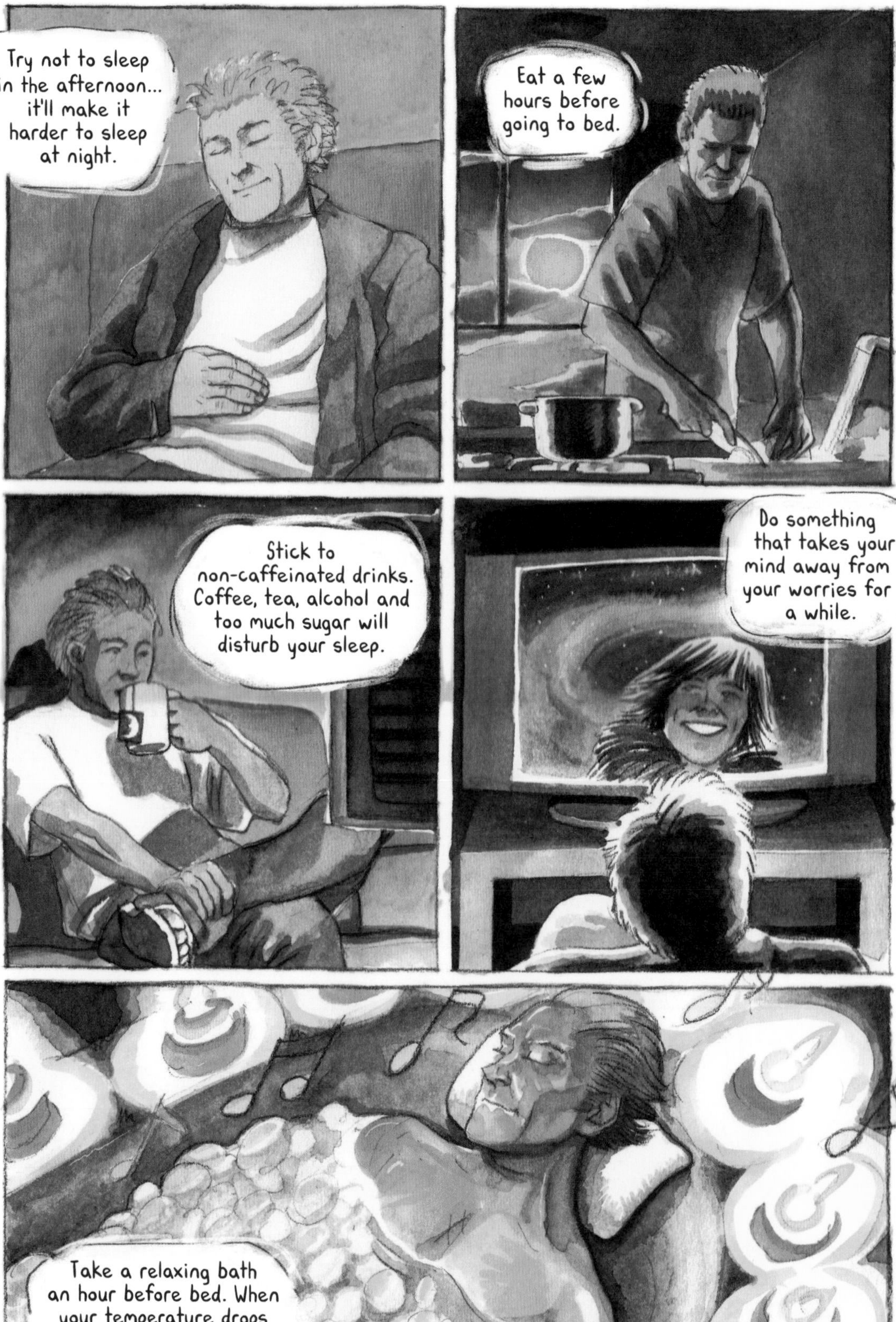
Try not to sleep in the afternoon... it'll make it harder to sleep at night.
Eat a few hours before going to bed.
Stick to non-caffeinated drinks. Coffee, tea, alcohol and too much sugar will disturb your sleep.
Do something that takes your mind away from your worries for a while.
Take a relaxing bath an hour before bed. When your temperature drops later it will help you get to sleep.

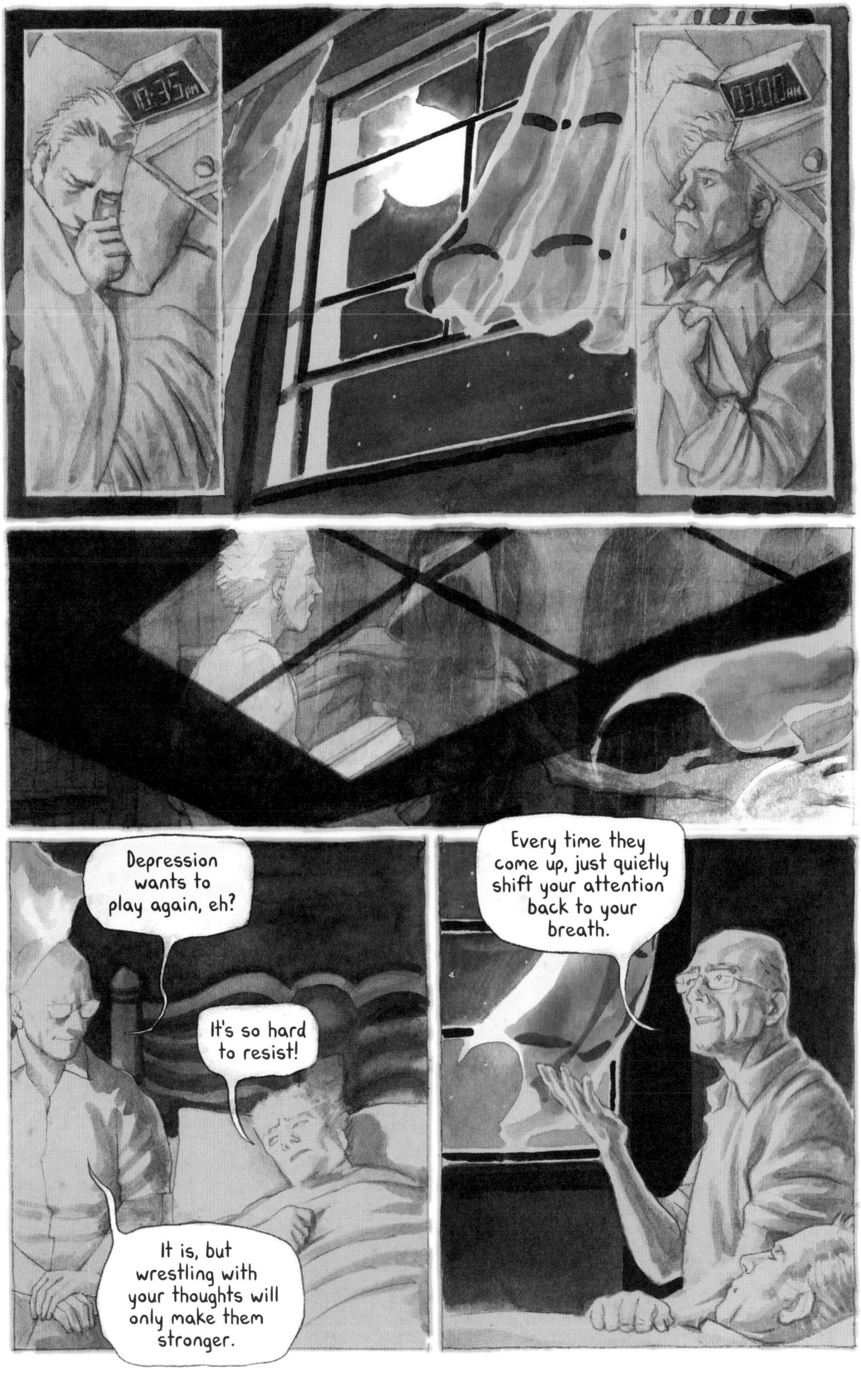
Depression wants to play again, eh?
It's so hard to resist!
It is, but wrestling with your thoughts will only make them stronger.
Every time they come up, just quietly shift your attention back to your breath.

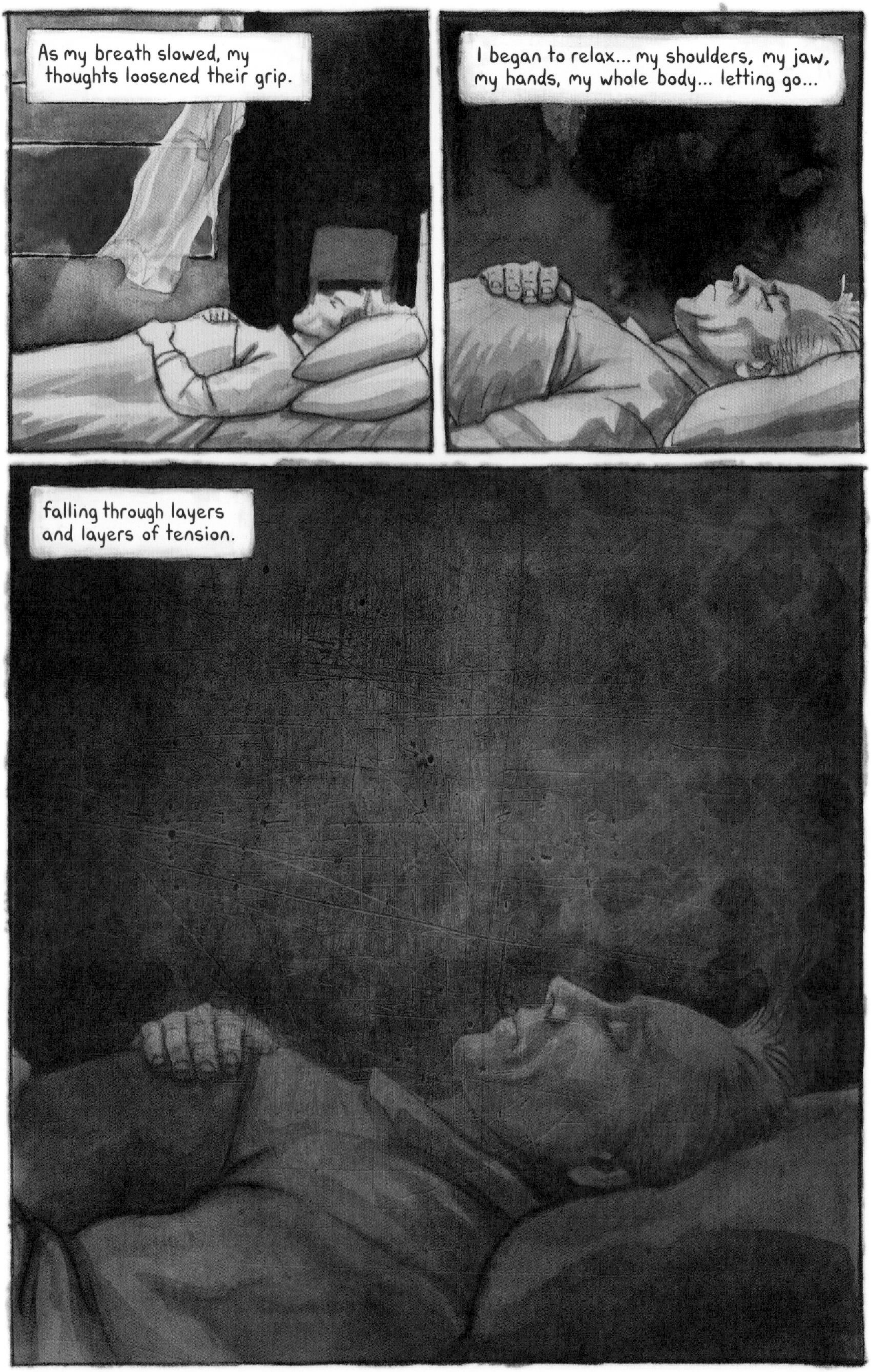
As my breath slowed, my thoughts loosened their grip.
I began to relax... my shoulders, my jaw, my hands, my whole body... letting go...
falling through layers and layers of tension.

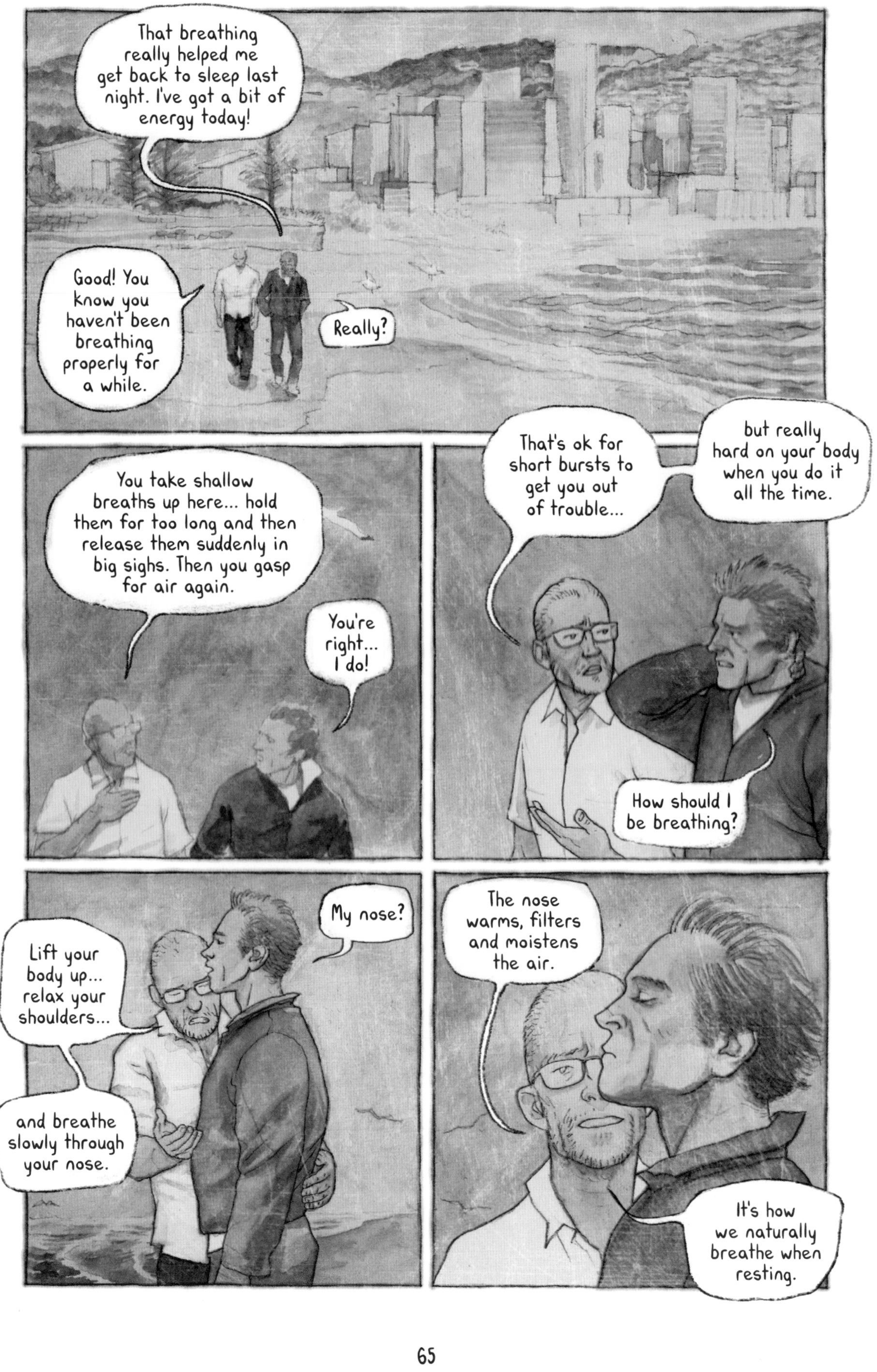

That breathing really helped me get back to sleep last night. I've got a bit of energy today!
Good! You know you haven't been breathing properly for a while.
Really?
You take shallow breaths up here... hold them for too long and then release them suddenly in big sighs. Then you gasp for air again.
You're right... I do!
That's ok for short bursts to get you out of trouble...
but really hard on your body when you do it all the time.
How should I be breathing?
Lift your body up... relax your shoulders...
and breathe slowly through your nose.
My nose?
The nose warms, filters and moistens the air.
It's how we naturally breathe when resting.

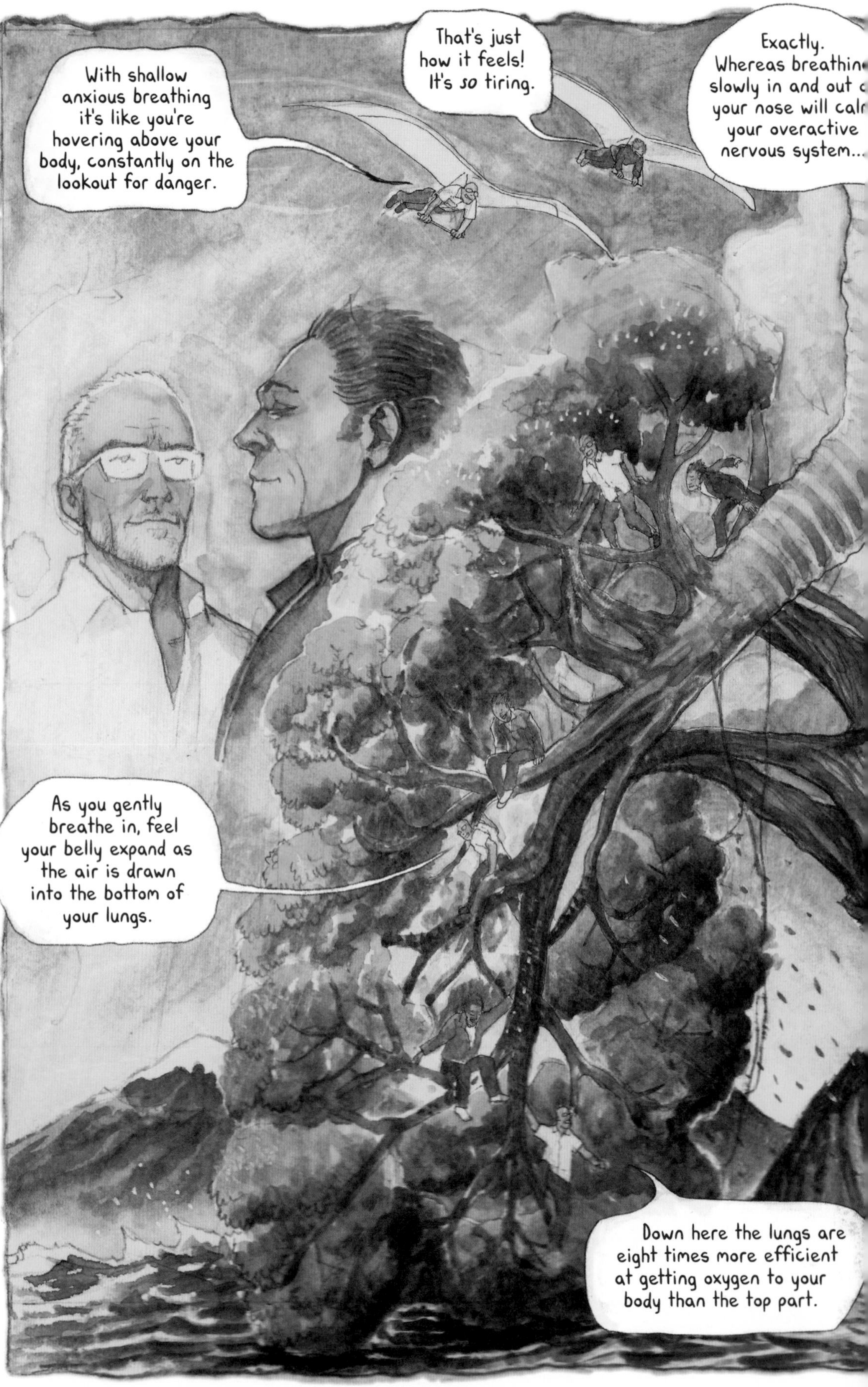
With shallow anxious breathing it's like you're hovering above your body, constantly on the lookout for danger.
That's just how it feels! It's so tiring.
Exactly. Whereas breathin slowly in and out your nose will cal your overactive nervous system...
As you gently breathe in, feel your belly expand as the air is drawn into the bottom of your lungs.
Down here the lungs are eight times more efficient at getting oxygen to your body than the top part.

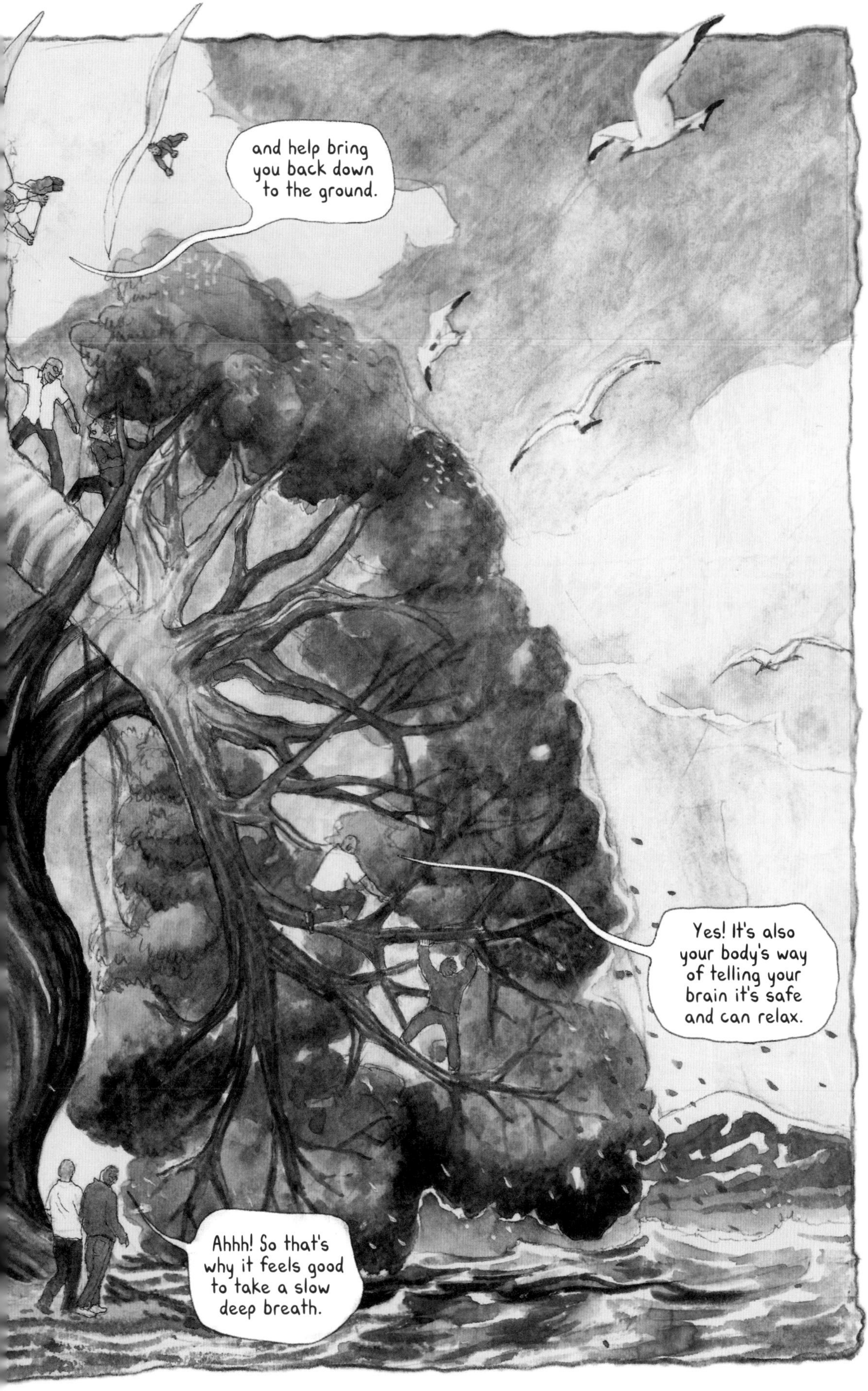
and help bring you back down to the ground.
Yes! It's also your body's way of telling your brain it's safe and can relax.
Ahhh! So that's why it feels good to take a slow deep breath.

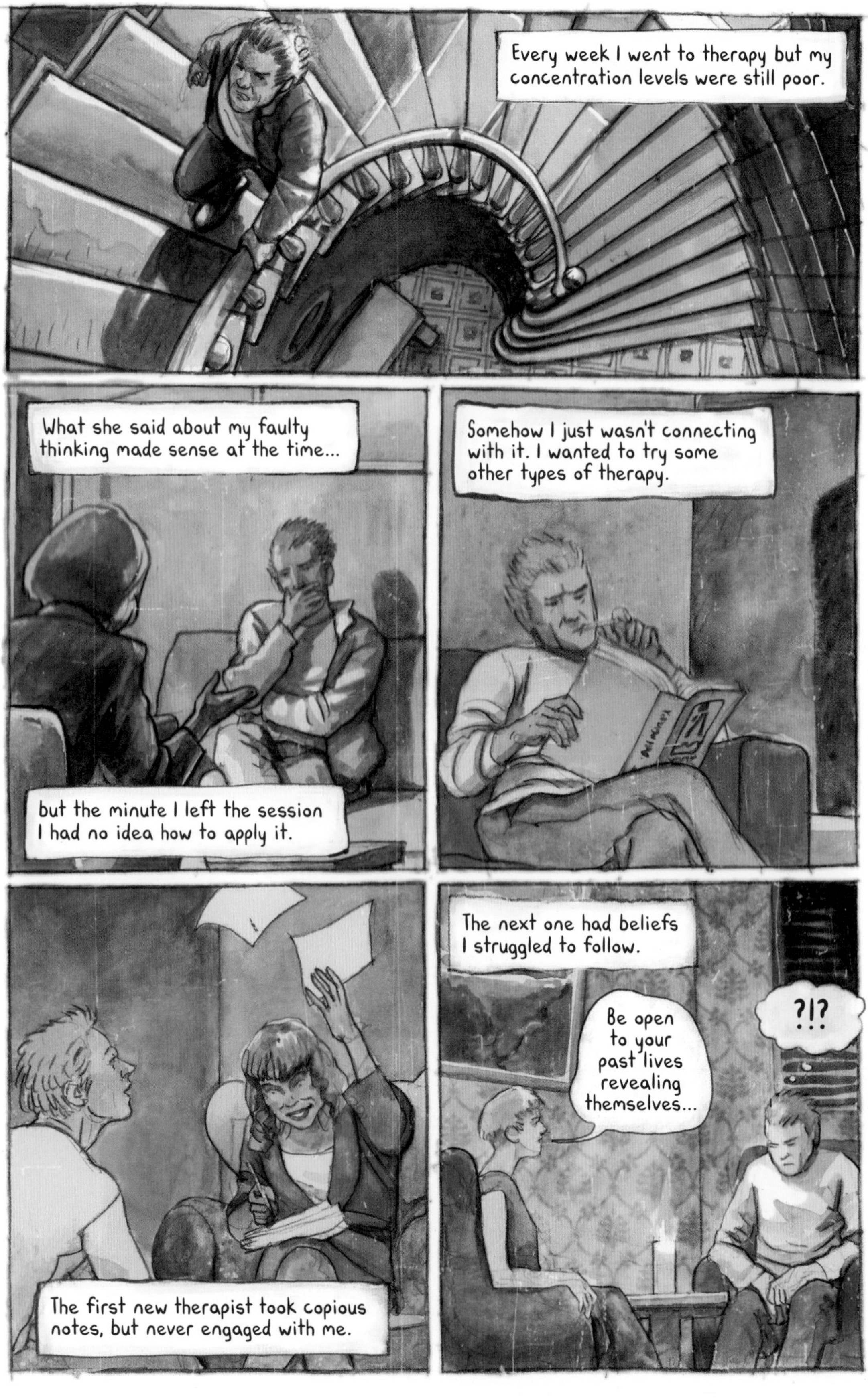
Every week I went to therapy but my concentration levels were still poor.
What she said about my faulty thinking made sense at the time...
but the minute I left the session I had no idea how to apply it.
Somehow I just wasn't connecting with it. I wanted to try some other types of therapy.
The first new therapist took copious notes, but never engaged with me.
The next one had beliefs I struggled to follow.
Be open to your past lives revealing themselves...
?!?

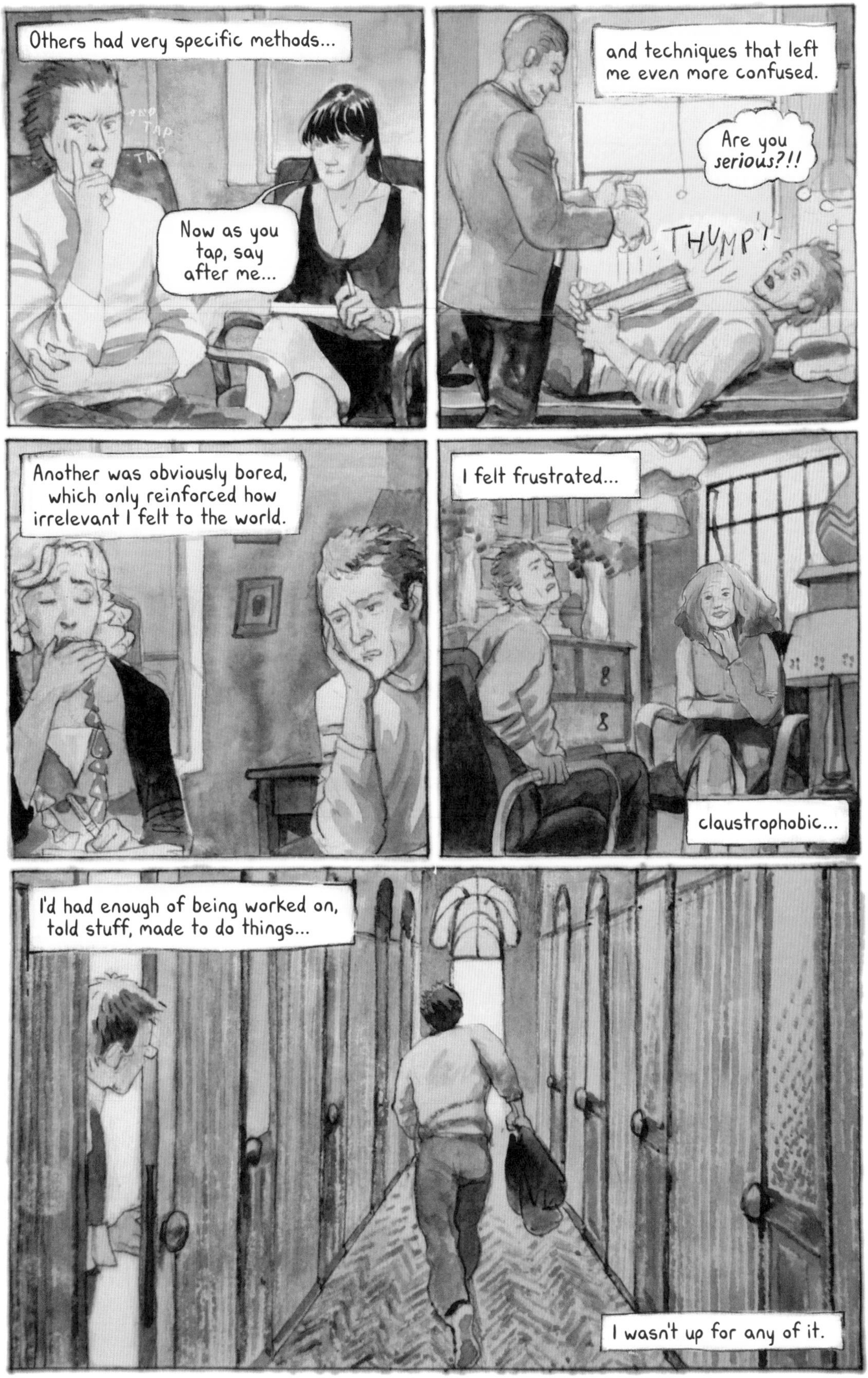
Others had very specific methods...
TAP
TAP
Now as you tap, say after me...
and techniques that left me even more confused.
Are you *serious?!!*
THUMP!
Another was obviously bored, which only reinforced how irrelevant I felt to the world.
I felt frustrated...
claustrophobic...
I'd had enough of being worked on, told stuff, made to do things...
I wasn't up for any of it.

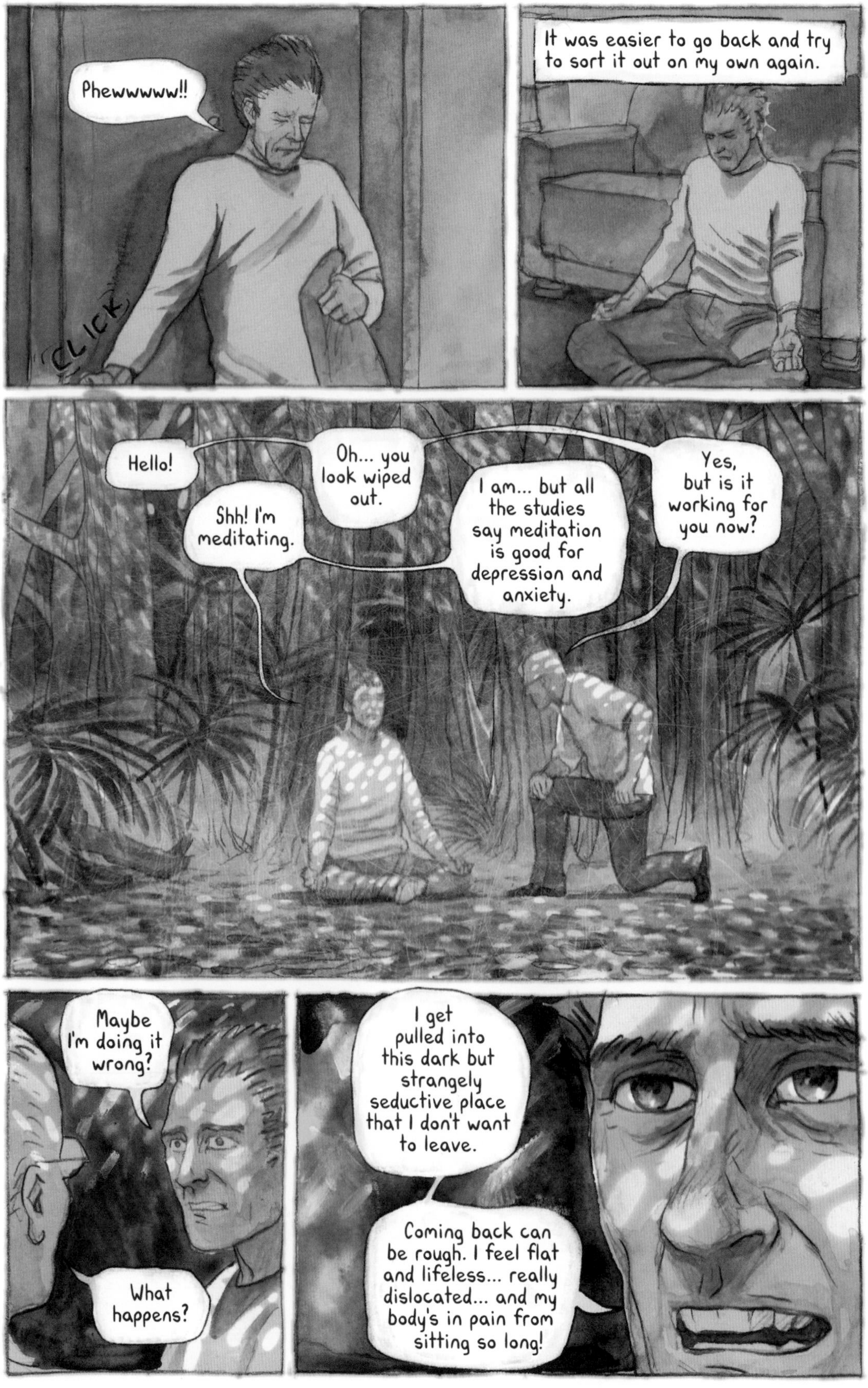
Phewwwww!!
CLICK
It was easier to go back and try to sort it out on my own again.
Hello!
Shh! I'm meditating.
Oh... you look wiped out.
I am... but all the studies say meditation is good for depression and anxiety.
Yes, but is it working for you now?
Maybe I'm doing it wrong?
What happens?
I get pulled into this dark but strangely seductive place that I don't want to leave.
Coming back can be rough. I feel flat and lifeless... really dislocated... and my body's in pain from sitting so long!

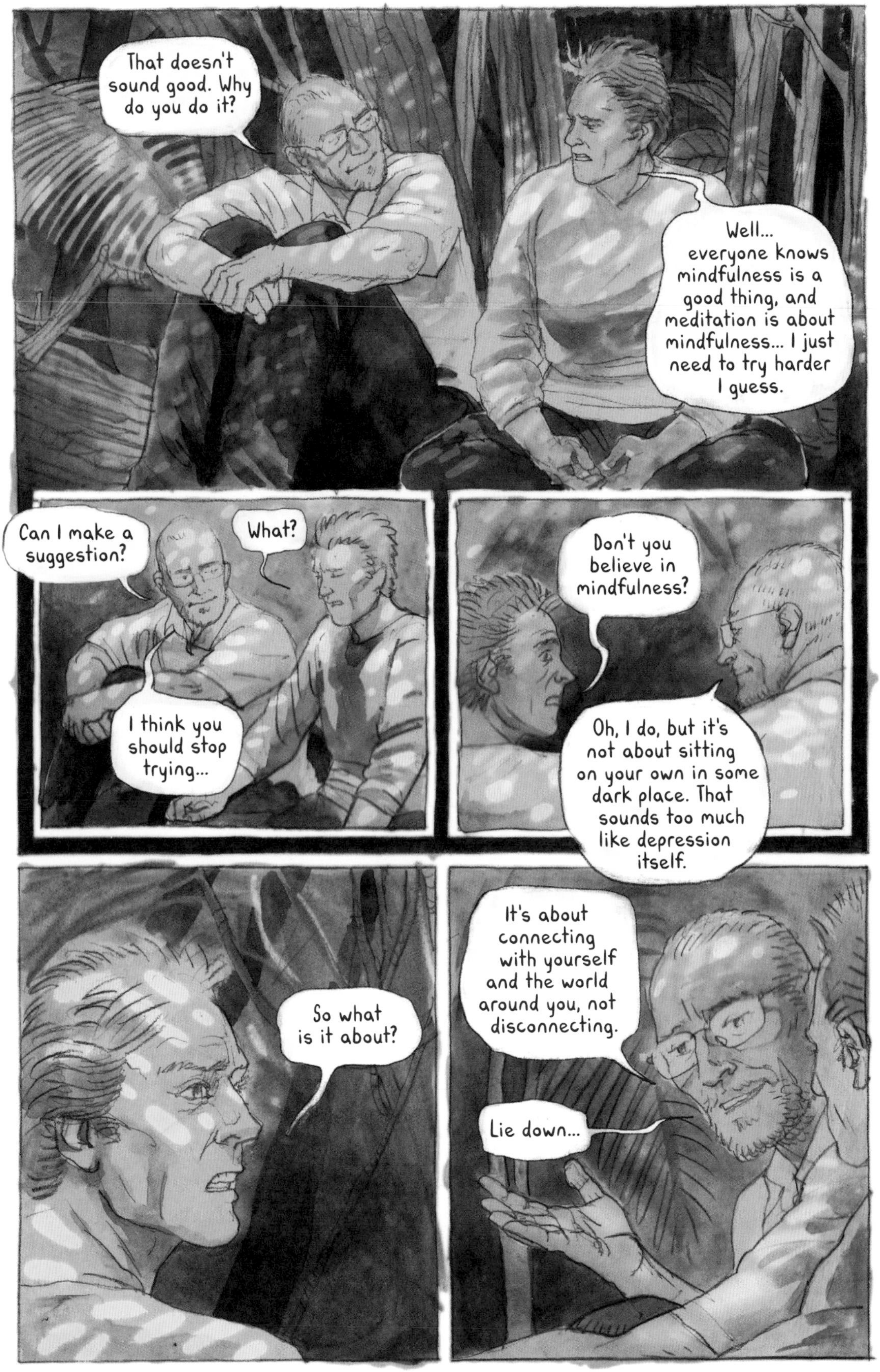
That doesn't sound good. Why do you do it?
Well... everyone knows mindfulness is a good thing, and meditation is about mindfulness... I just need to try harder I guess.
Can I make a suggestion?
What?
I think you should stop trying...
Don't you believe in mindfulness?
Oh, I do, but it's not about sitting on your own in some dark place. That sounds too much like depression itself.
So what is it about?
It's about connecting with yourself and the world around you, not disconnecting.
Lie down...

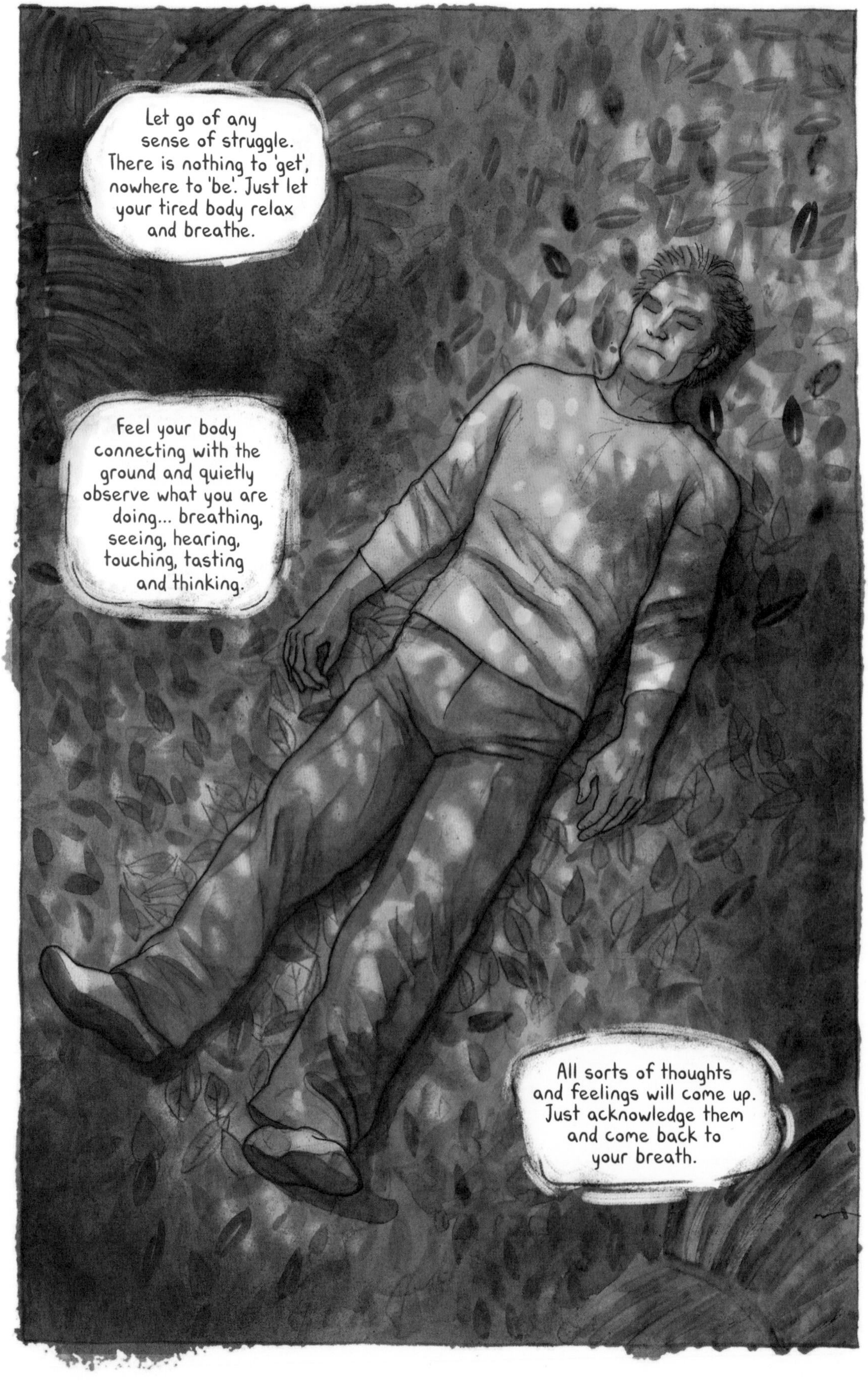
Let go of any sense of struggle. There is nothing to 'get', nowhere to 'be'. Just let your tired body relax and breathe.
Feel your body connecting with the ground and quietly observe what you are doing... breathing, seeing, hearing, touching, tasting and thinking.
All sorts of thoughts and feelings will come up. Just acknowledge them and come back to your breath.

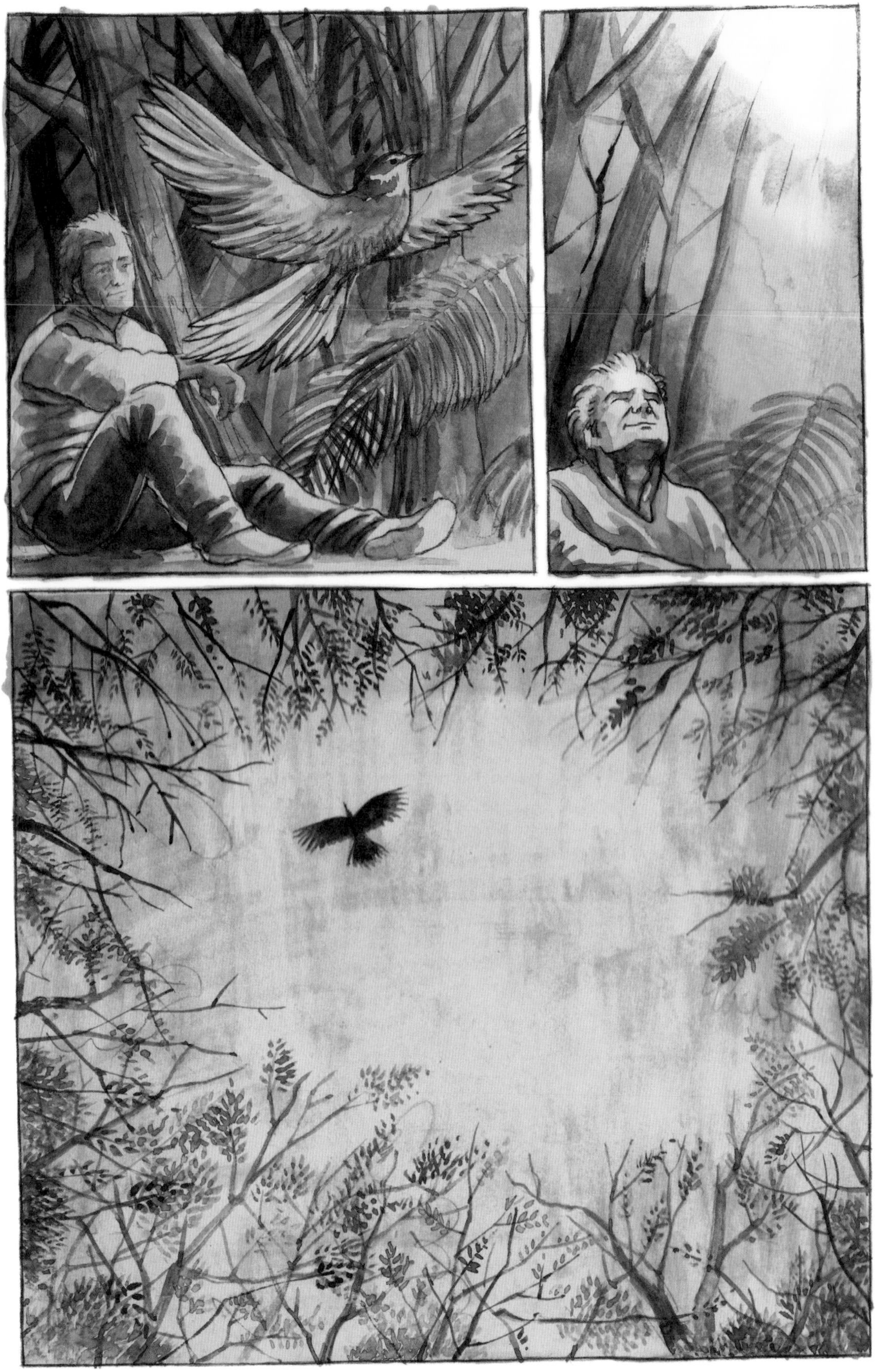

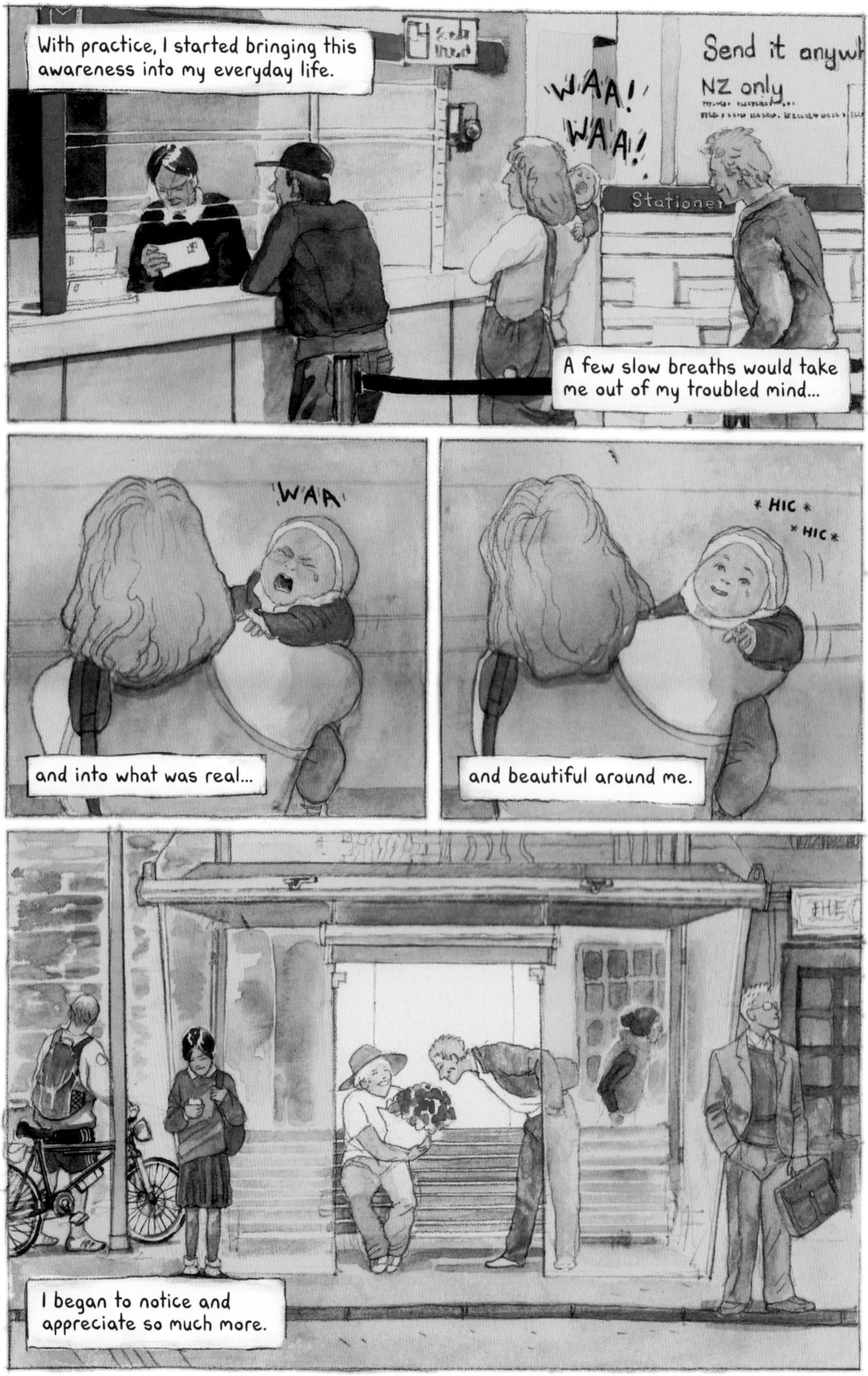
With practice, I started bringing this awareness into my everyday life.
WAA! WAA!
Send it anywh
NZ only
Stationer
A few slow breaths would take me out of my troubled mind...
WAA
and into what was real...
HIC
HIC
and beautiful around me.
I began to notice and appreciate so much more.

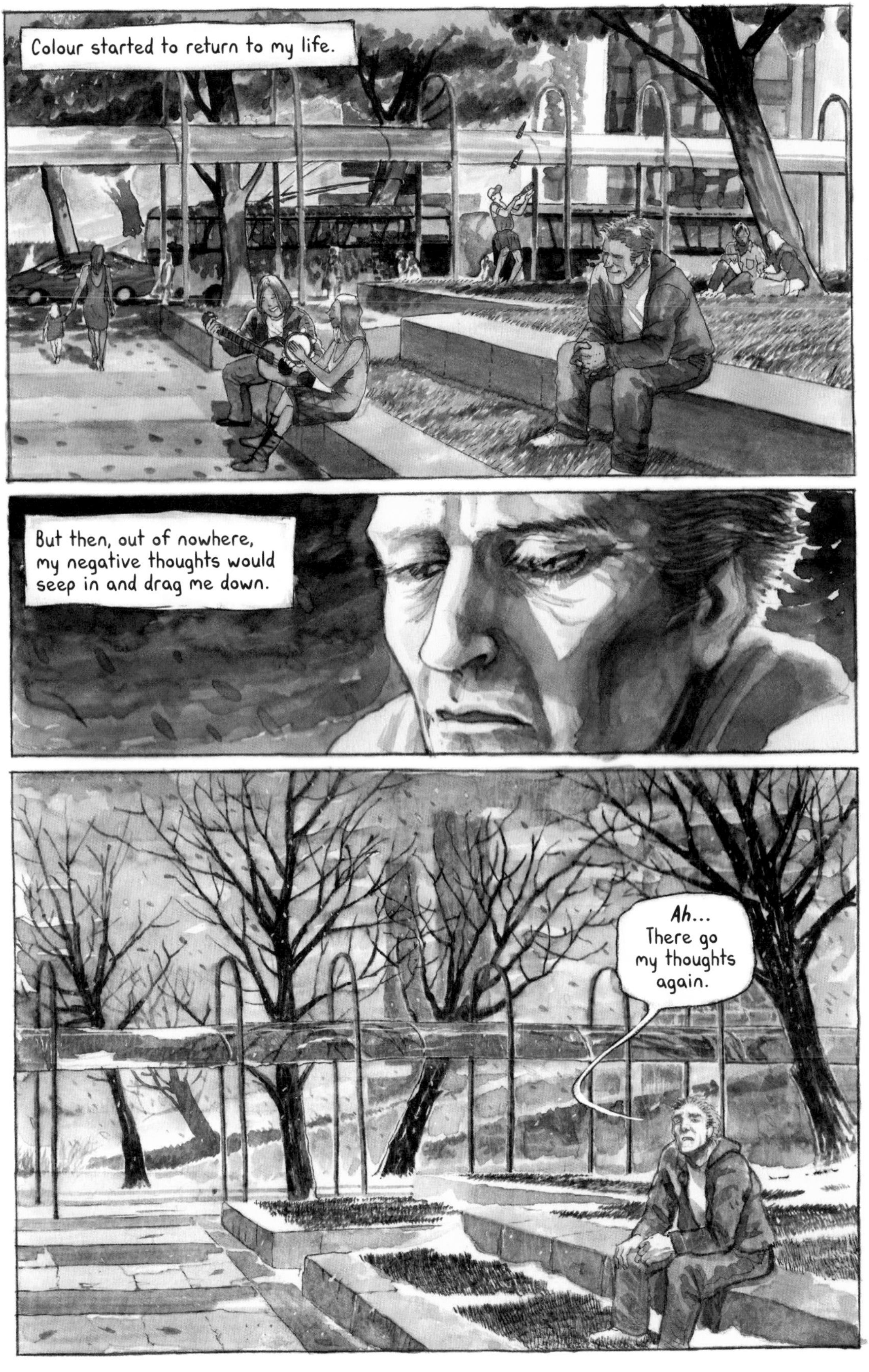
Colour started to return to my life.
But then, out of nowhere, my negative thoughts would seep in and drag me down.
Ah... There go my thoughts again.

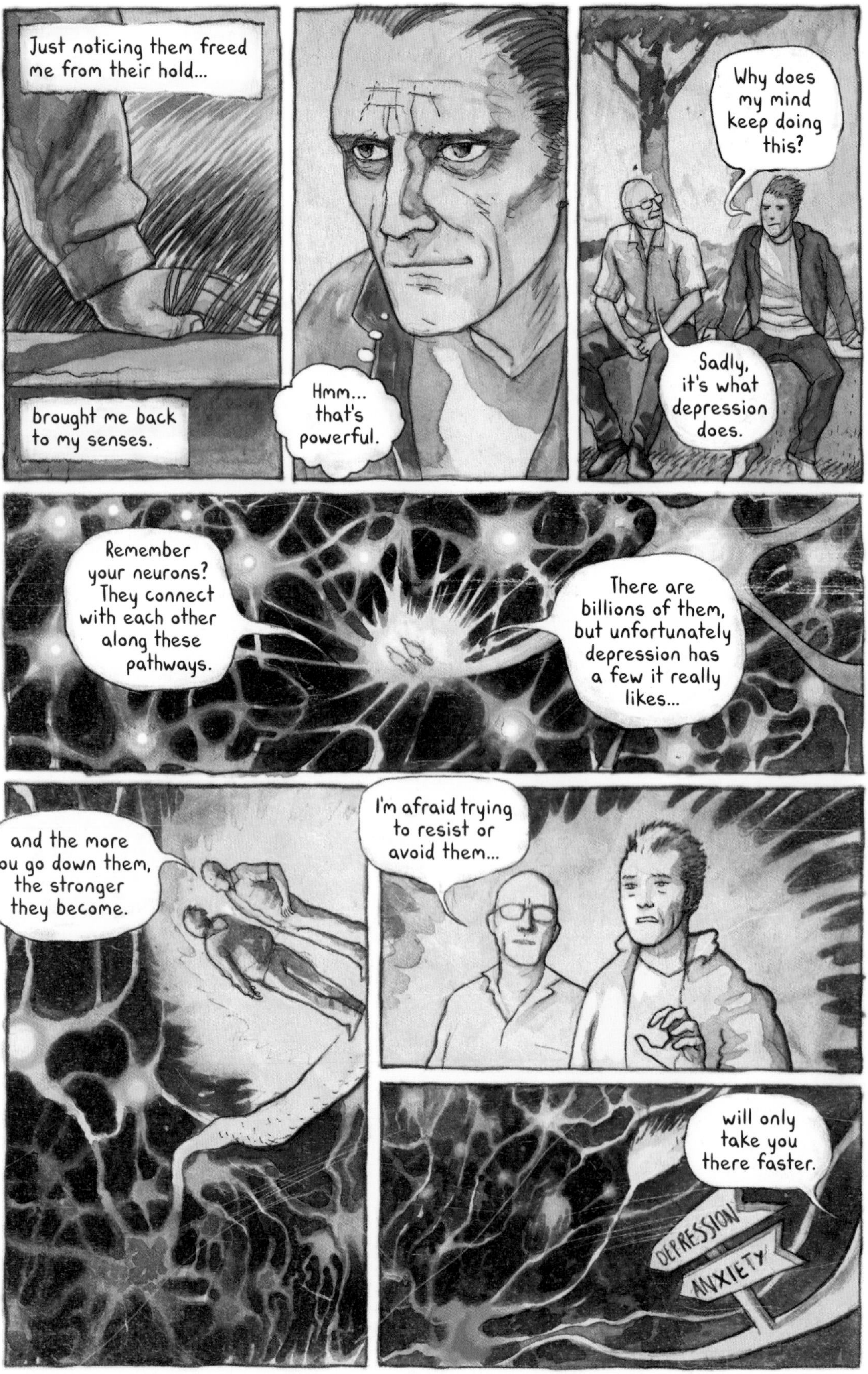
Just noticing them freed me from their hold...
brought me back to my senses.
Hmm... that's powerful.
Why does my mind keep doing this?
Sadly, it's what depression does.
Remember your neurons? They connect with each other along these pathways.
There are billions of them, but unfortunately depression has a few it really likes...
and the more you go down them, the stronger they become.
I'm afraid trying to resist or avoid them...
will only take you there faster.
DEPRESSION
ANXIETY

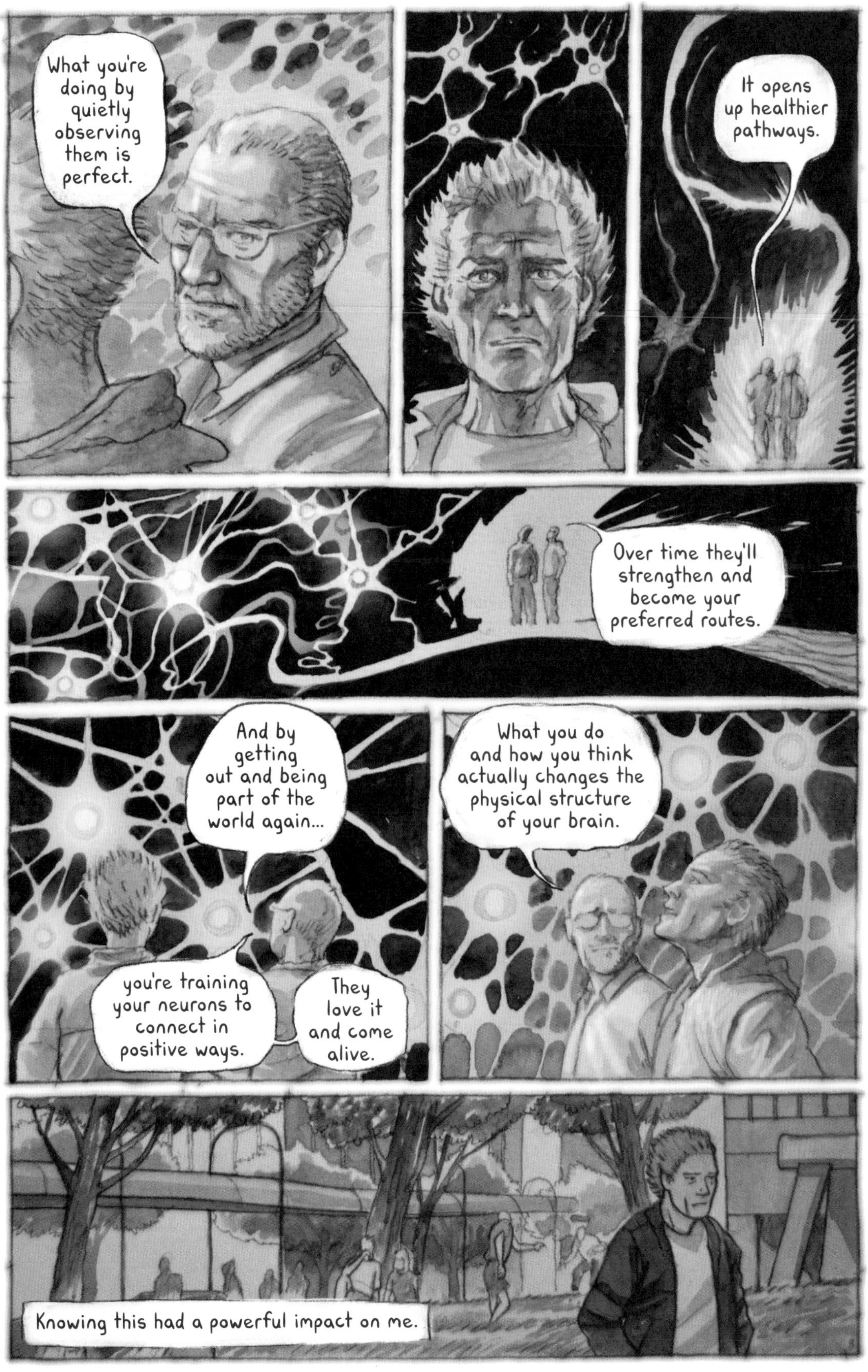
What you're doing by quietly observing them is perfect.
It opens up healthier pathways.
Over time they'll strengthen and become your preferred routes.
And by getting out and being part of the world again...
you're training your neurons to connect in positive ways.
They love it and come alive.
What you do and how you think actually changes the physical structure of your brain.
Knowing this had a powerful impact on me.

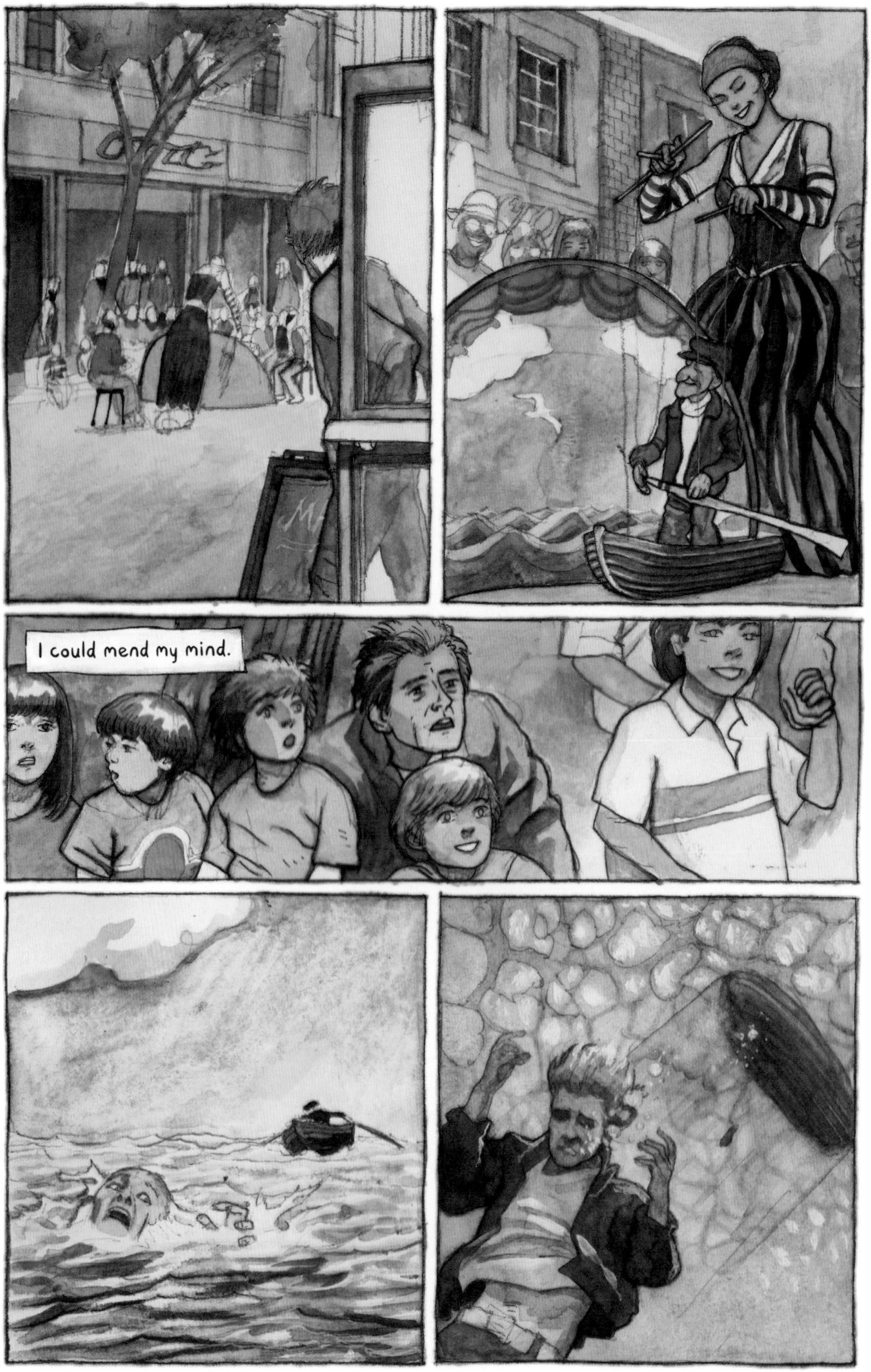
I could mend my mind.

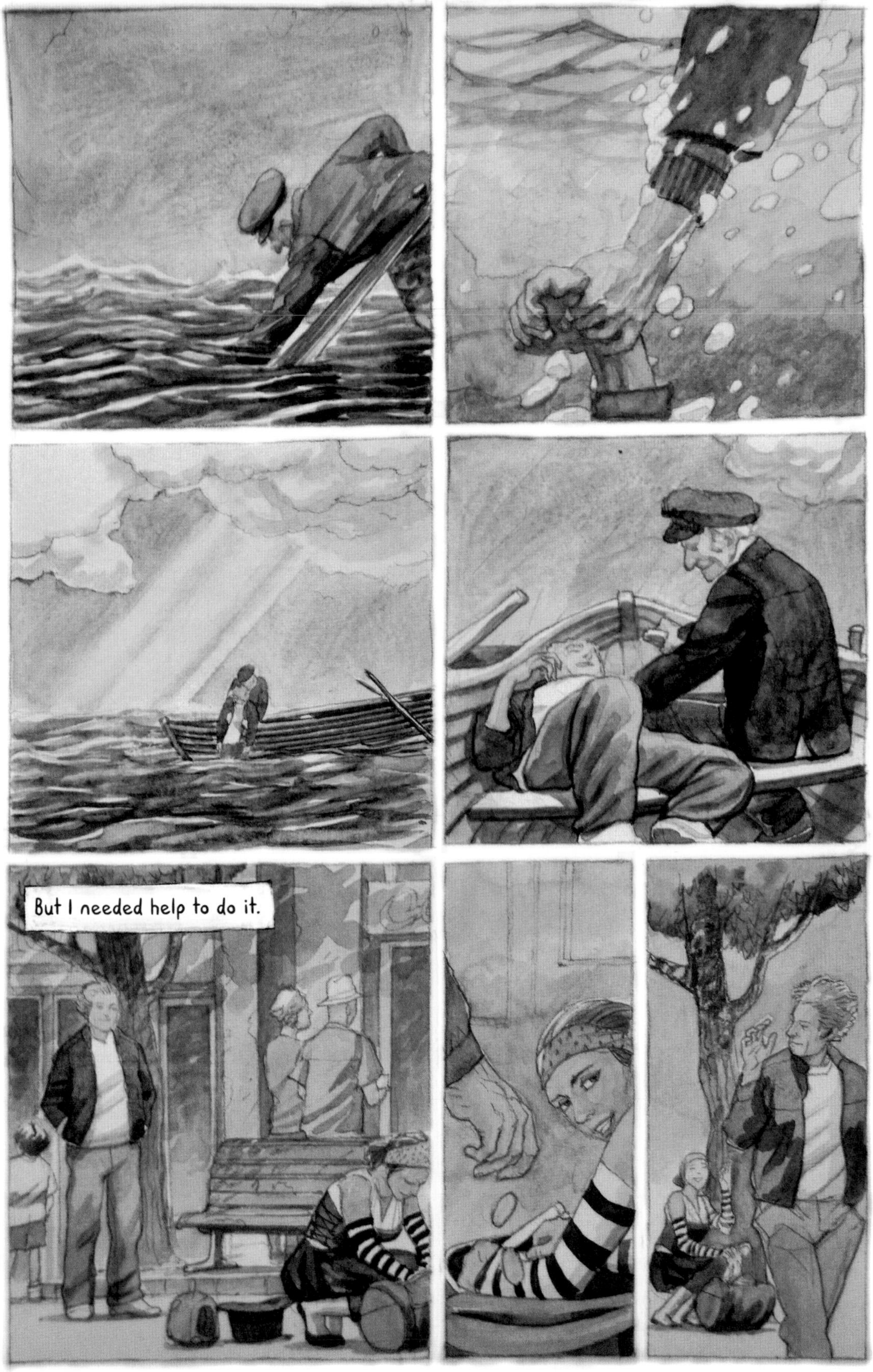
But I needed help to do it.

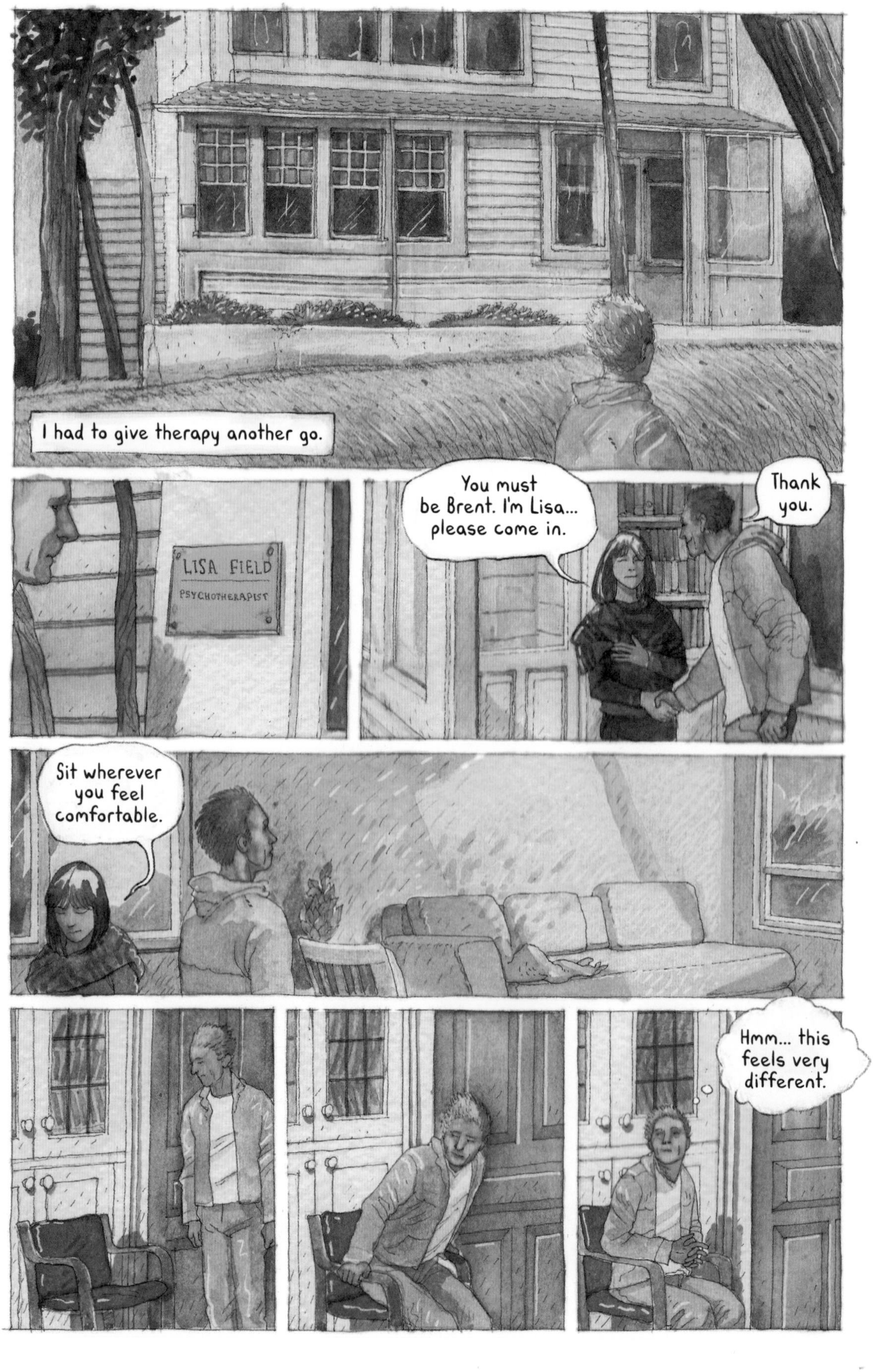
I had to give therapy another go.
LISA FIELD
PSYCHOTHERAPIST
You must be Brent. I'm Lisa... please come in.
Thank you.
Sit wherever you feel comfortable.
Hmm... this feels very different.

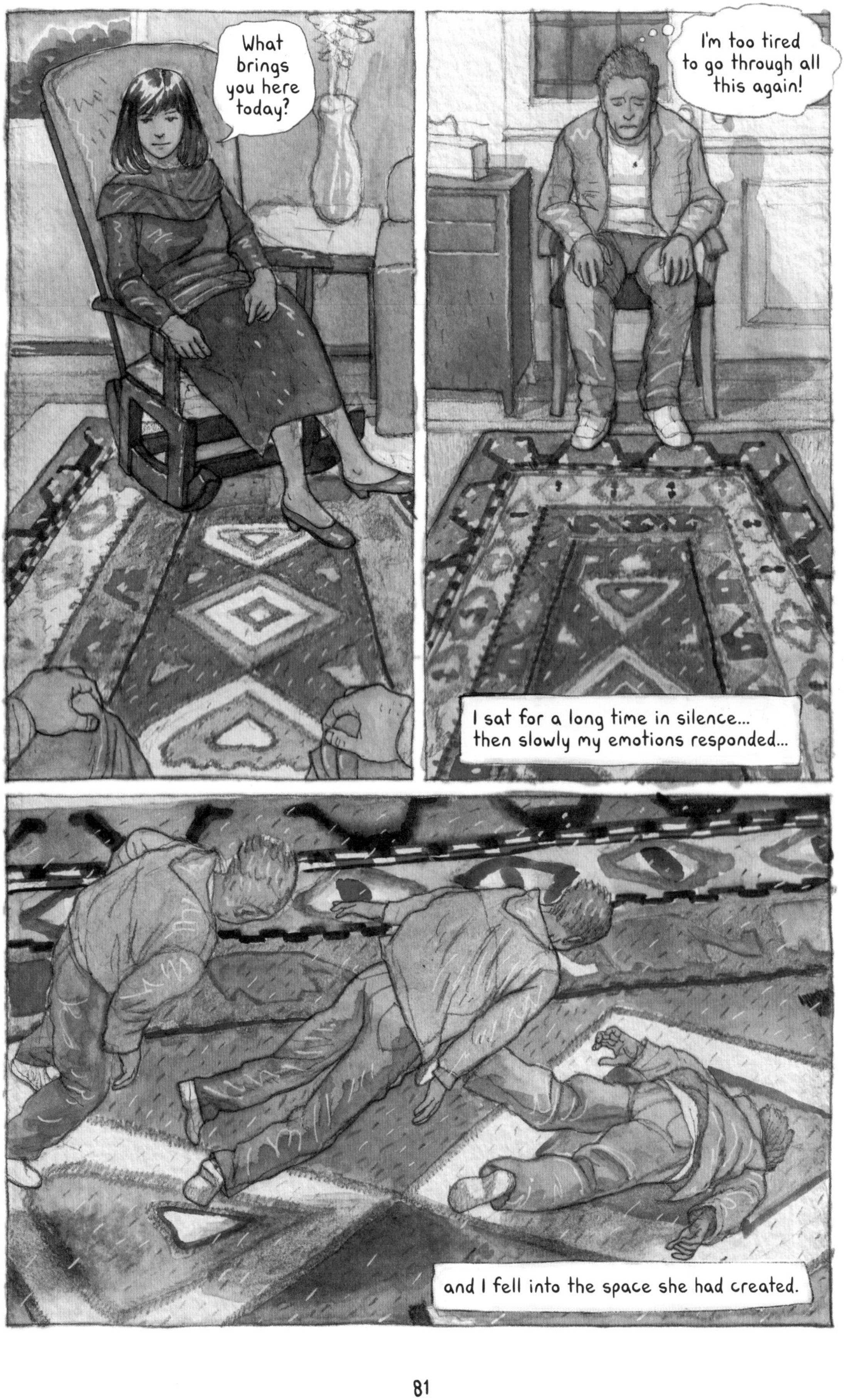
What brings you here today?
I'm too tired to go through all this again!
I sat for a long time in silence... then slowly my emotions responded...
and I fell into the space she had created.

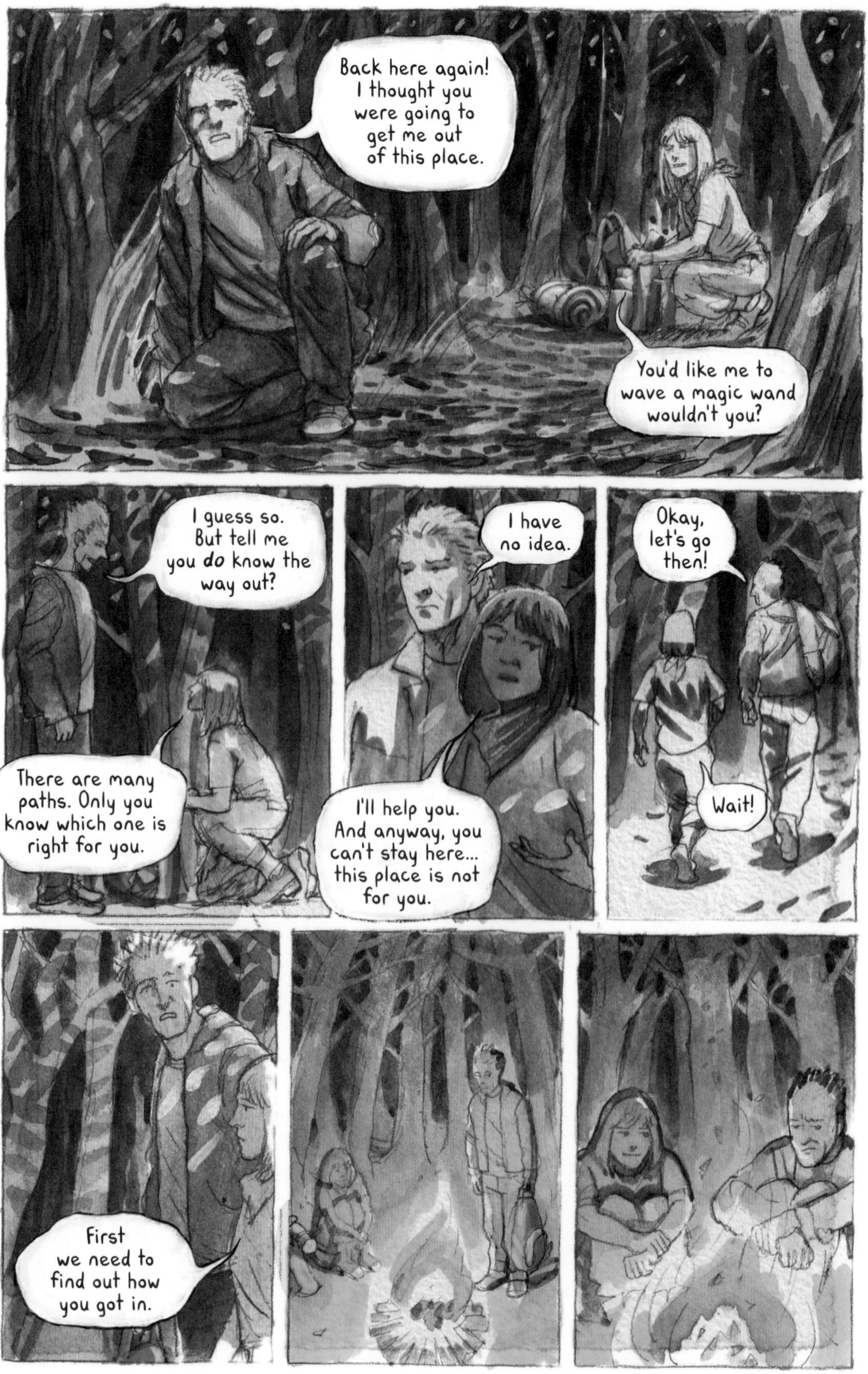
Back here again! I thought you were going to get me out of this place.
You'd like me to wave a magic wand wouldn't you?
I guess so. But tell me you *do* know the way out?
There are many paths. Only you know which one is right for you.
I have no idea.
I'll help you. And anyway, you can't stay here... this place is not for you.
Okay, let's go then!
Wait!
First we need to find out how you got in.

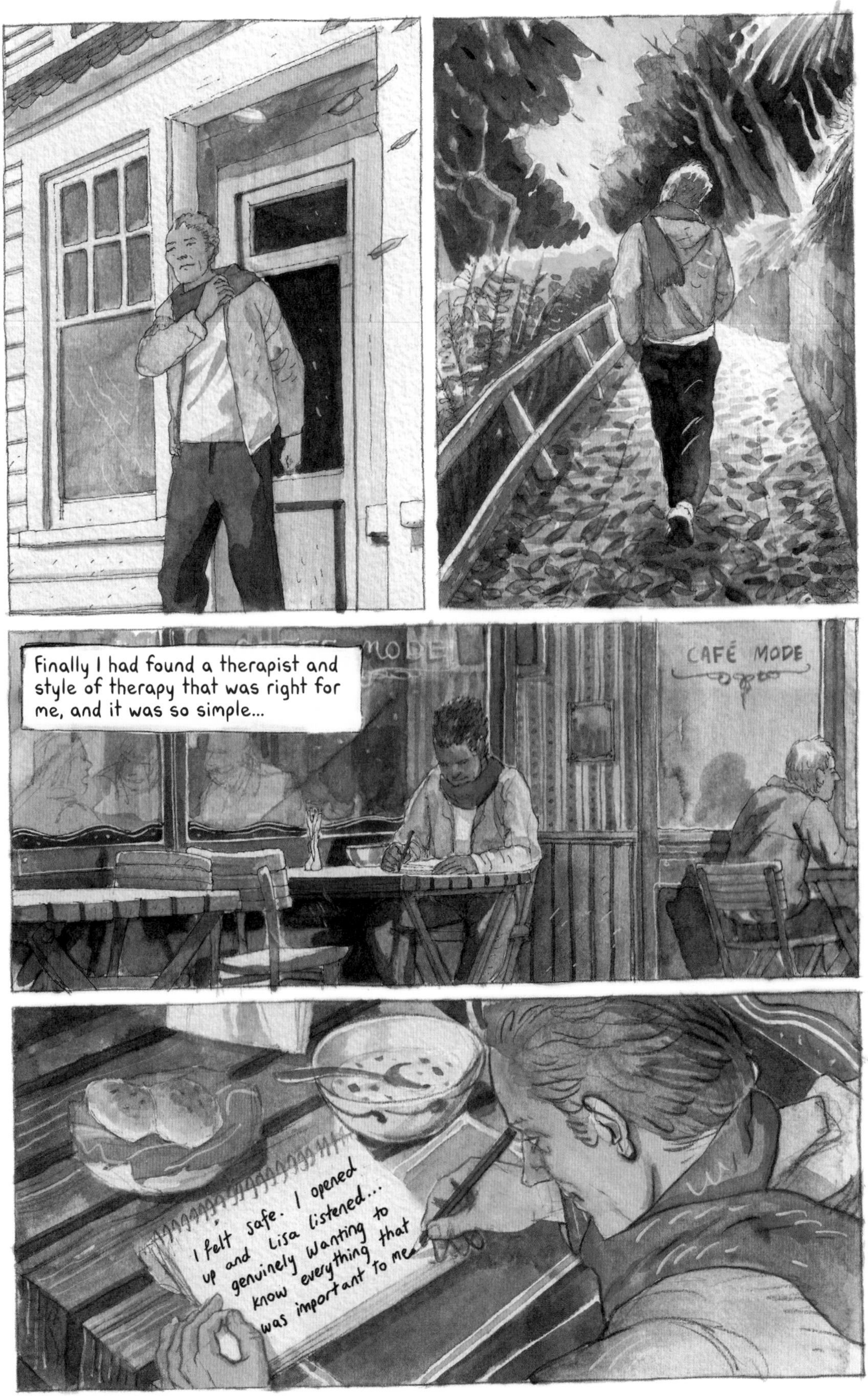
Finally I had found a therapist and style of therapy that was right for me, and it was so simple...
CAFÉ MODE
I felt safe. I opened up and Lisa listened... genuinely wanting to know everything that was important to me.

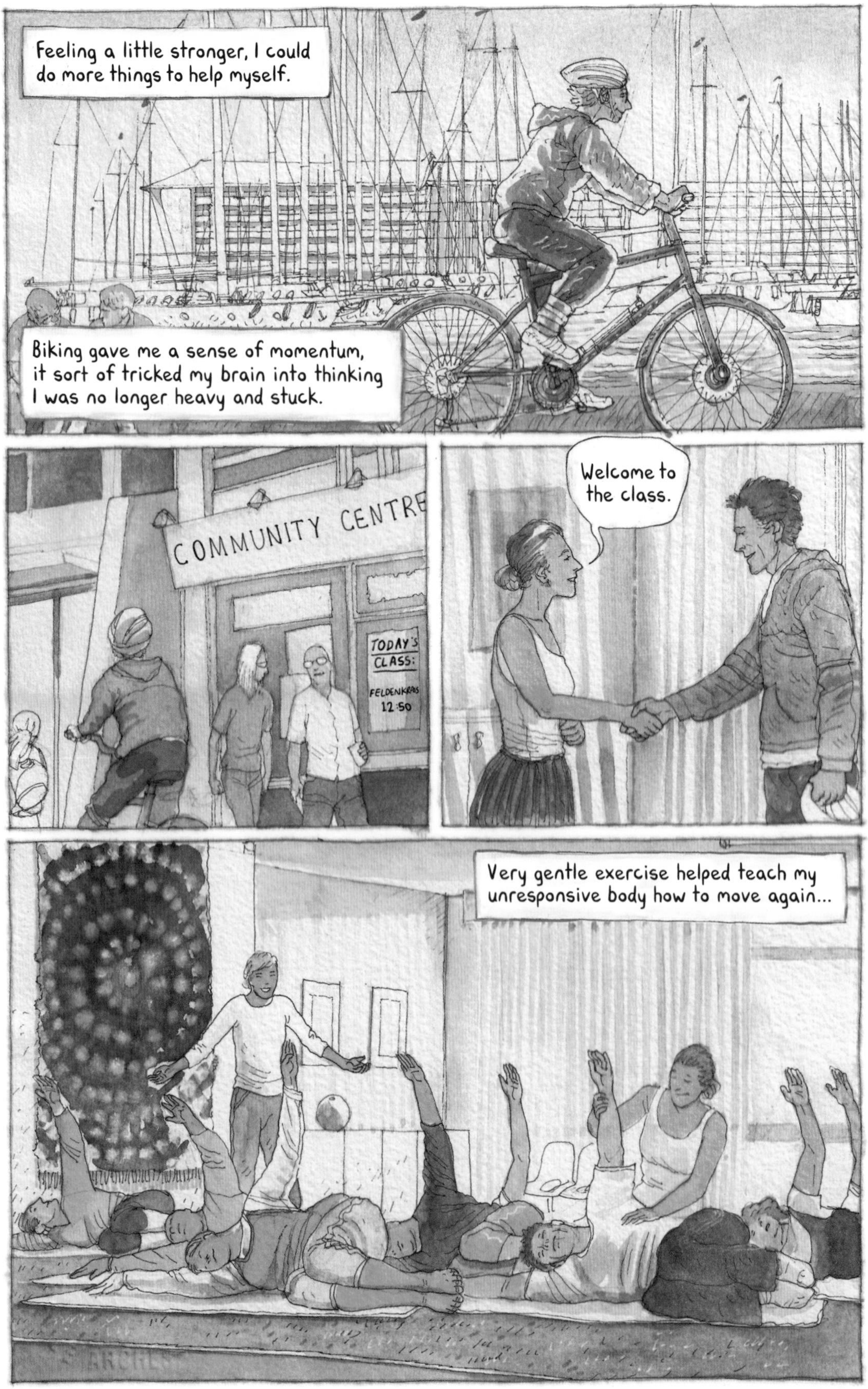
Feeling a little stronger, I could do more things to help myself.
Biking gave me a sense of momentum, it sort of tricked my brain into thinking I was no longer heavy and stuck.
COMMUNITY CENTRE
TODAY'S CLASS:
FELDENKRAIS 12:50
Welcome to the class.
Very gentle exercise helped teach my unresponsive body how to move again...

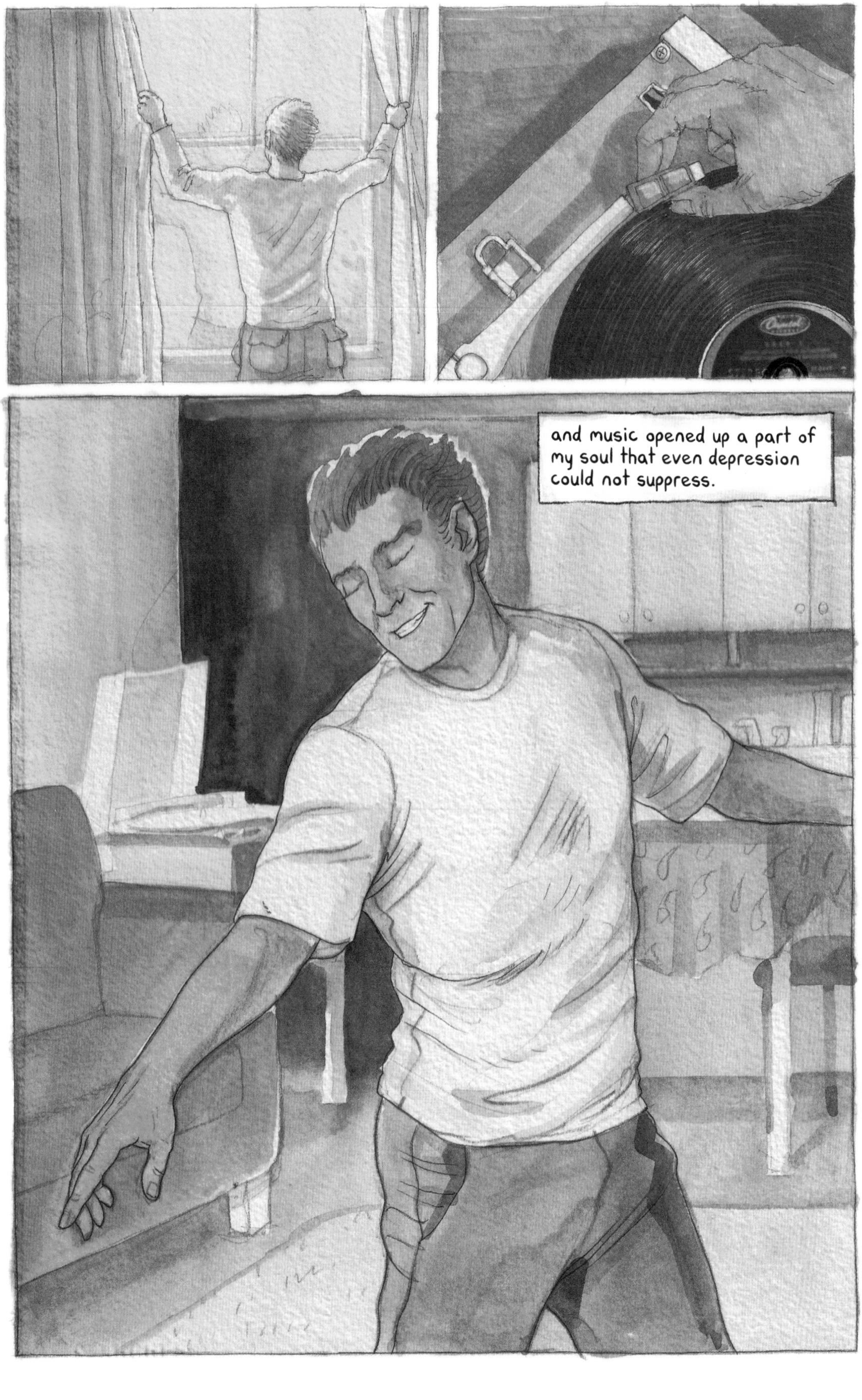
and music opened up a part of
my soul that even depression
could not suppress.

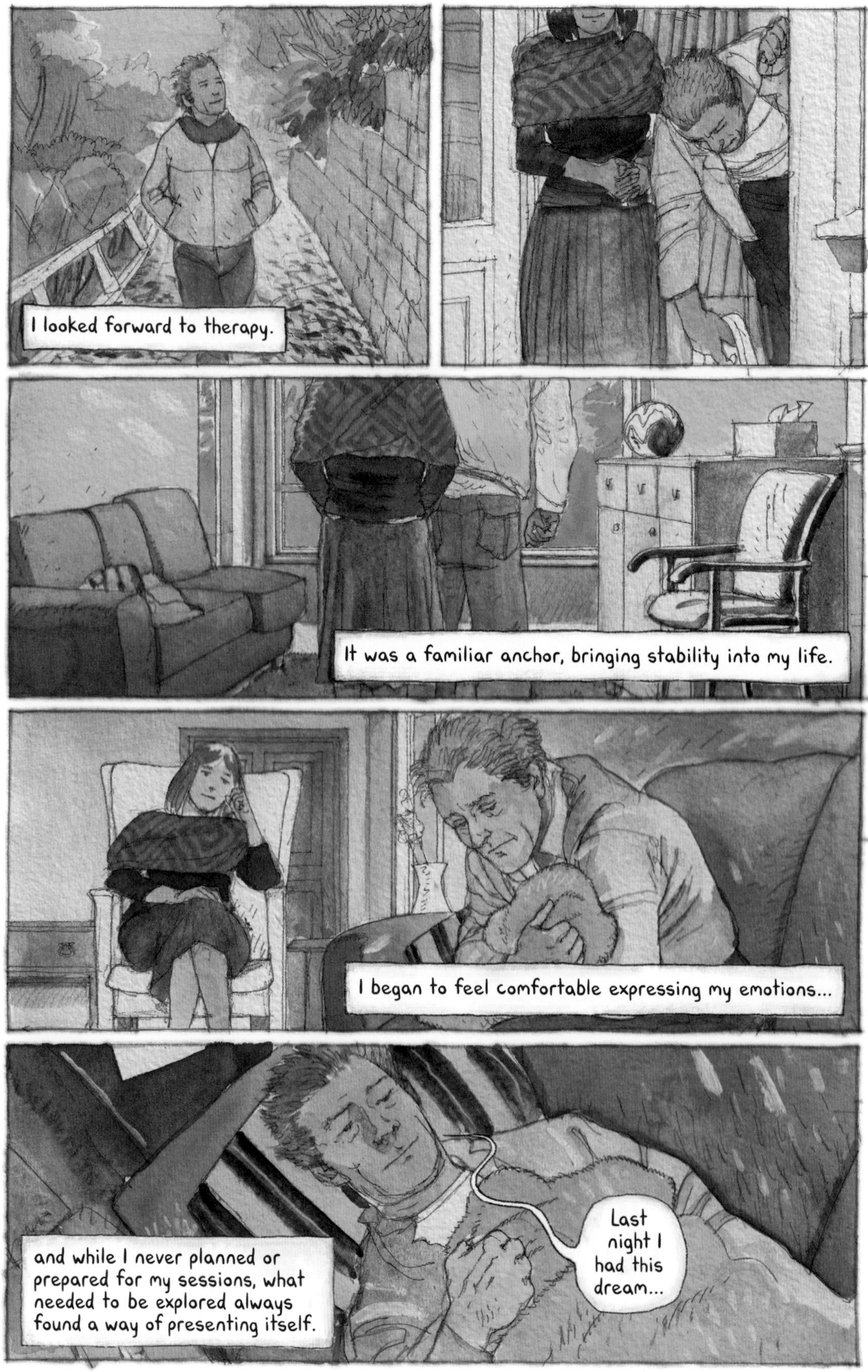
I looked forward to therapy.
It was a familiar anchor, bringing stability into my life.
I began to feel comfortable expressing my emotions...
and while I never planned or prepared for my sessions, what needed to be explored always found a way of presenting itself.
Last night I had this dream...

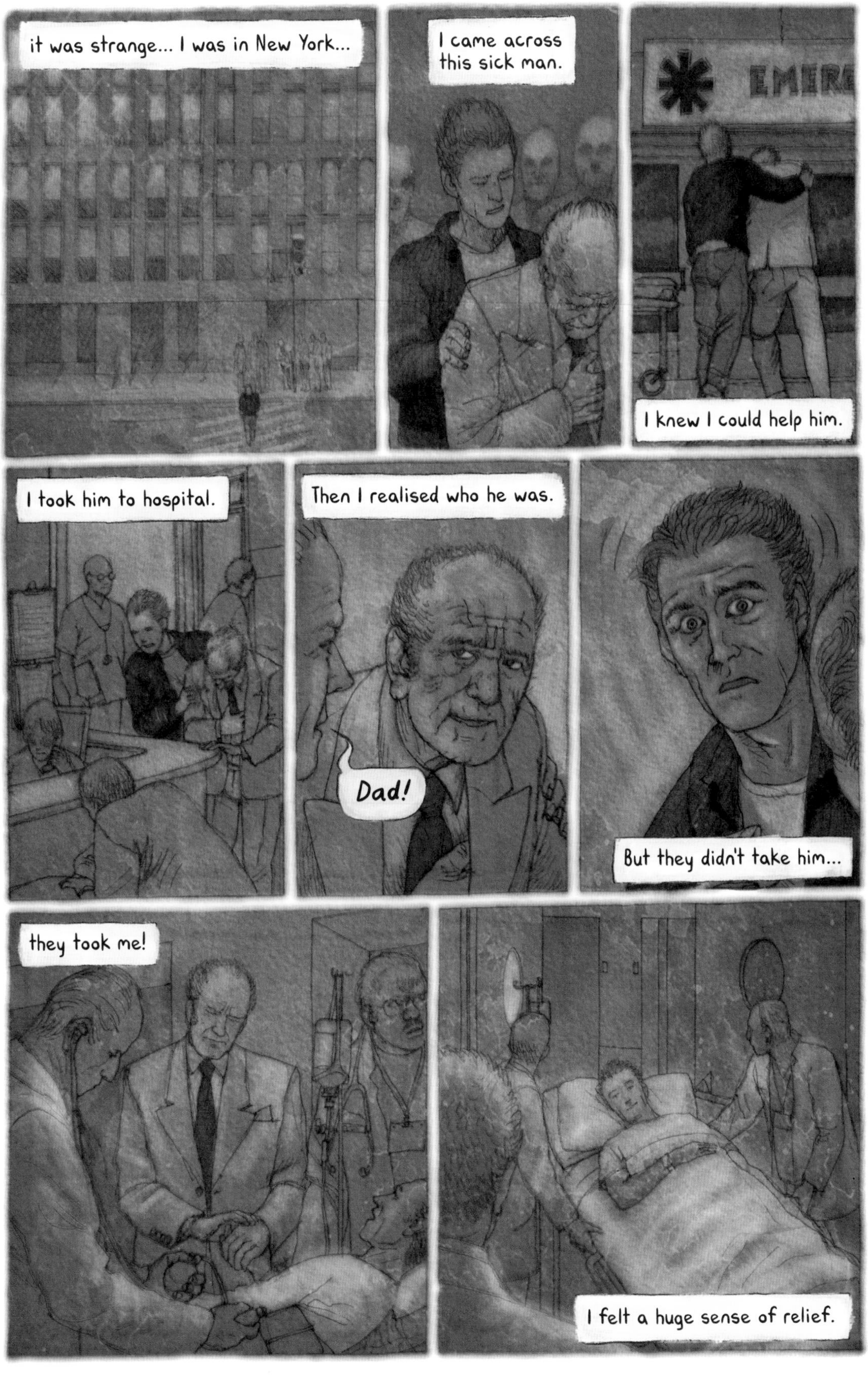
it was strange... I was in New York...
I came across this sick man.
EMERG
I knew I could help him.
I took him to hospital.
Then I realised who he was.
Dad!
But they didn't take him...
they took me!
I felt a huge sense of relief.

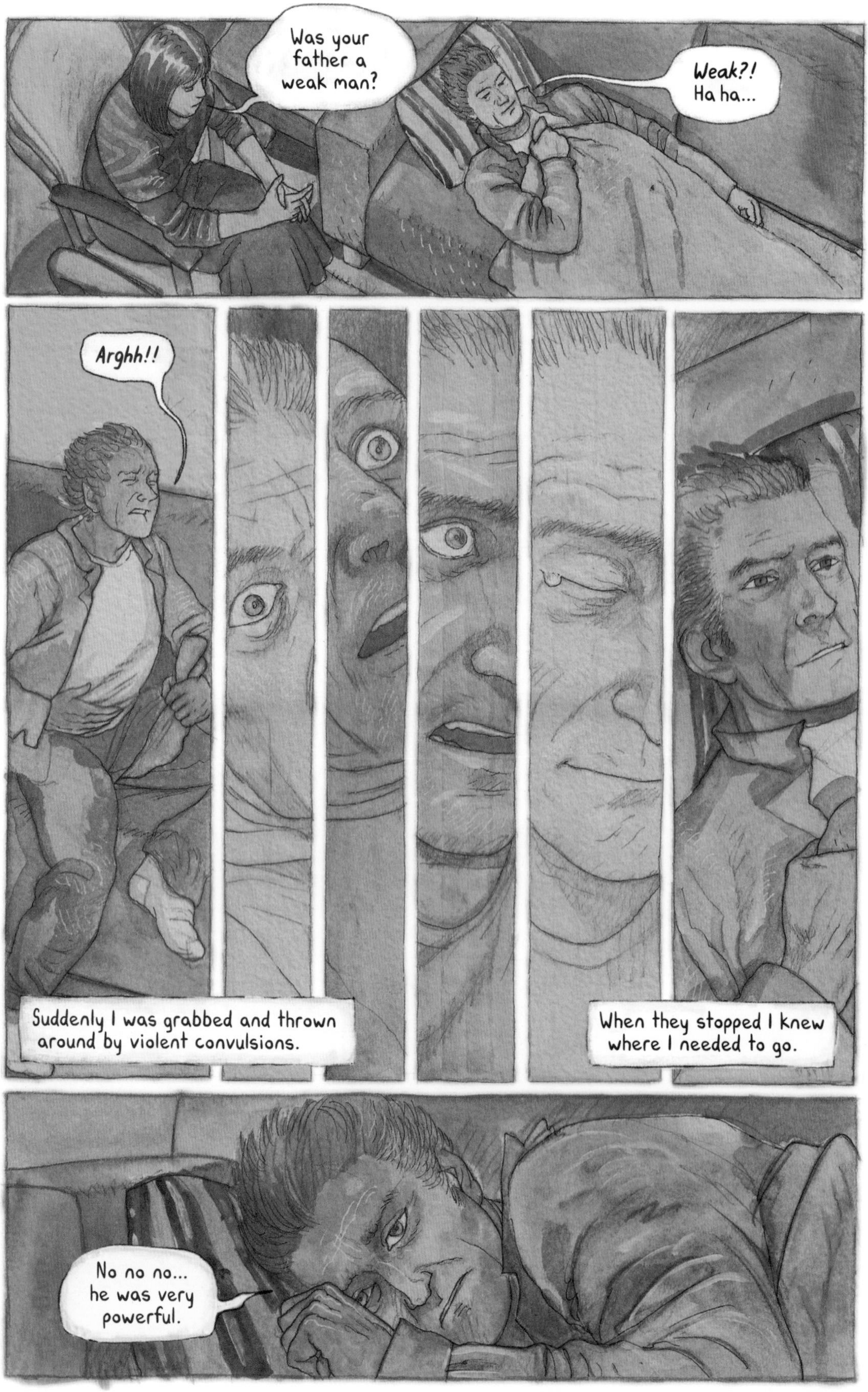

Was your father a weak man?
Weak?! Ha ha...
Arghh!!
Suddenly I was grabbed and thrown around by violent convulsions.
When they stopped I knew where I needed to go.
No no no... he was very powerful.

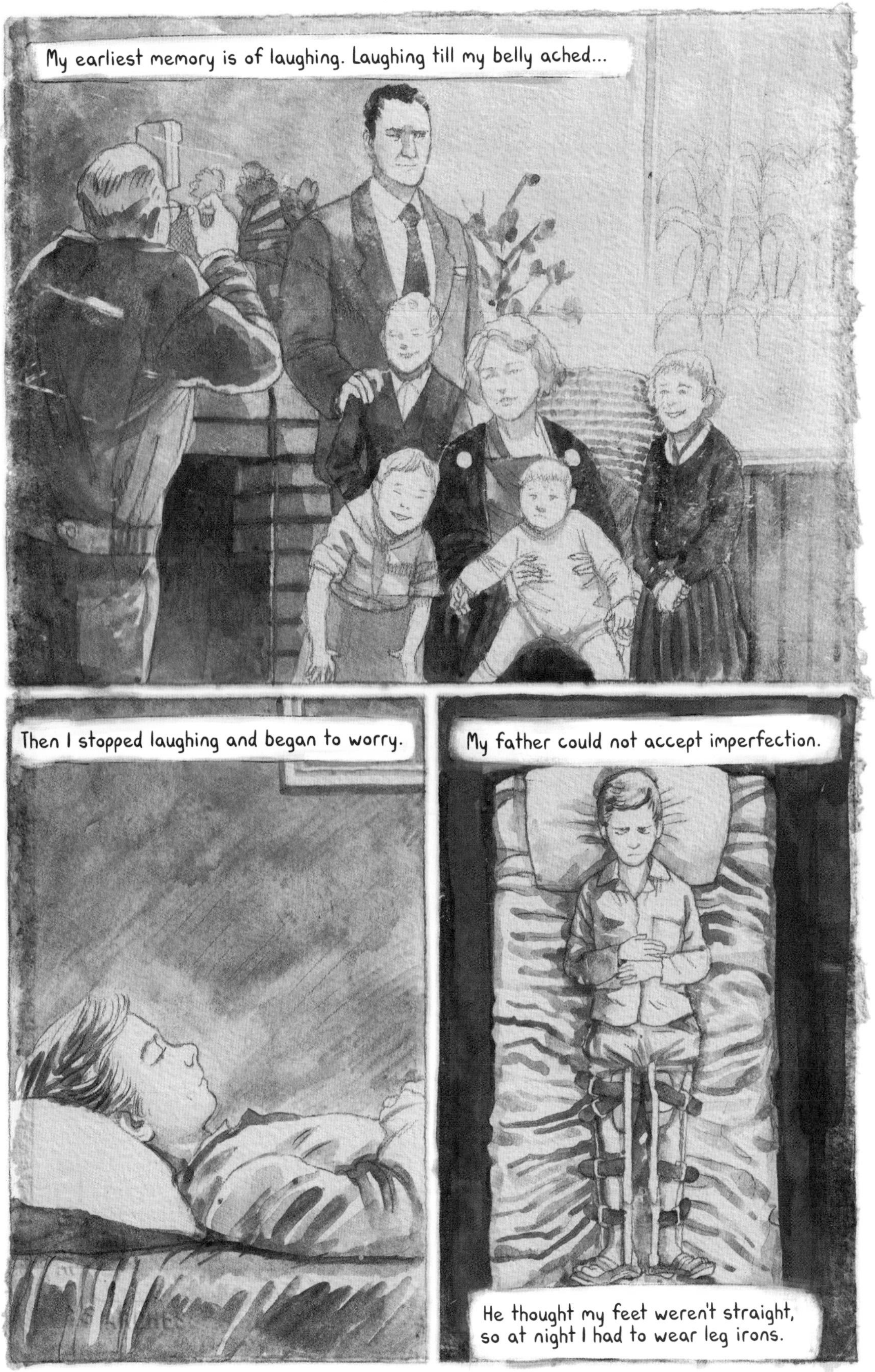
My earliest memory is of laughing. Laughing till my belly ached...
Then I stopped laughing and began to worry.
My father could not accept imperfection.
He thought my feet weren't straight, so at night I had to wear leg irons.

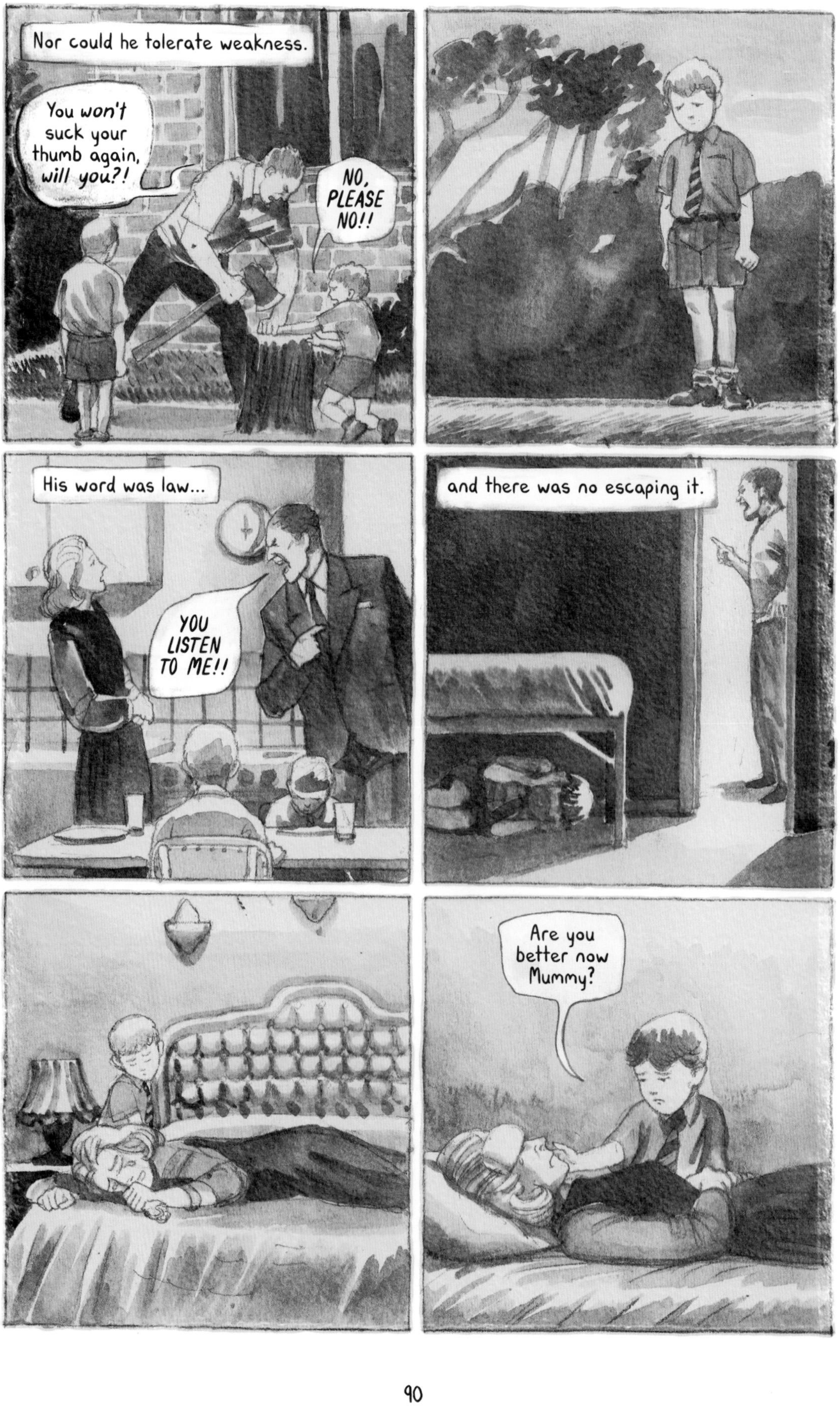

Nor could he tolerate weakness.
You won't suck your thumb again, will you?!
NO, PLEASE NO!!
His word was law...
YOU LISTEN TO ME!!
and there was no escaping it.
Are you better now Mummy?

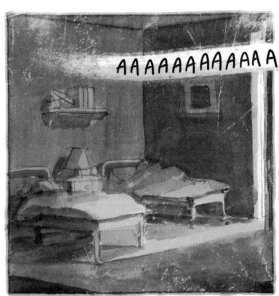

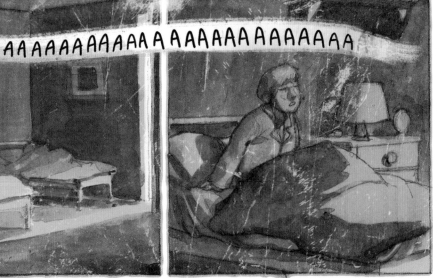

AAAAAAAAAAAAA AAAAA AAAAAAAA

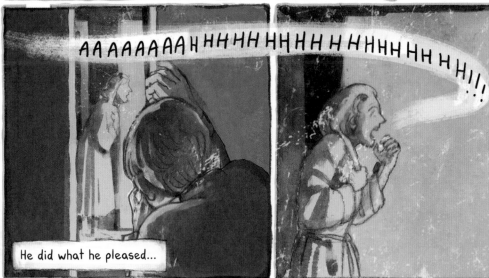

AAAAAAAAHHHHH HHHHH H HHHHHHH HHI!!

He did what he pleased...

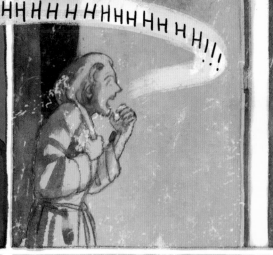

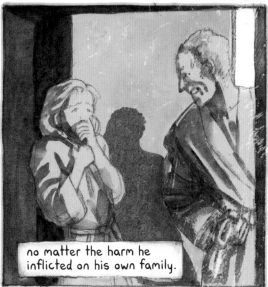

no matter the harm he inflicted on his own family.

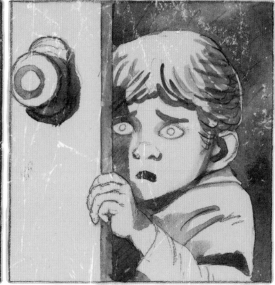

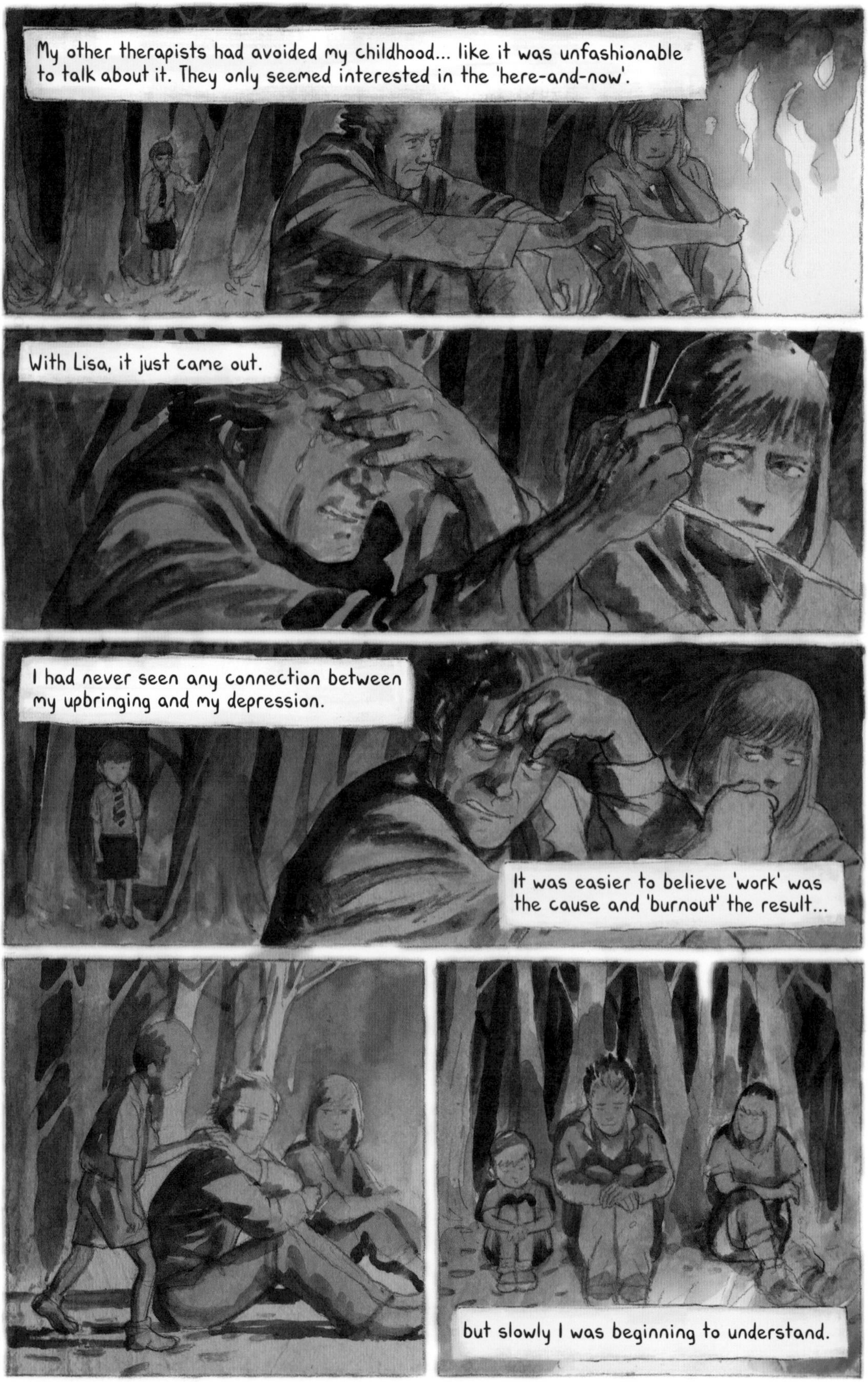
My other therapists had avoided my childhood... like it was unfashionable to talk about it. They only seemed interested in the 'here-and-now'.
With Lisa, it just came out.
I had never seen any connection between my upbringing and my depression.
It was easier to believe 'work' was the cause and 'burnout' the result...
but slowly I was beginning to understand.

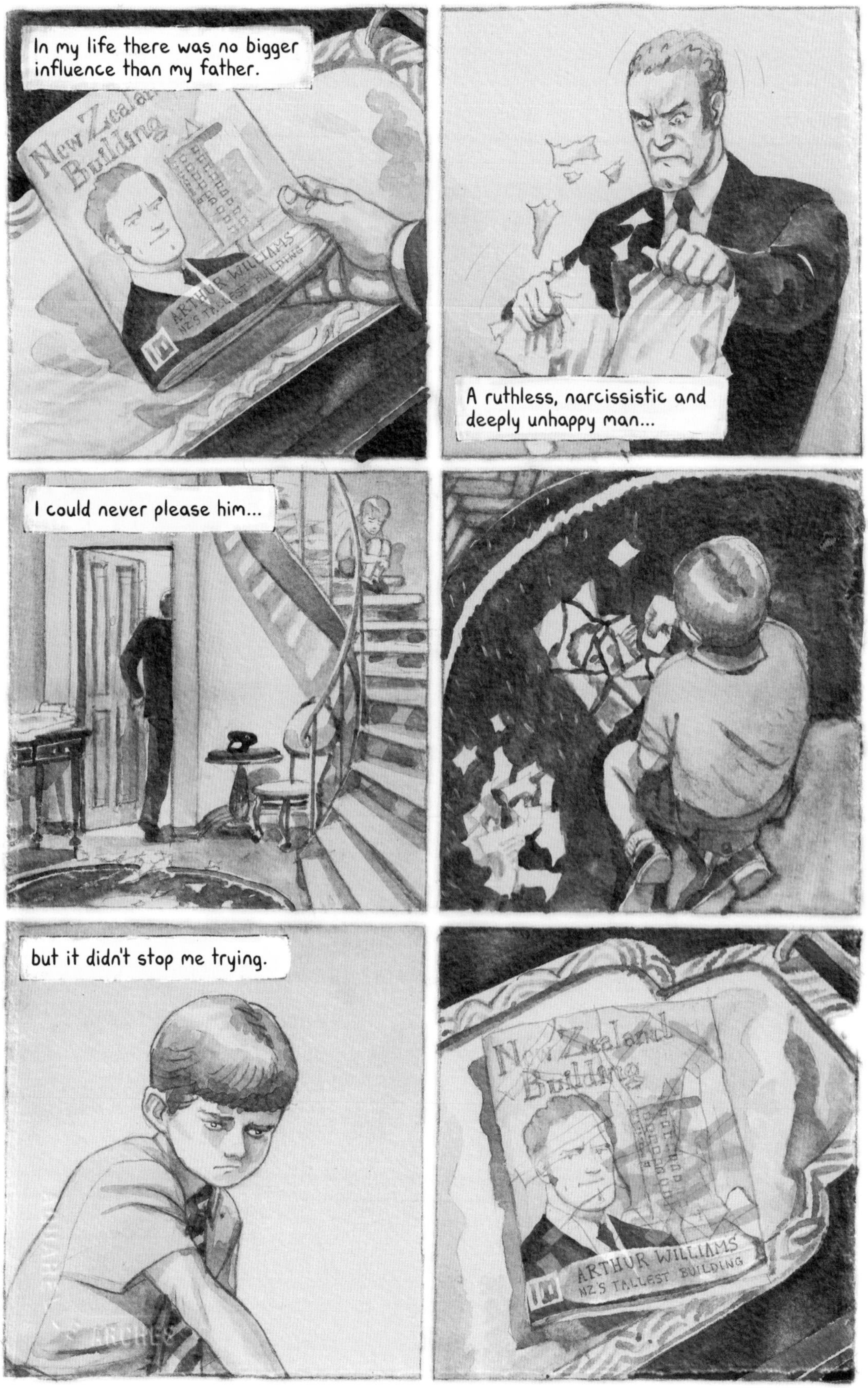
In my life there was no bigger influence than my father.
New Zealand Building
ARTHUR WILLIAMS
NZ'S TALLEST BUILDING
A ruthless, narcissistic and deeply unhappy man...
I could never please him...
but it didn't stop me trying.
New Zealand Building
ARTHUR WILLIAMS
NZ'S TALLEST BUILDING

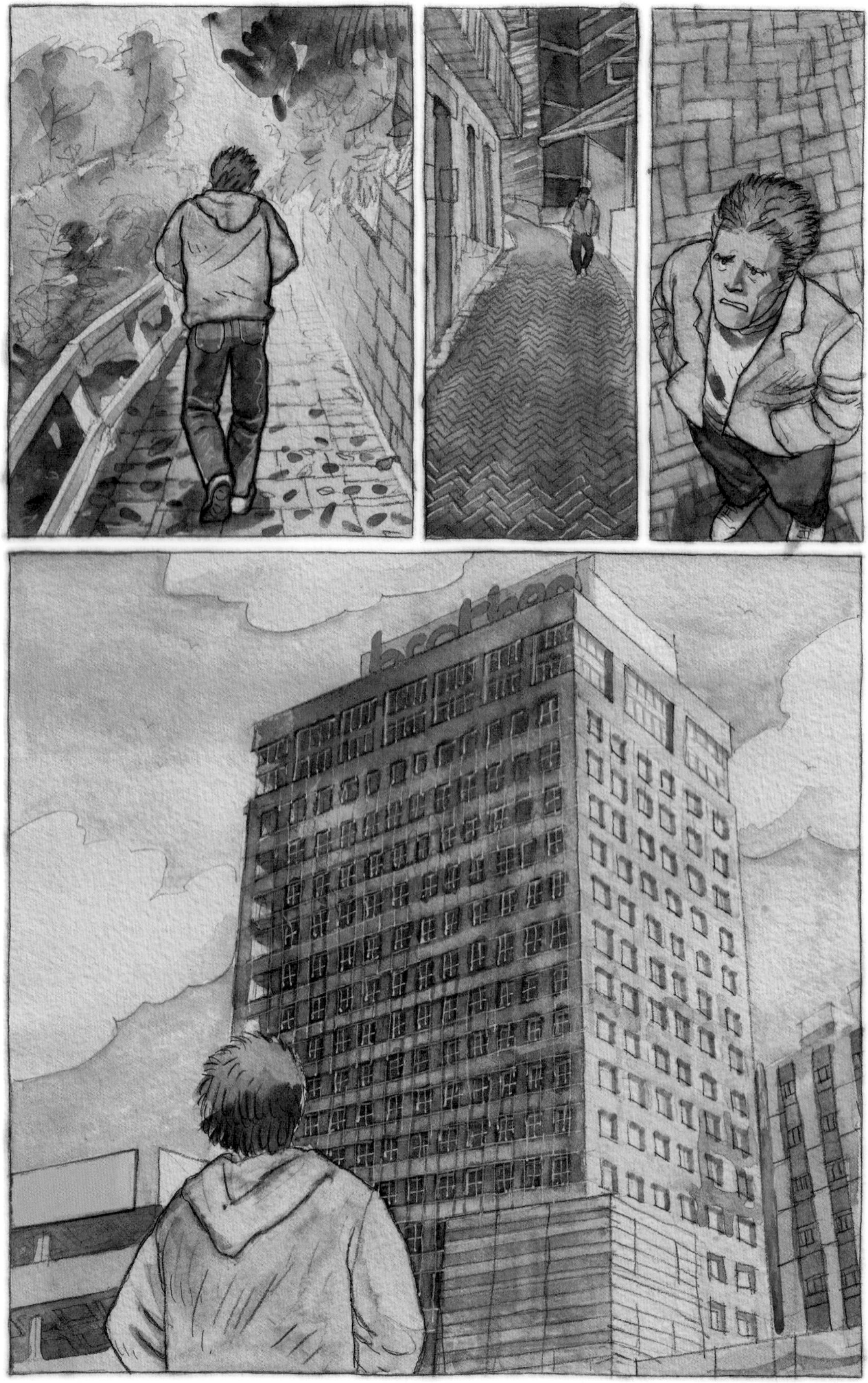

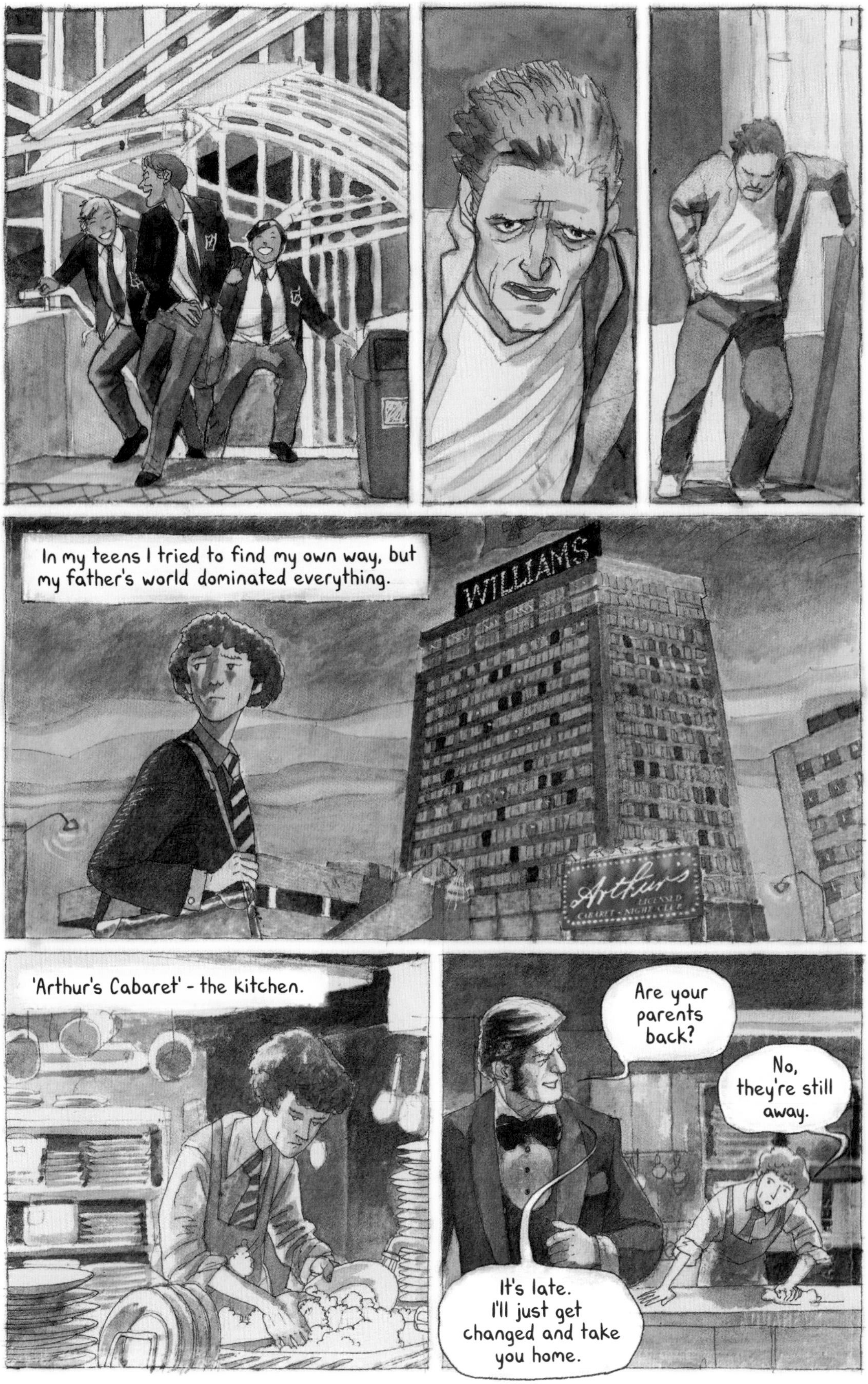
In my teens I tried to find my own way, but my father's world dominated everything.
WILLIAMS
Arthur's
LICENSED
CABARET · NIGHT CLUB
'Arthur's Cabaret' - the kitchen.
Are your parents back?
No, they're still away.
It's late. I'll just get changed and take you home.

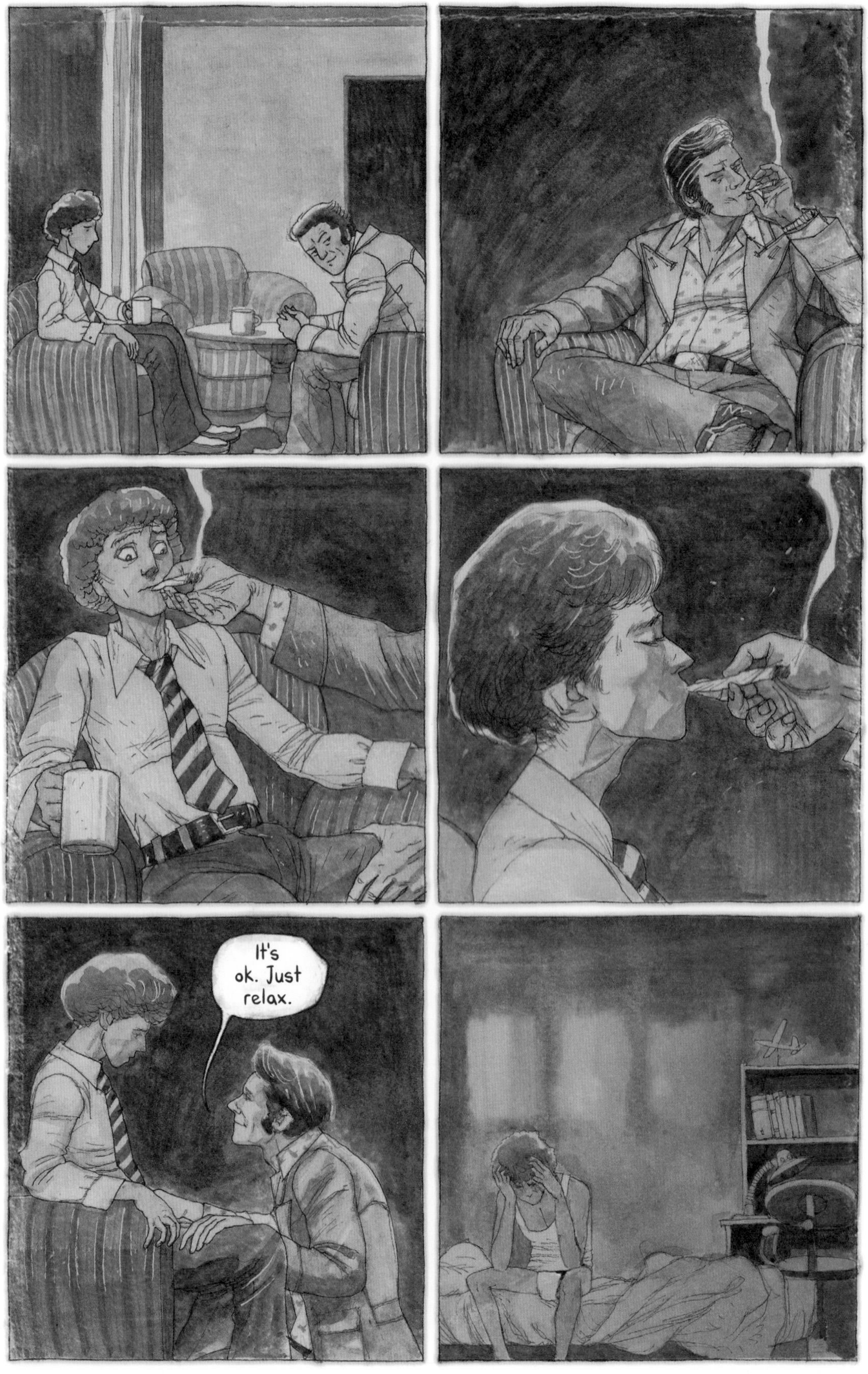
It's ok. Just relax.

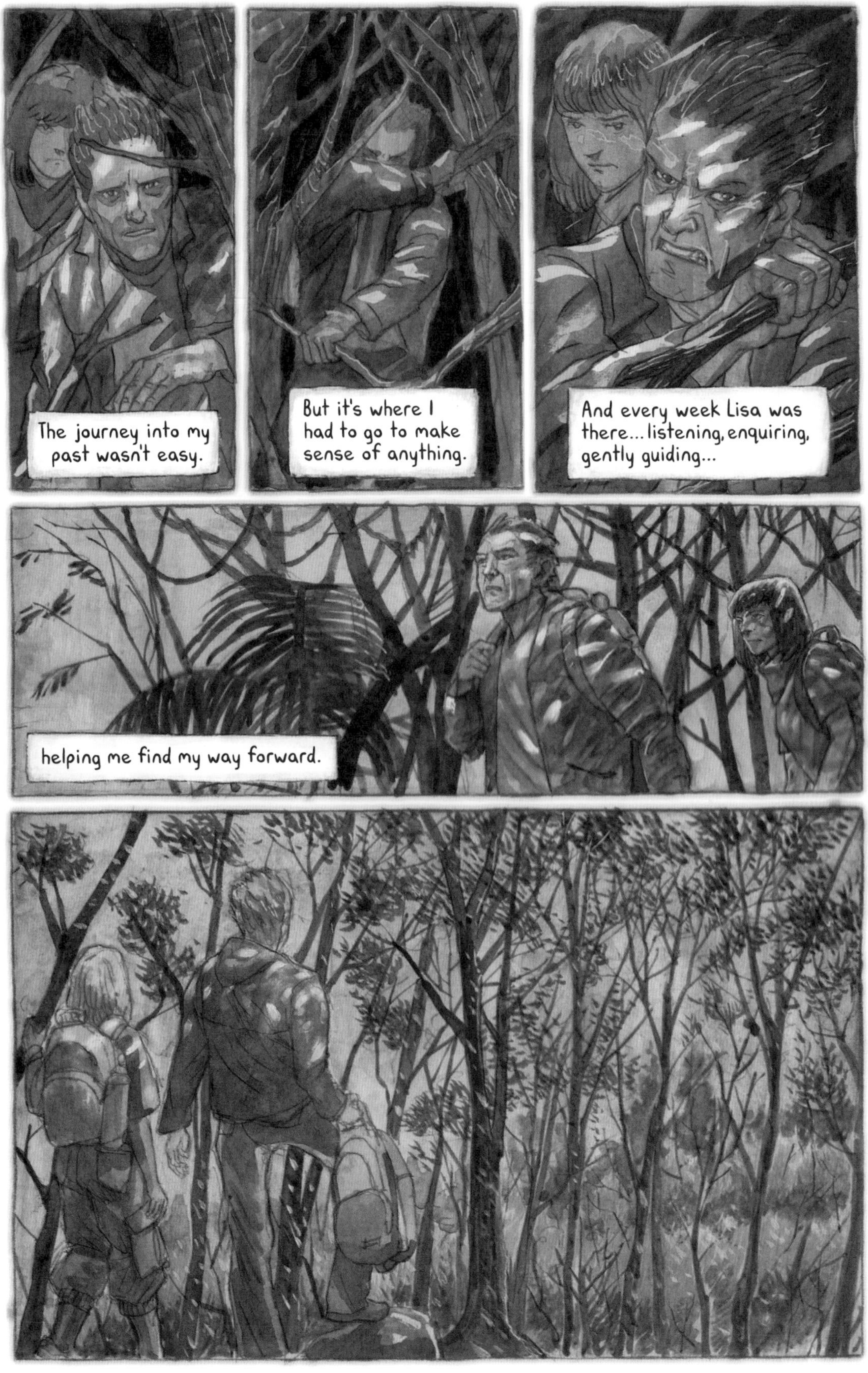
The journey into my past wasn't easy.
But it's where I had to go to make sense of anything.
And every week Lisa was there... listening, enquiring, gently guiding...
helping me find my way forward.

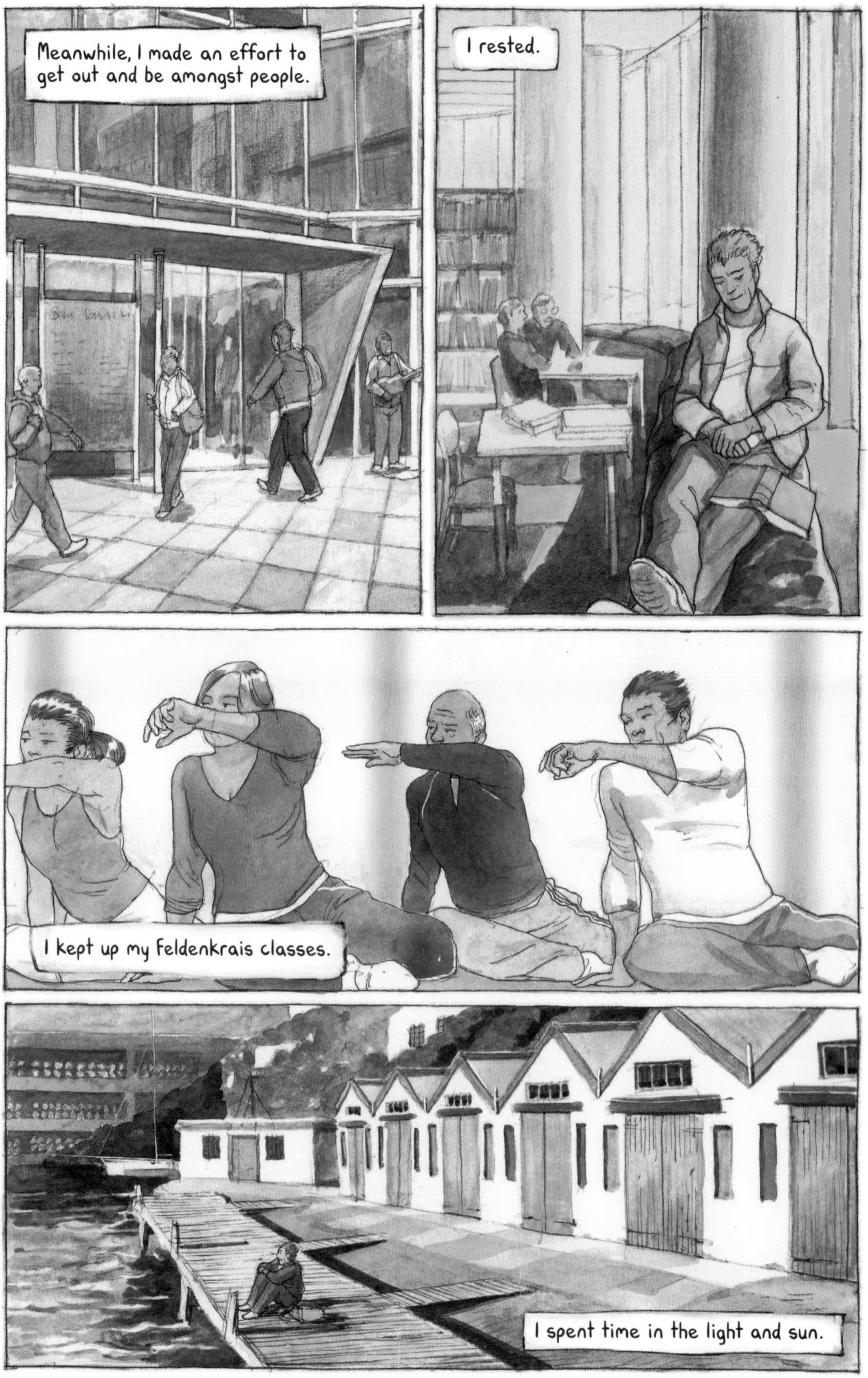
Meanwhile, I made an effort to get out and be amongst people.
I rested.
I kept up my Feldenkrais classes.
I spent time in the light and sun.

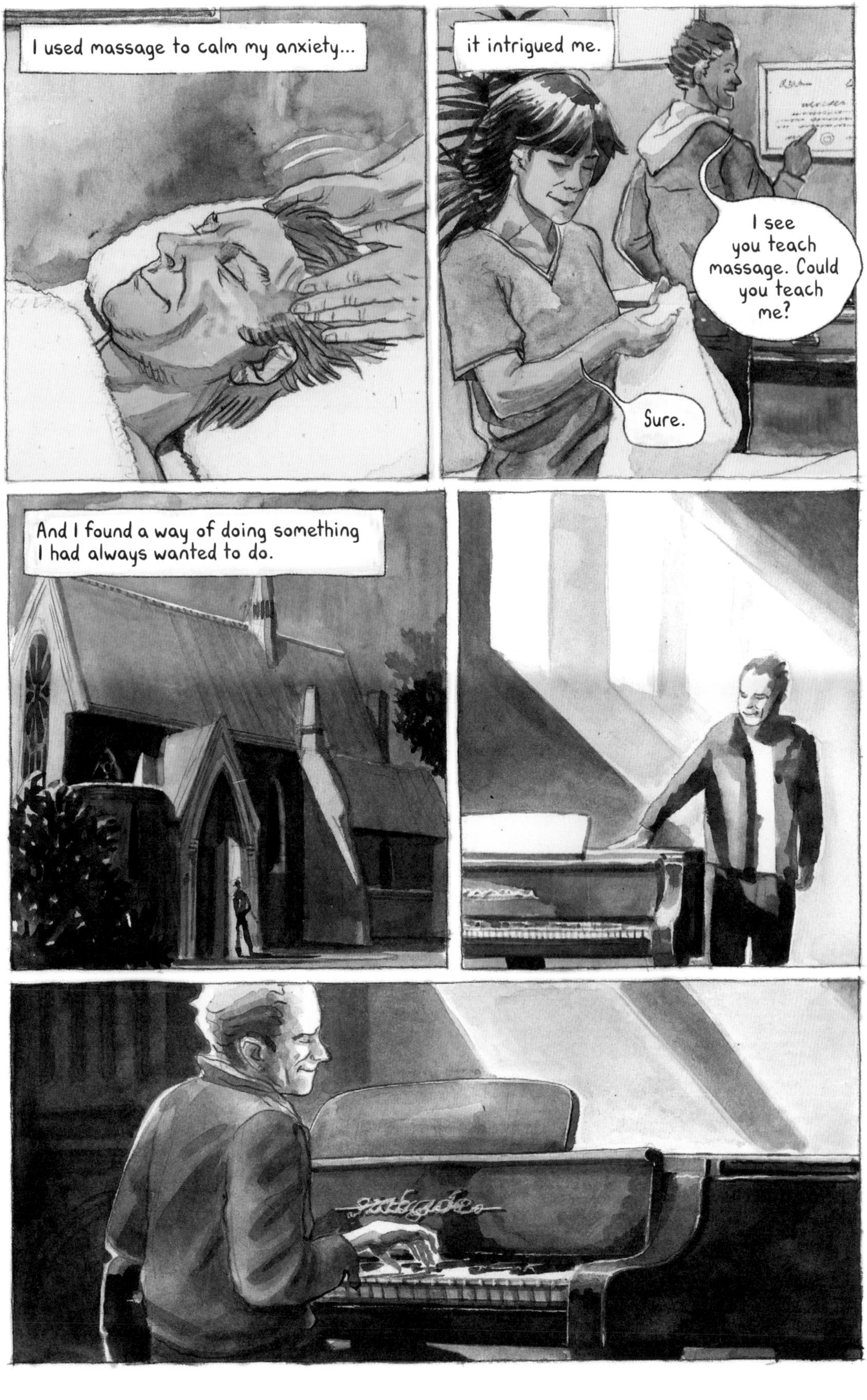
I used massage to calm my anxiety...
it intrigued me.
I see you teach massage. Could you teach me?
Sure.
And I found a way of doing something I had always wanted to do.

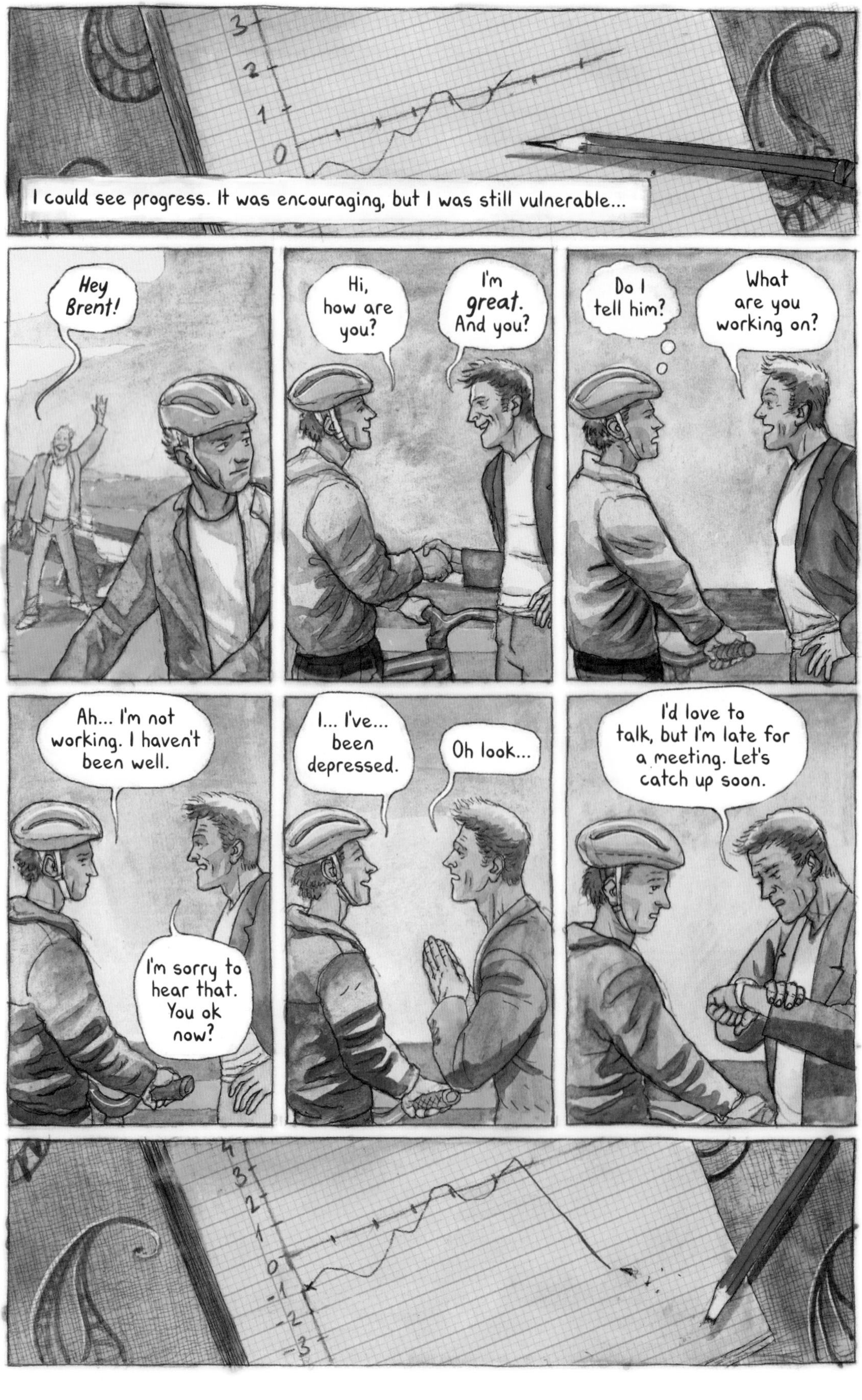
3
2
1
0
I could see progress. It was encouraging, but I was still vulnerable...
Hey Brent!
Hi, how are you?
I'm great. And you?
Do I tell him?
What are you working on?
Ah... I'm not working. I haven't been well.
I'm sorry to hear that. You ok now?
I... I've... been depressed.
Oh look...
I'd love to talk, but I'm late for a meeting. Let's catch up soon.
4
3
2
1
0
-1
-2
-3

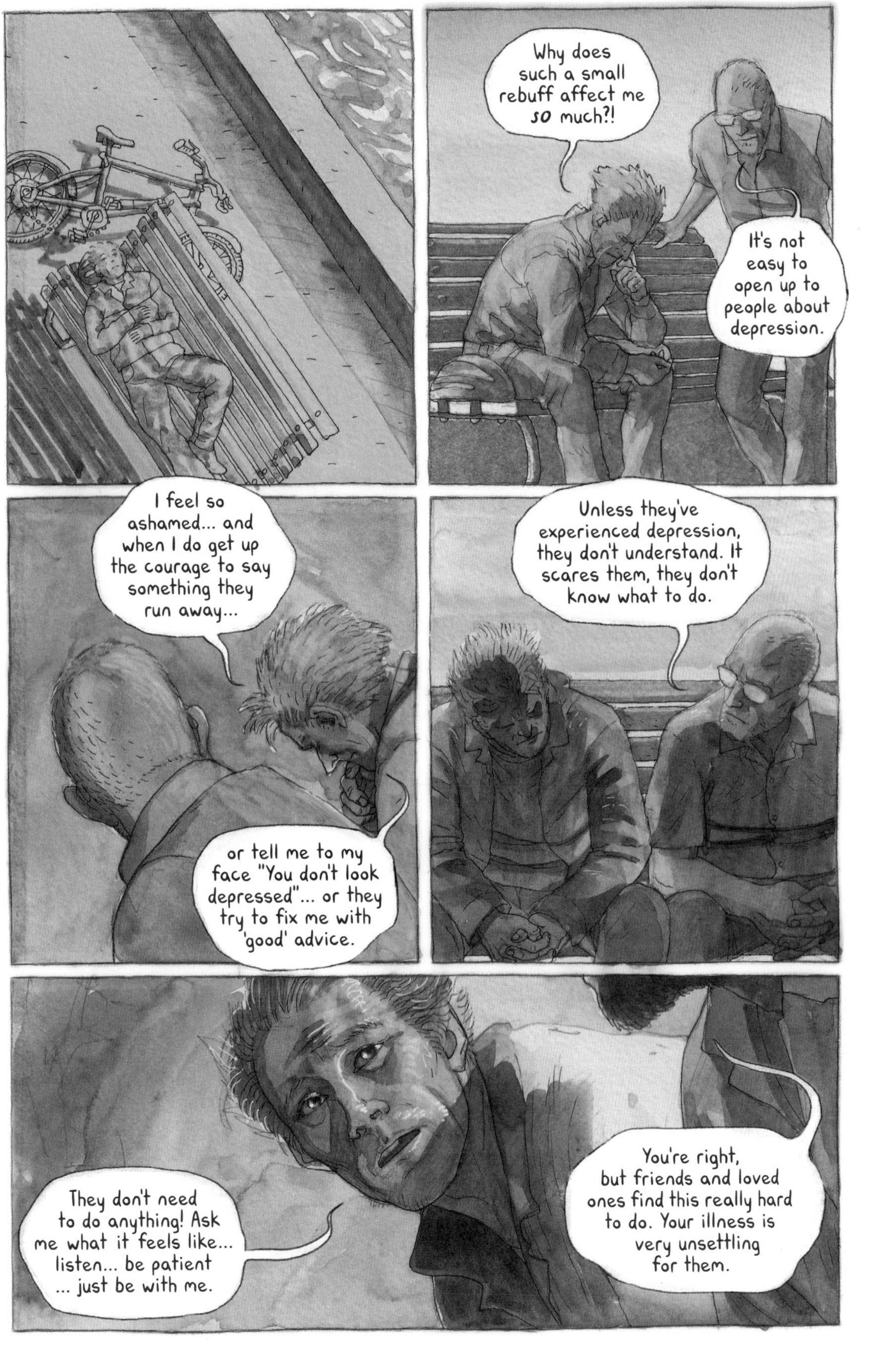
Why does such a small rebuff affect me so much?!
It's not easy to open up to people about depression.
I feel so ashamed... and when I do get up the courage to say something they run away...
or tell me to my face "You don't look depressed"... or they try to fix me with 'good' advice.
Unless they've experienced depression, they don't understand. It scares them, they don't know what to do.
They don't need to do anything! Ask me what it feels like... listen... be patient ... just be with me.
You're right, but friends and loved ones find this really hard to do. Your illness is very unsettling for them.

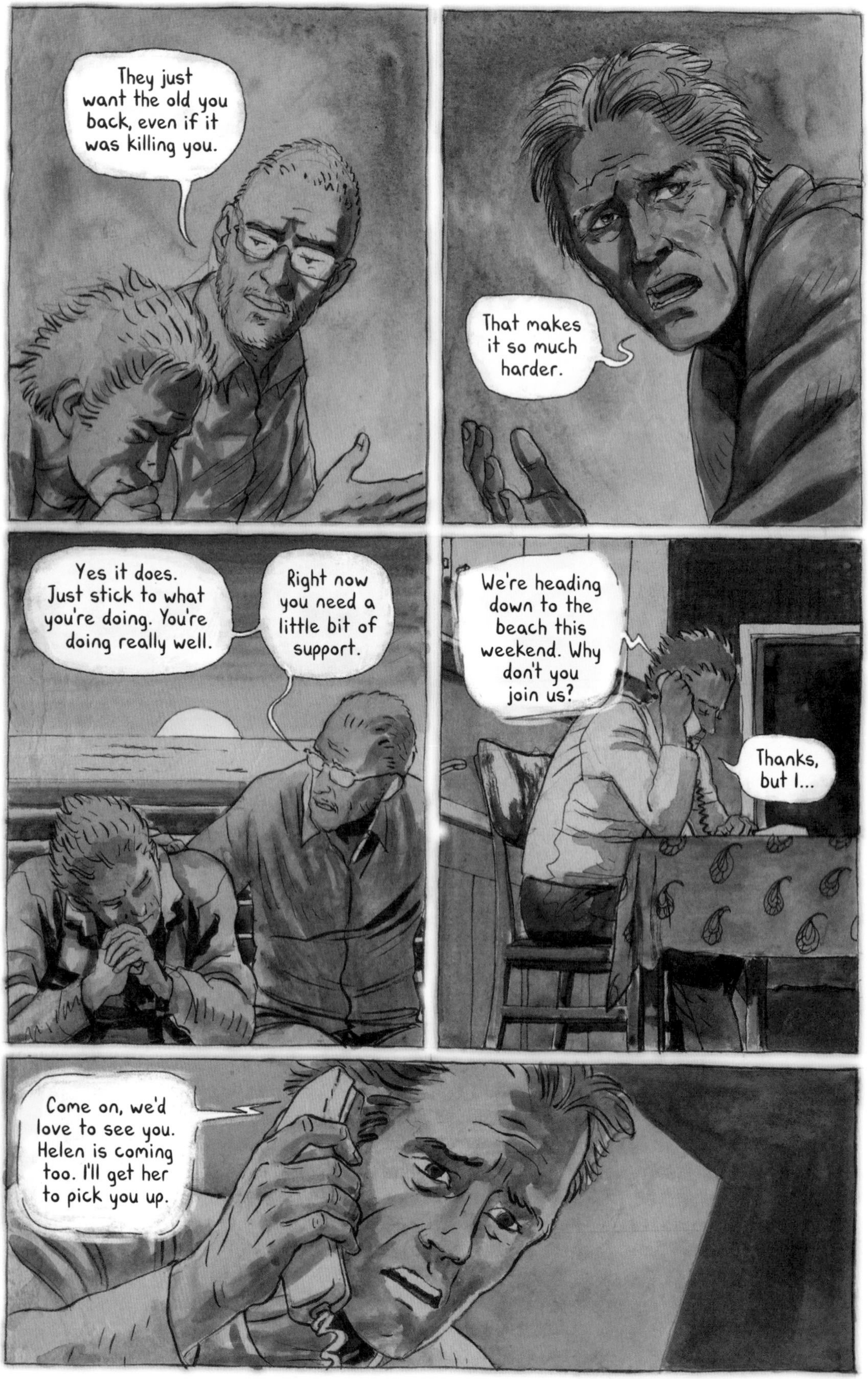
They just want the old you back, even if it was killing you.
That makes it so much harder.
Yes it does. Just stick to what you're doing. You're doing really well.
Right now you need a little bit of support.
We're heading down to the beach this weekend. Why don't you join us?
Thanks, but I...
Come on, we'd love to see you. Helen is coming too. I'll get her to pick you up.

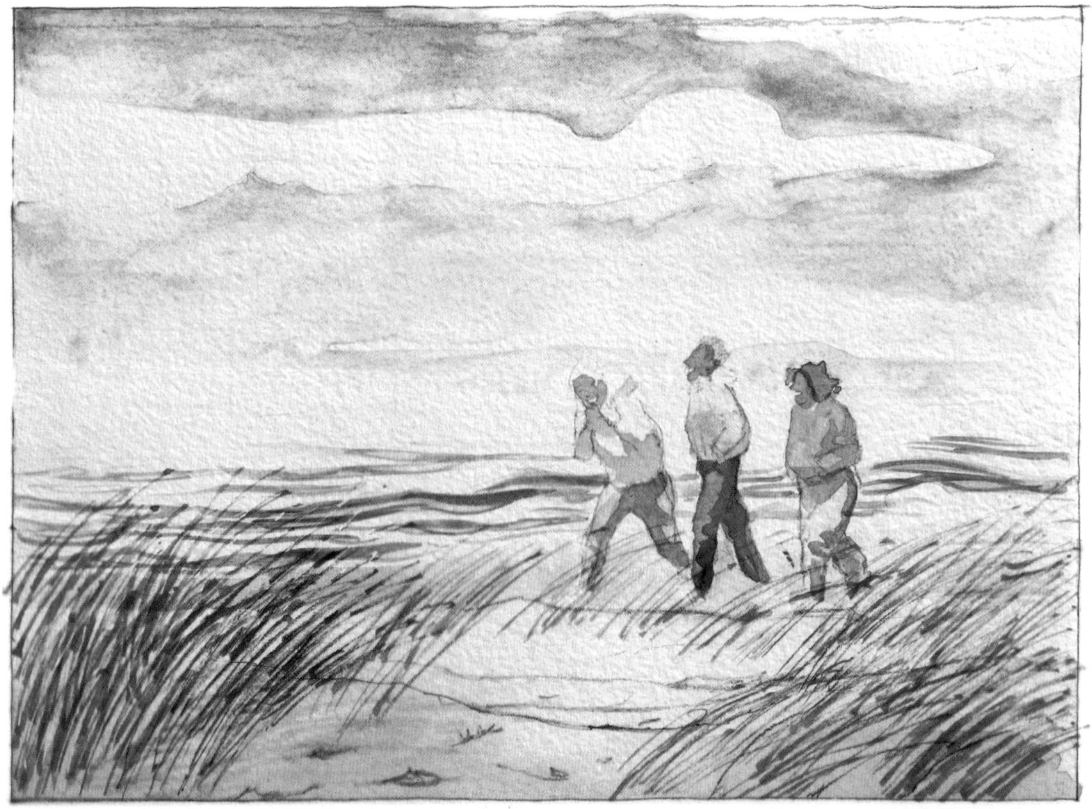

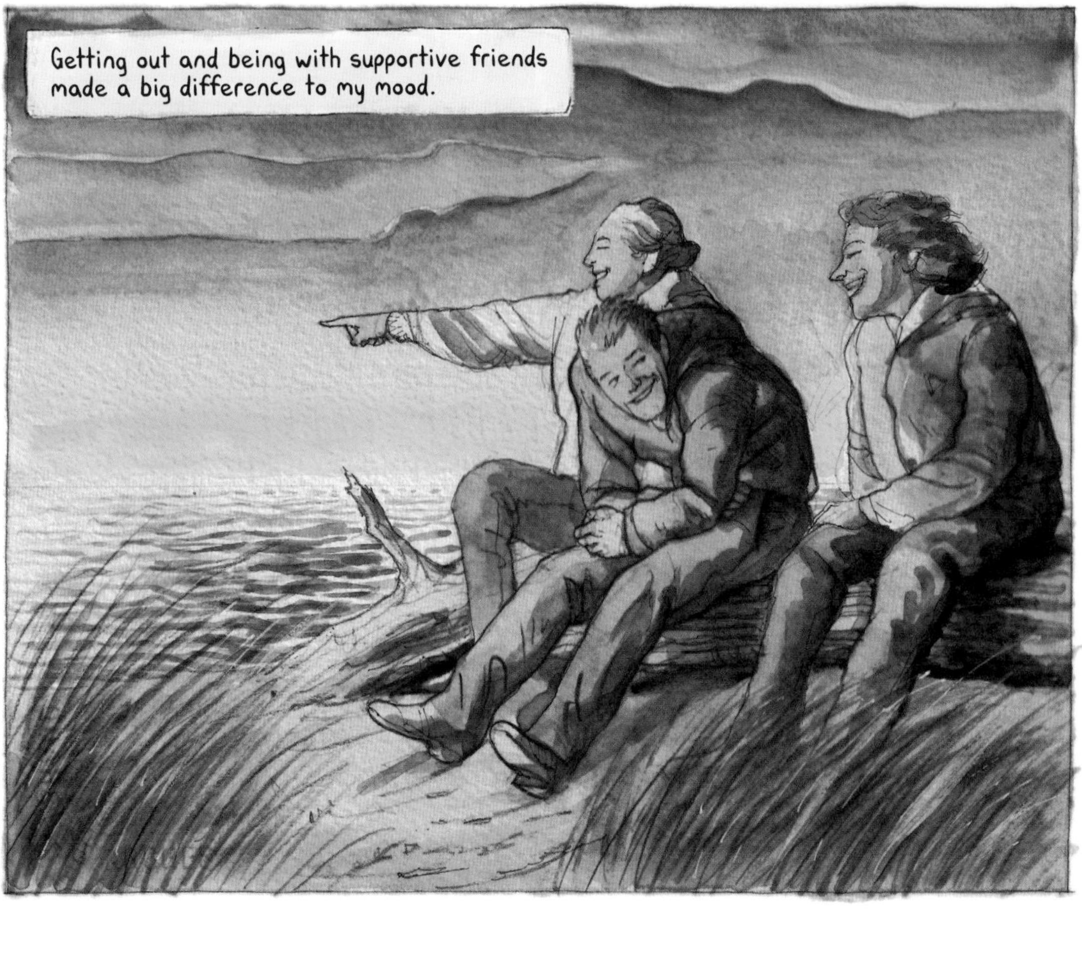
Getting out and being with supportive friends made a big difference to my mood.

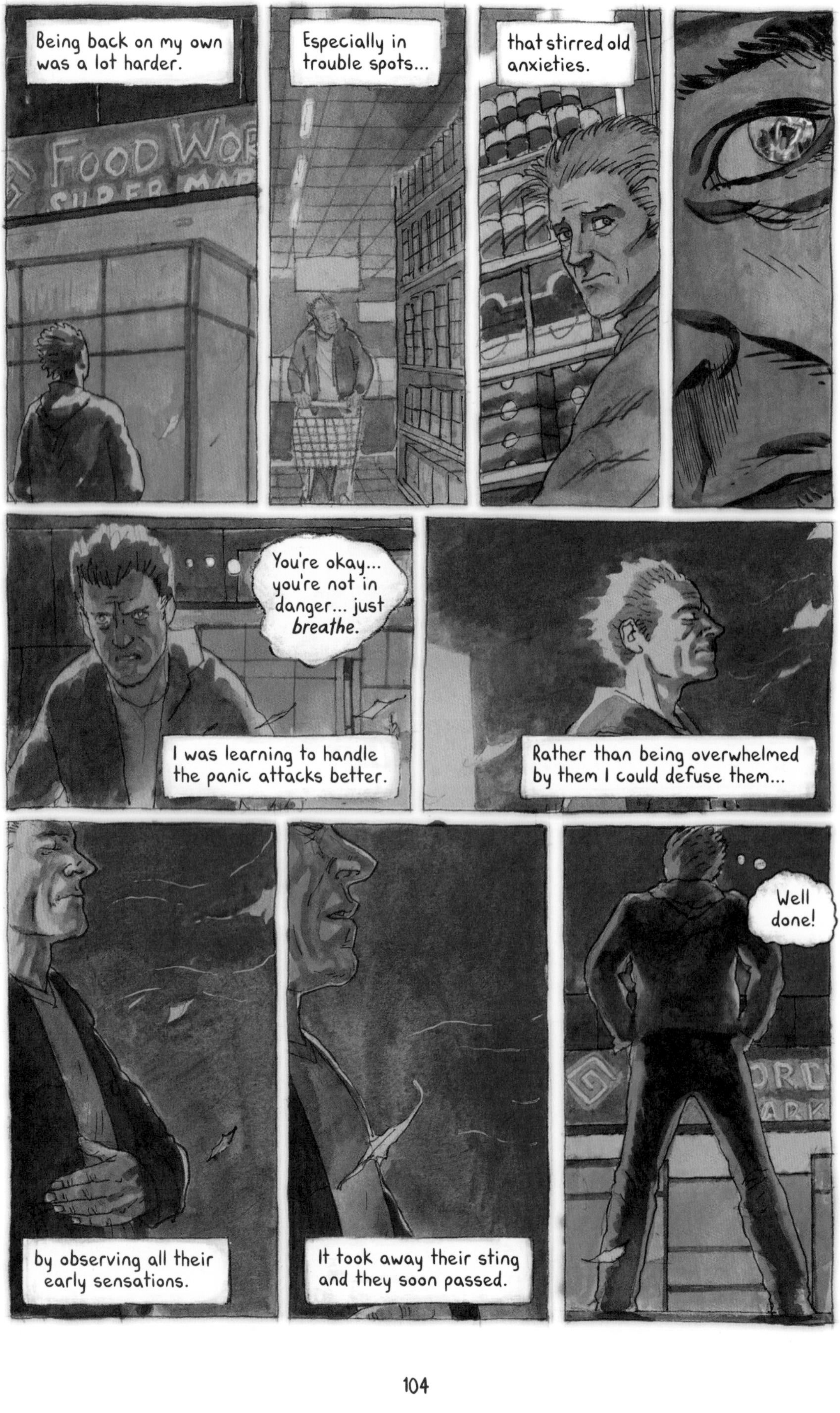
Being back on my own was a lot harder.
FOOD WOR
SUPER MAR
Especially in trouble spots...
that stirred old anxieties.
You're okay... you're not in danger... just *breathe*.
I was learning to handle the panic attacks better.
Rather than being overwhelmed by them I could defuse them...
by observing all their early sensations.
It took away their sting and they soon passed.
Well done!

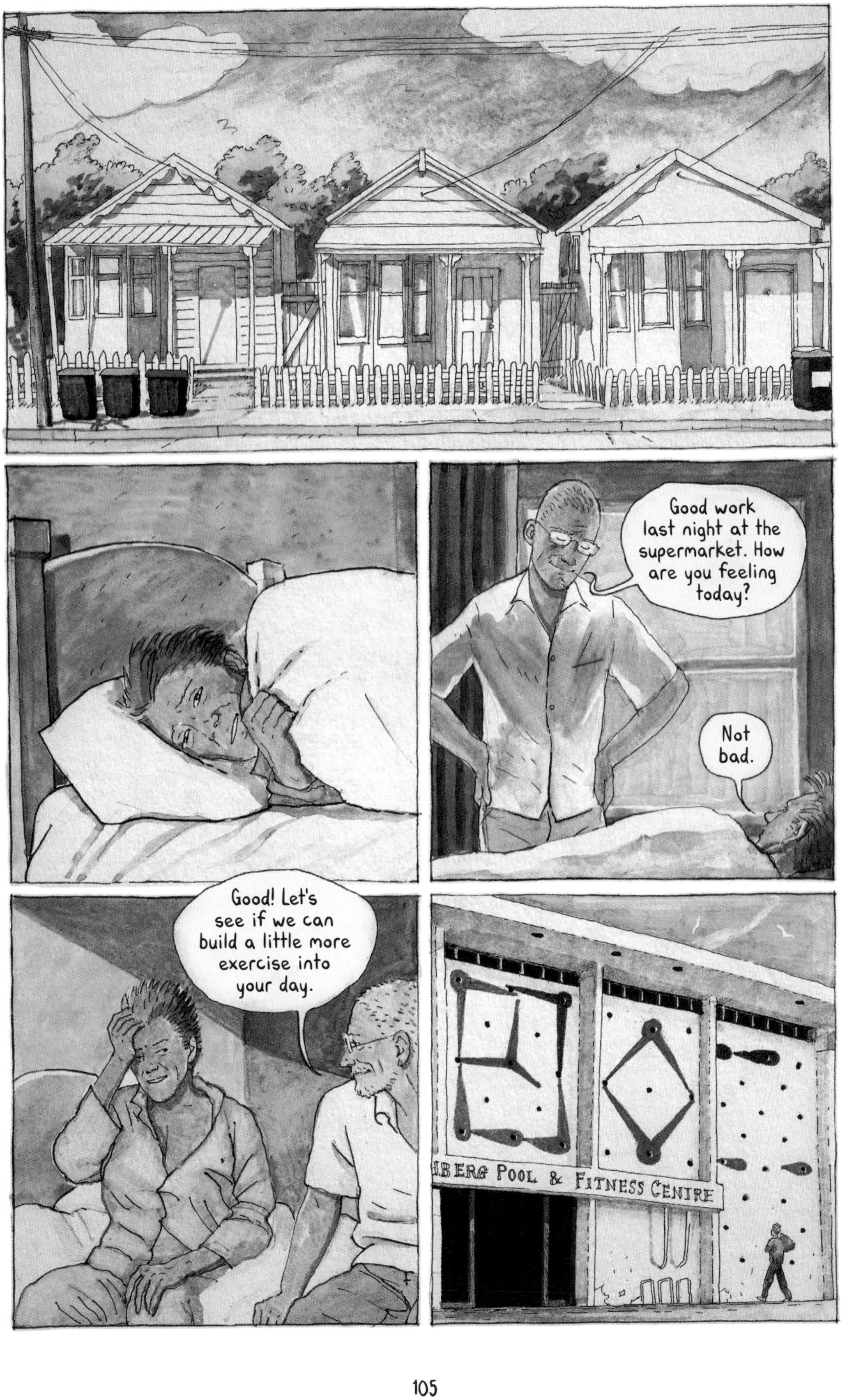
Good work last night at the supermarket. How are you feeling today?
Not bad.
Good! Let's see if we can build a little more exercise into your day.
BERG POOL & FITNESS CENTRE

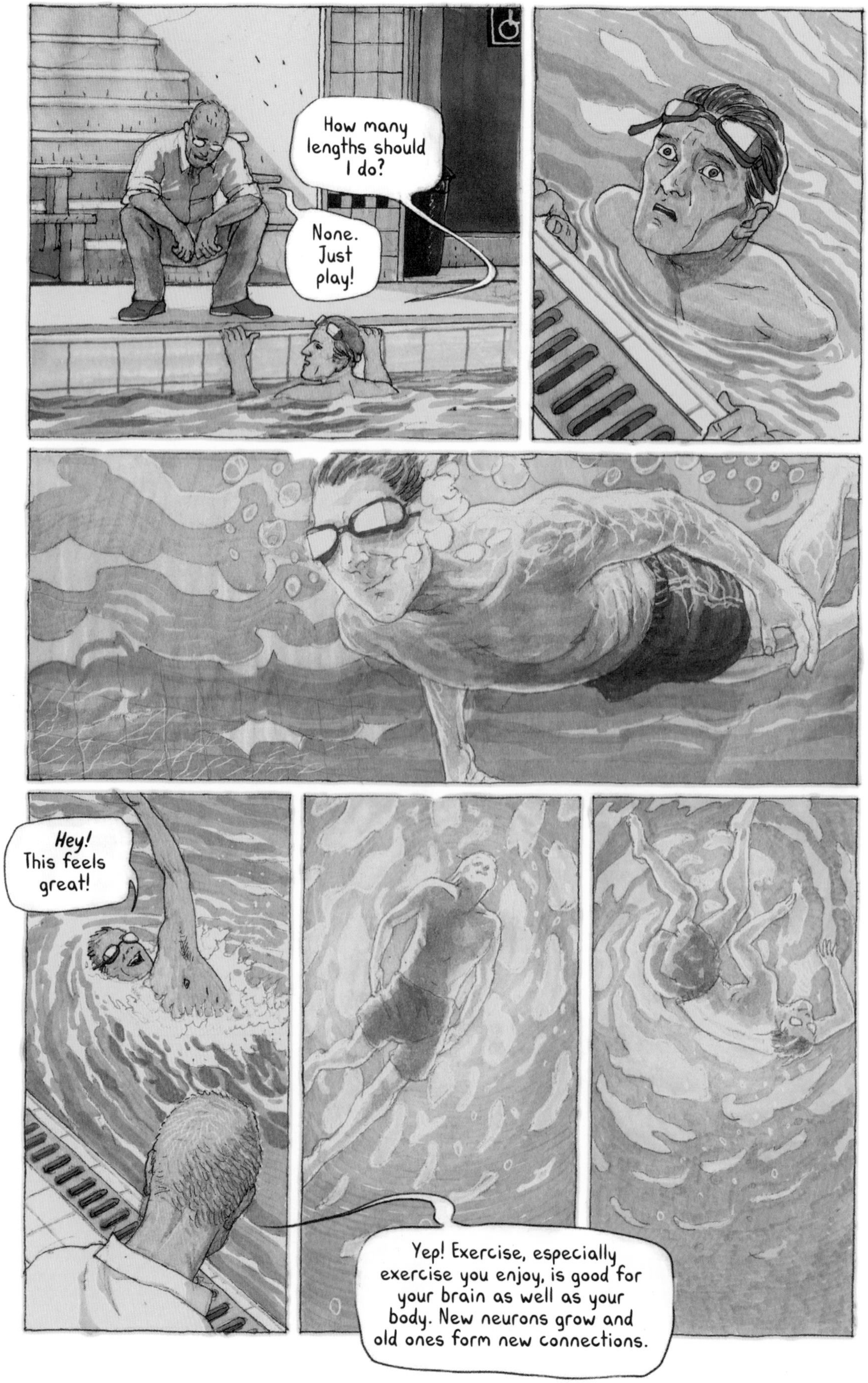
How many lengths should I do?
None. Just play!
Hey! This feels great!
Yep! Exercise, especially exercise you enjoy, is good for your brain as well as your body. New neurons grow and old ones form new connections.

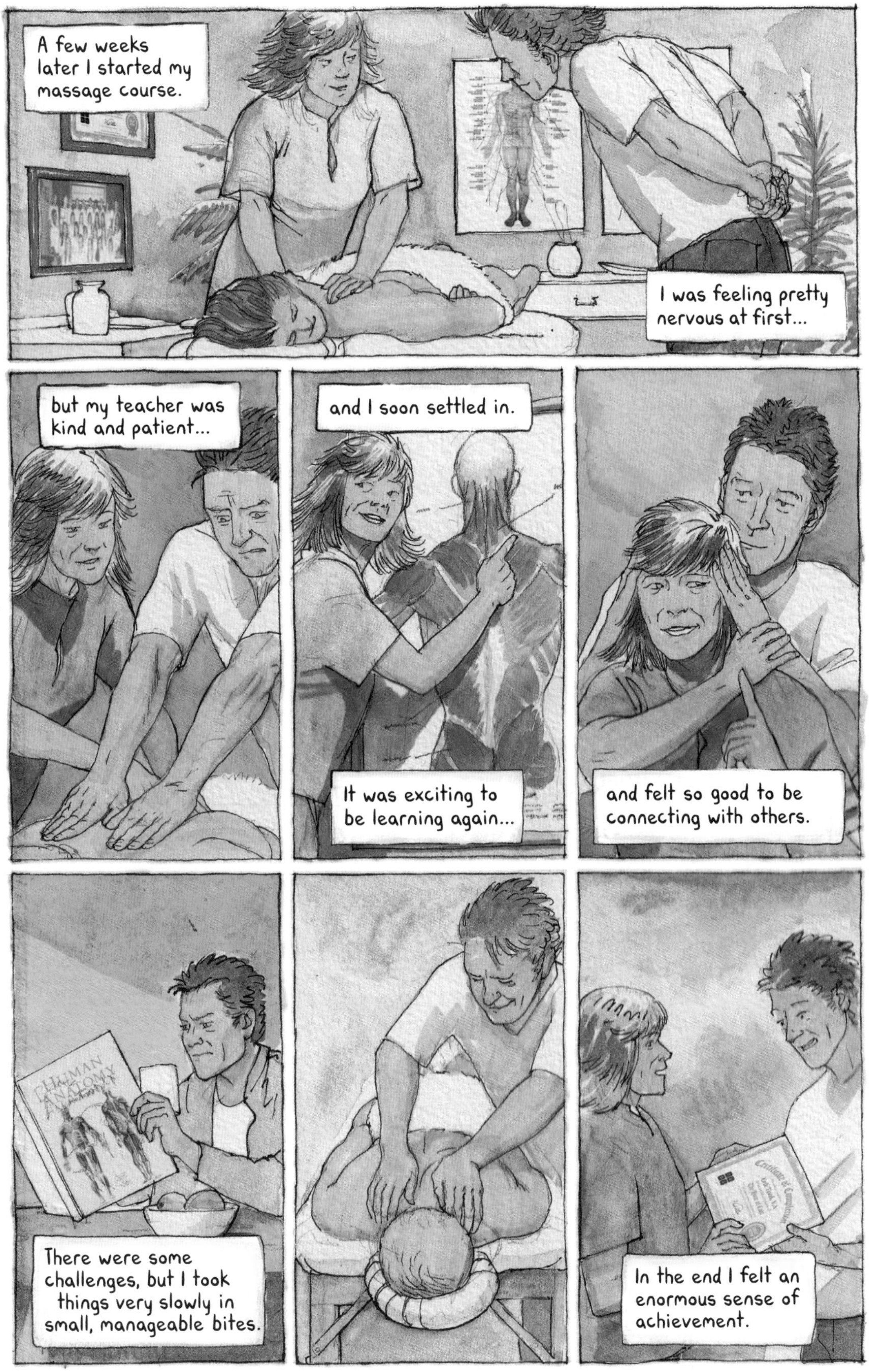
A few weeks later I started my massage course.
I was feeling pretty nervous at first...
but my teacher was kind and patient...
and I soon settled in.
It was exciting to be learning again...
and felt so good to be connecting with others.
There were some challenges, but I took things very slowly in small, manageable bites.
In the end I felt an enormous sense of achievement.

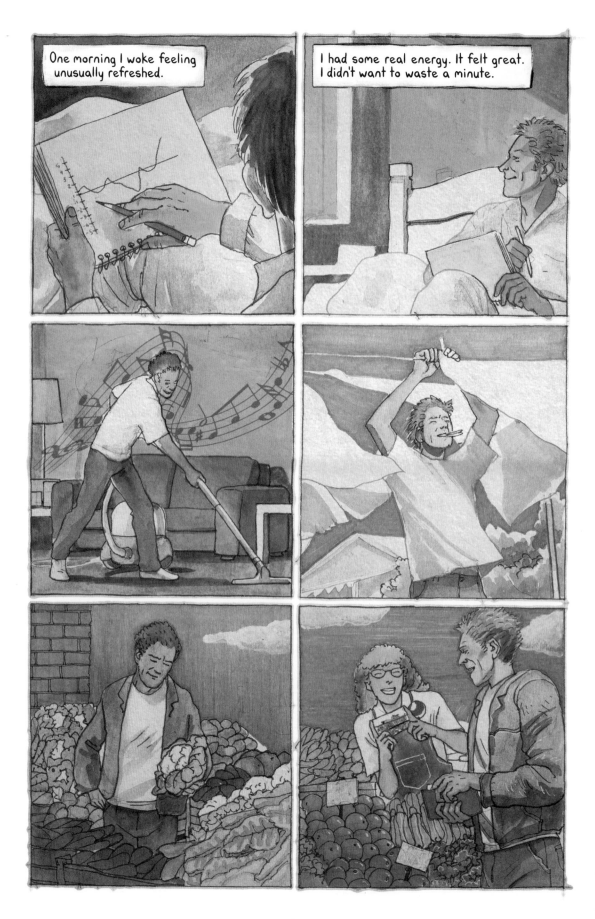

One morning I woke feeling unusually refreshed.

I had some real energy. It felt great. I didn't want to waste a minute.

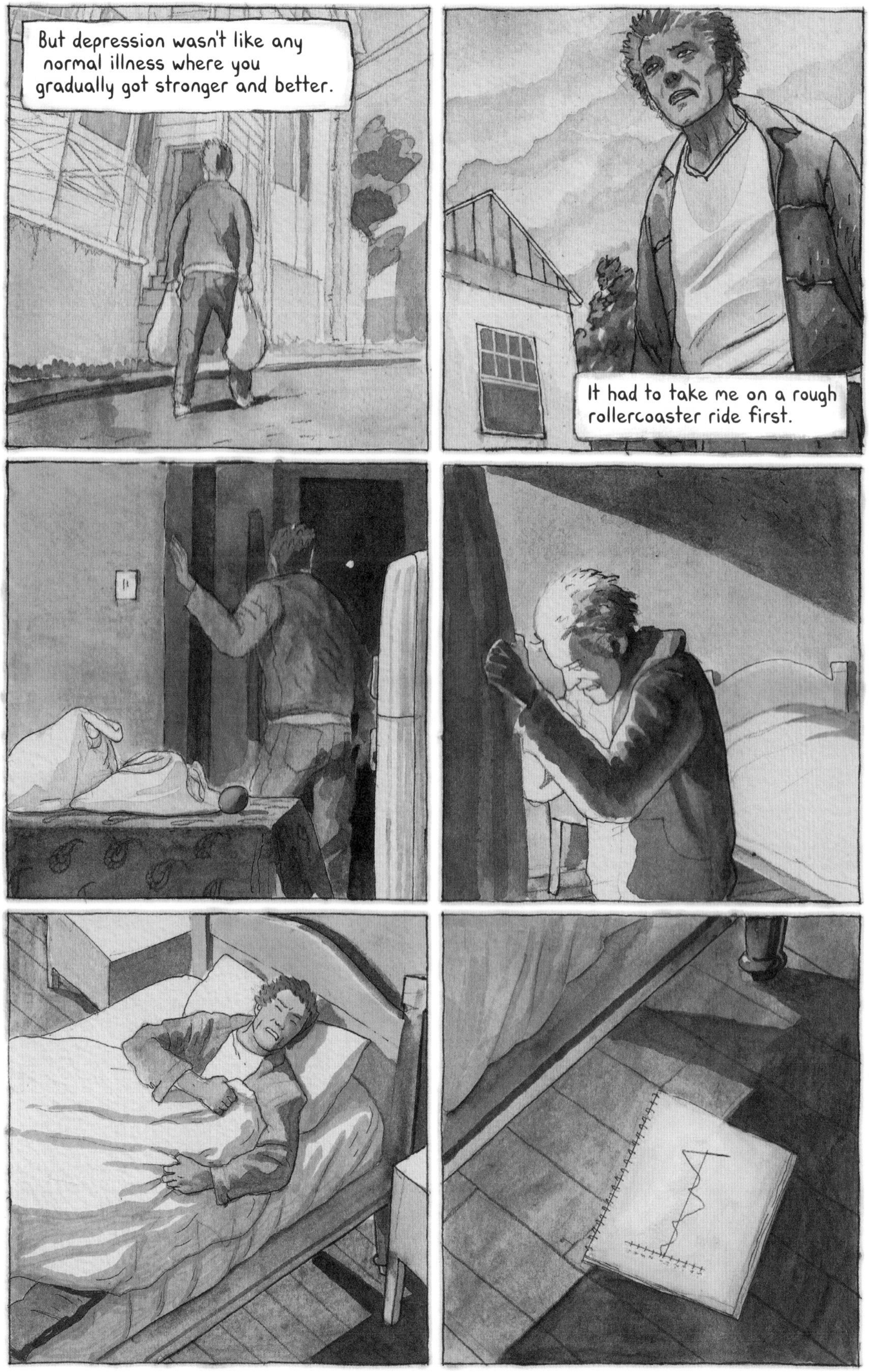
But depression wasn't like any normal illness where you gradually got stronger and better.
It had to take me on a rough rollercoaster ride first.

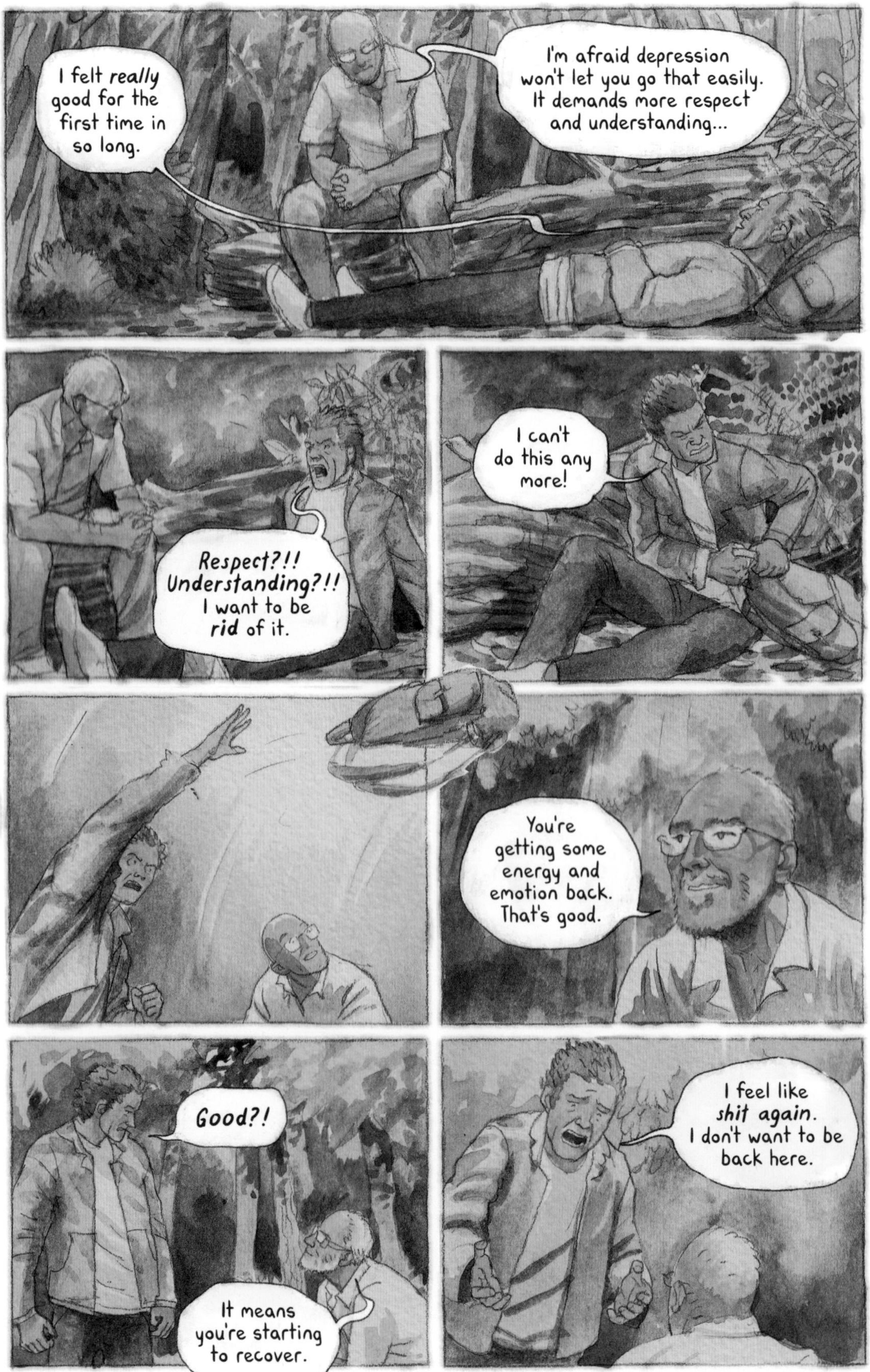
I felt *really* good for the first time in so long.
I'm afraid depression won't let you go that easily. It demands more respect and understanding...
Respect?!! Understanding?!! I want to be *rid* of it.
I can't do this any more!
You're getting some energy and emotion back. That's good.
Good?!
It means you're starting to recover.
I feel like *shit again*. I don't want to be back here.

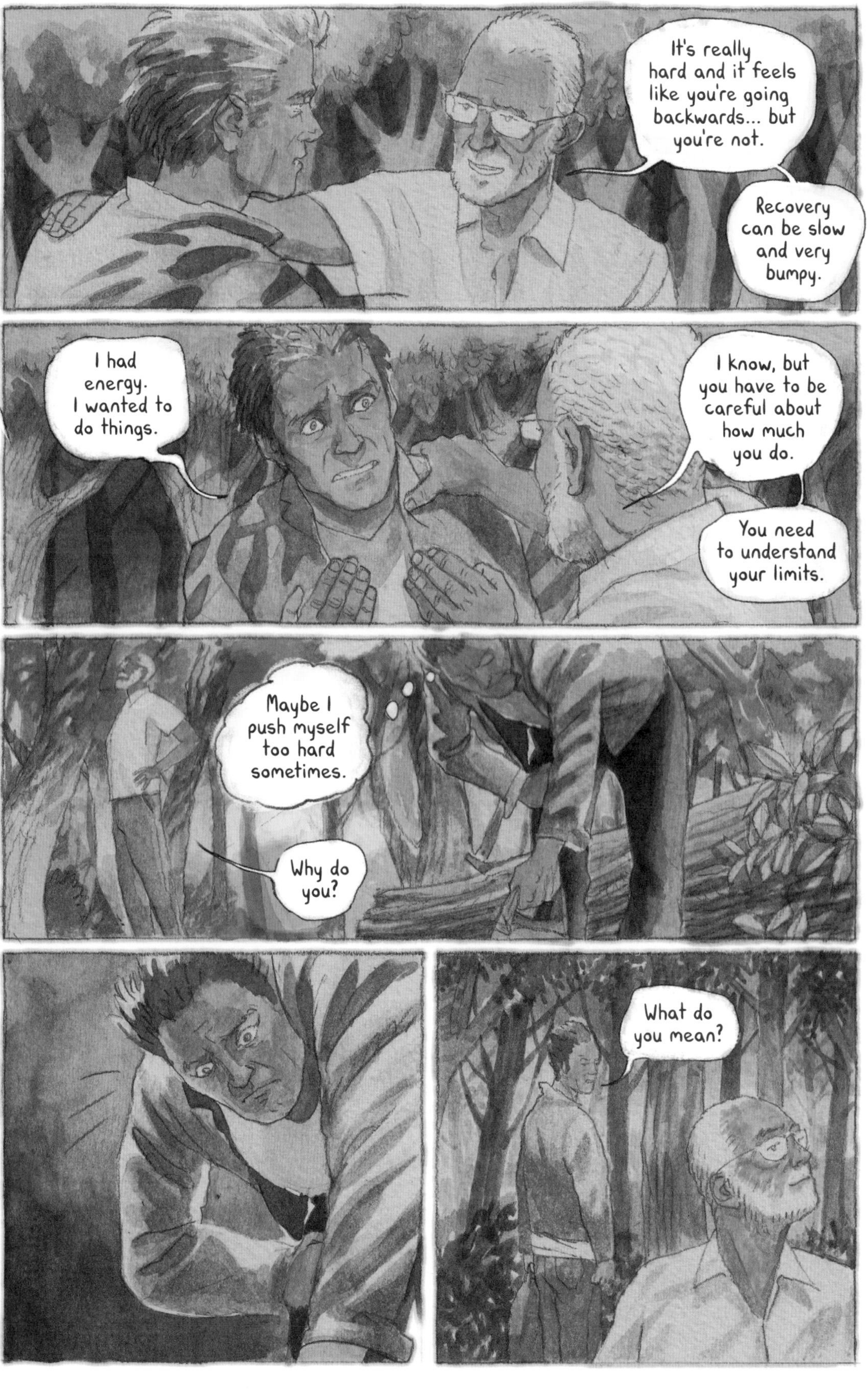
It's really hard and it feels like you're going backwards... but you're not.
Recovery can be slow and very bumpy.
I had energy. I wanted to do things.
I know, but you have to be careful about how much you do.
You need to understand your limits.
Maybe I push myself too hard sometimes.
Why do you?
What do you mean?

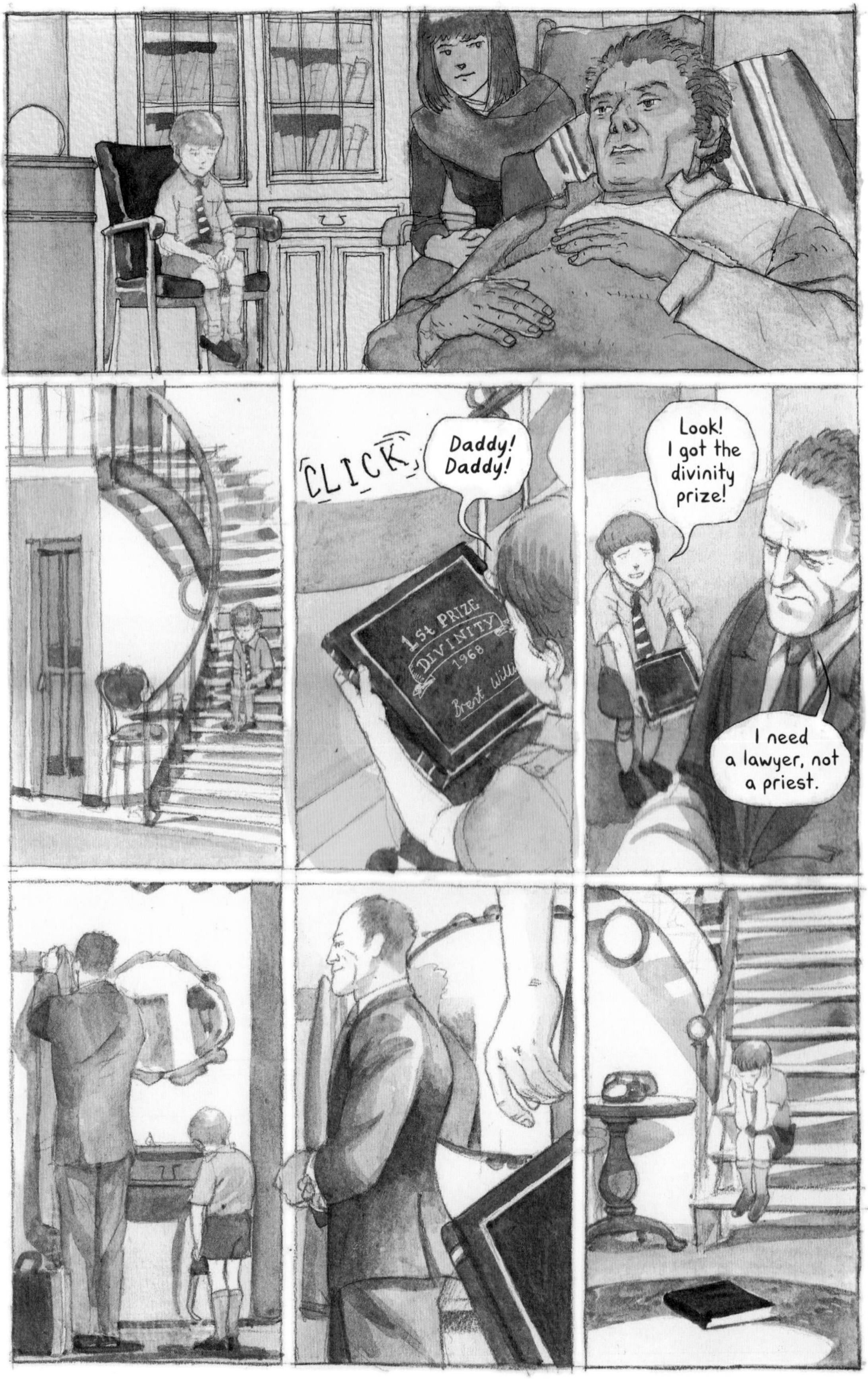
CLICK
Daddy! Daddy!
1st PRIZE
DIVINITY
1968
Look! I got the divinity prize!
I need a lawyer, not a priest.

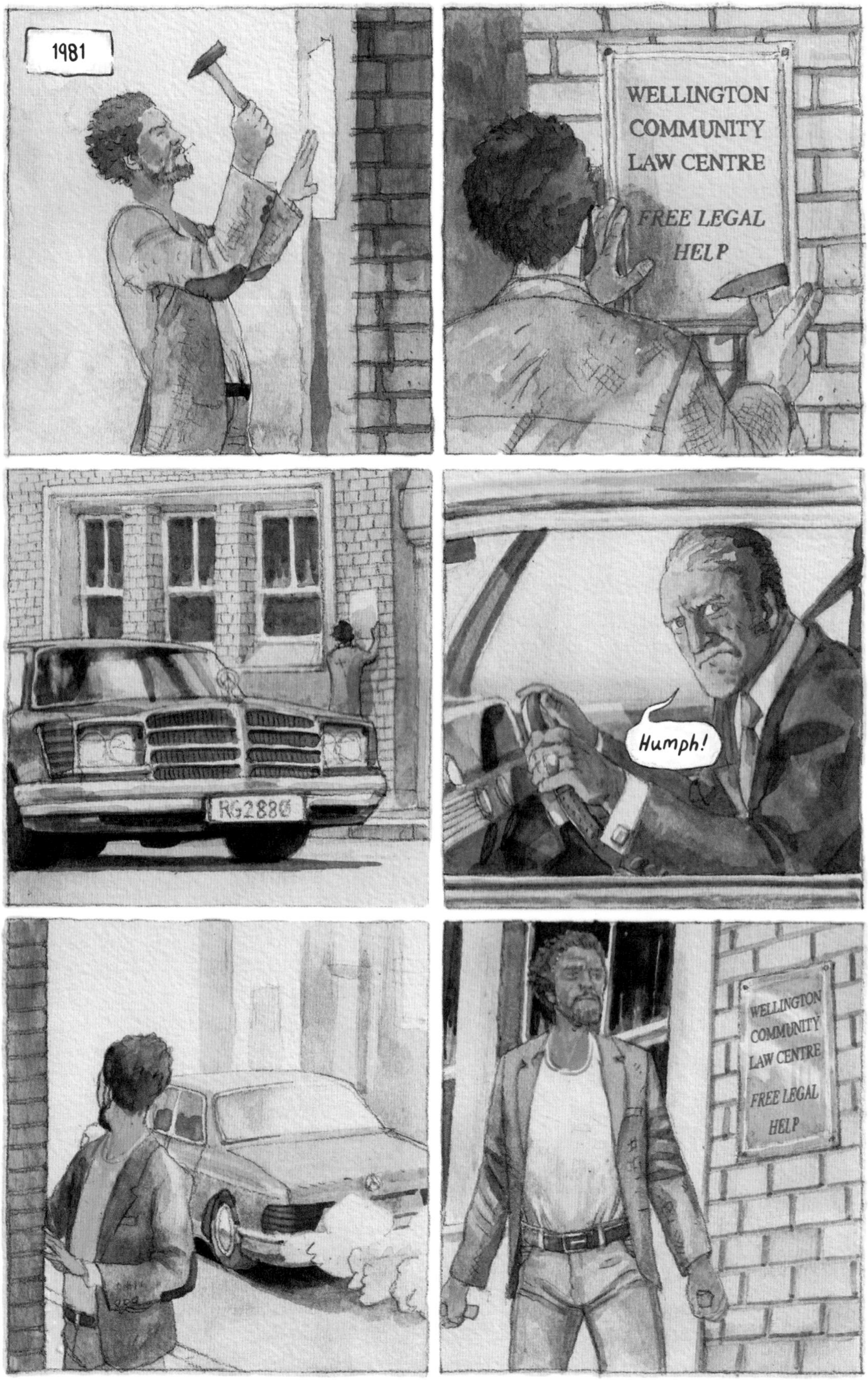
1981
WELLINGTON
COMMUNITY
LAW CENTRE
FREE LEGAL
HELP
RG2880
Humph!
WELLINGTON
COMMUNITY
LAW CENTRE
FREE LEGAL
HELP

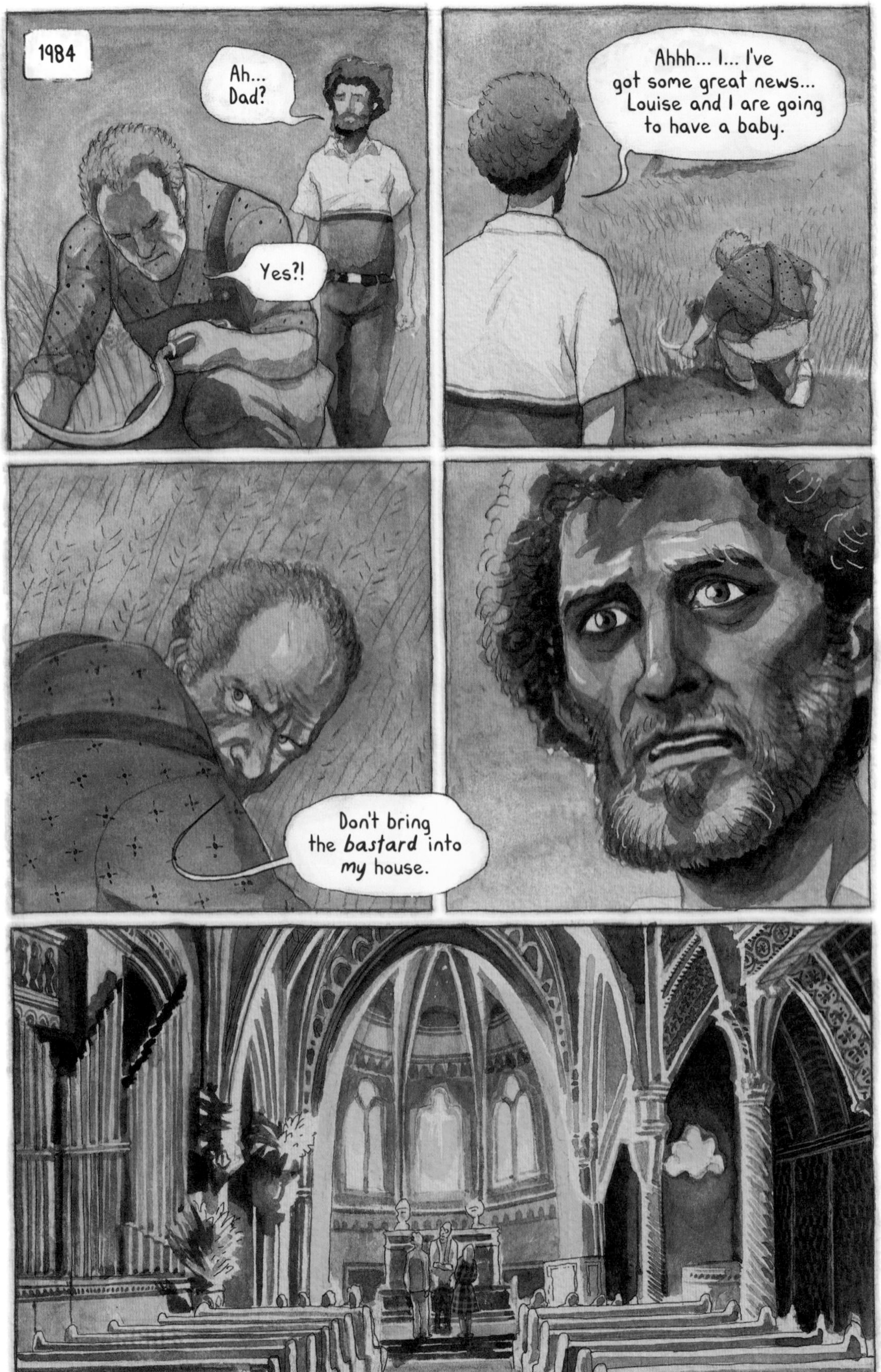
1984
Ah... Dad?
Yes?!
Ahhh... I... I've got some great news... Louise and I are going to have a baby.
Don't bring the *bastard* into *my* house.

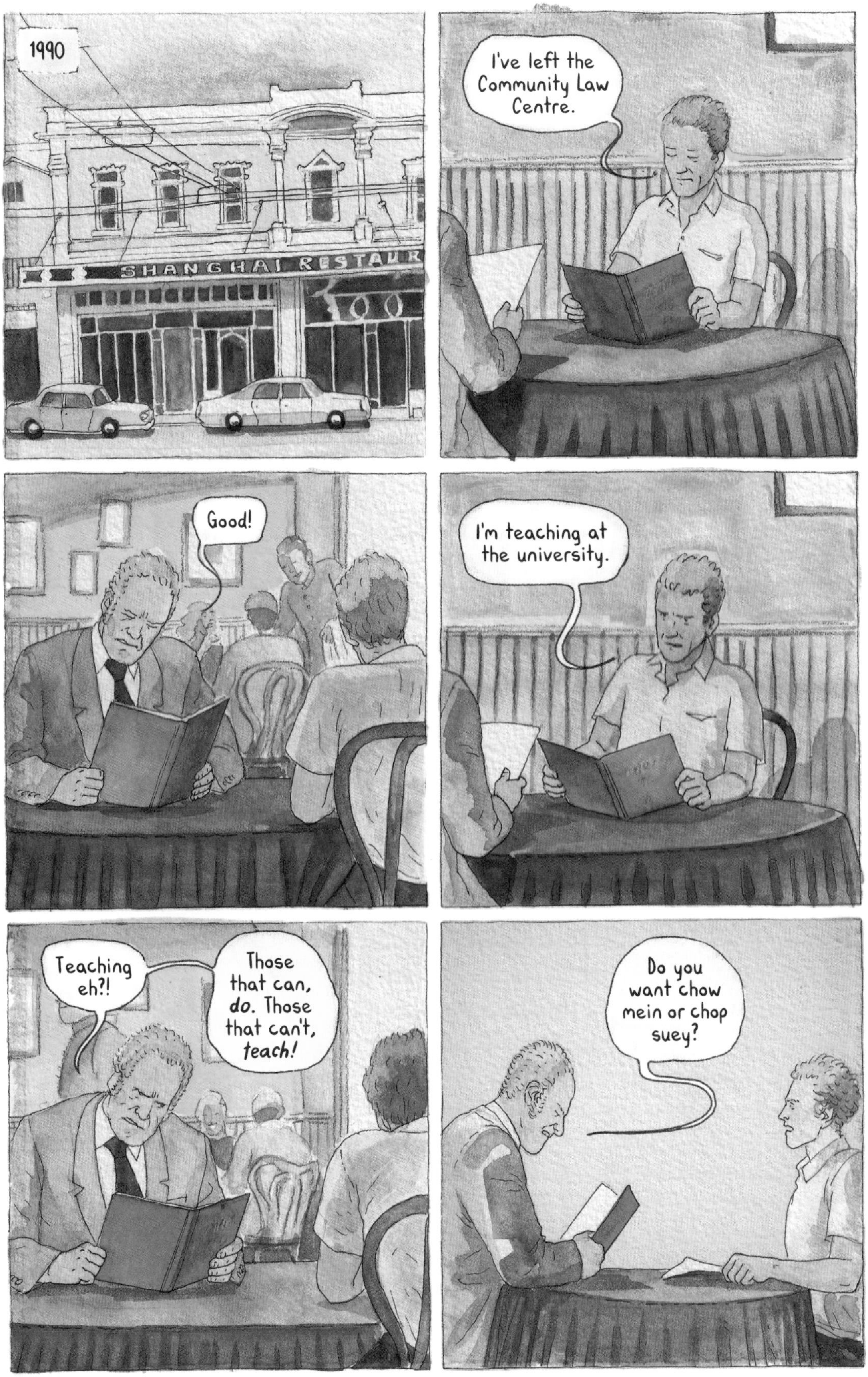
1990
SHANGHAI RESTAUR
I've left the Community Law Centre.
Good!
I'm teaching at the university.
Teaching eh?!
Those that can, *do.* Those that can't, *teach!*
Do you want chow mein or chop suey?

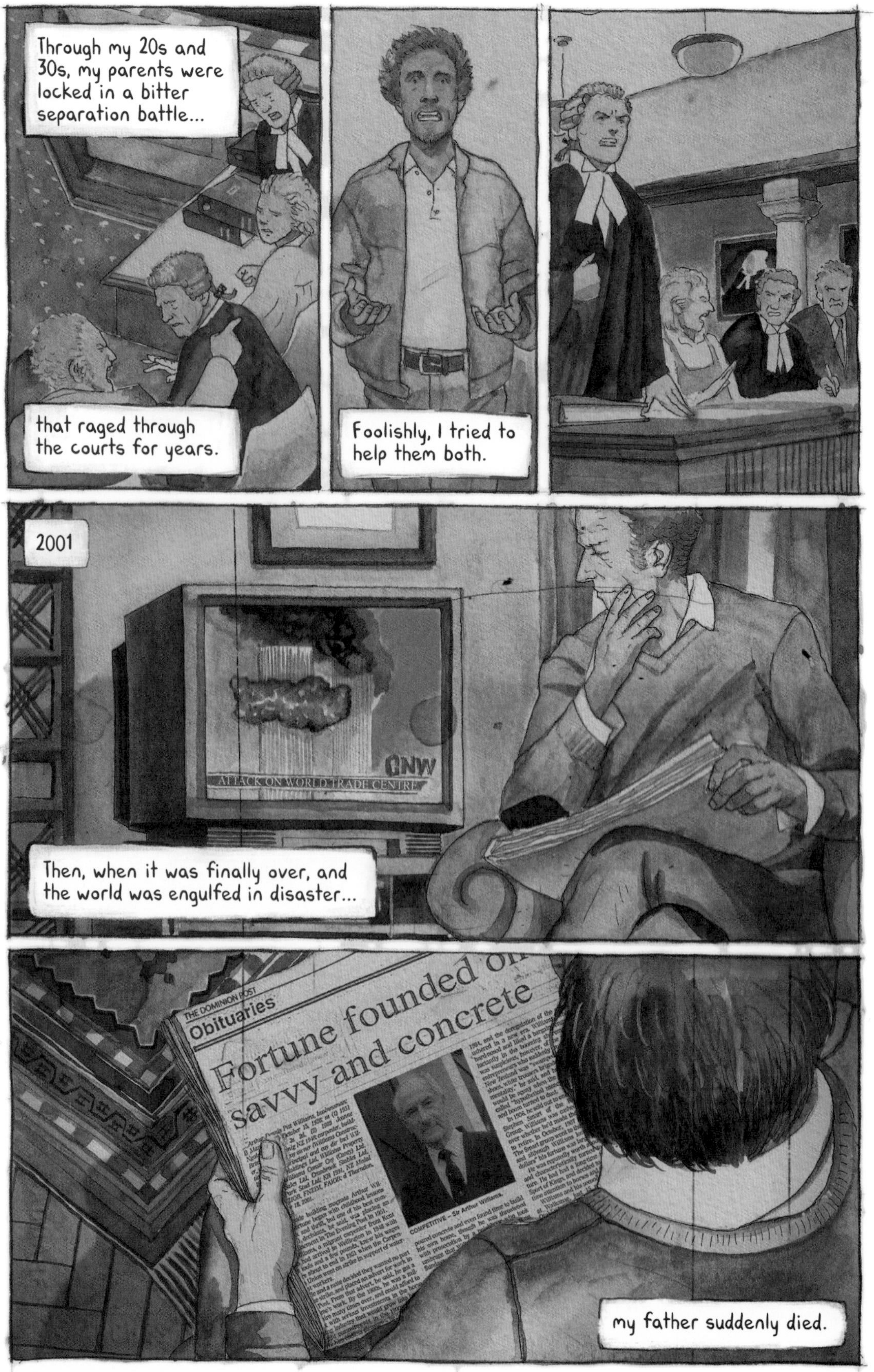
Through my 20s and 30s, my parents were locked in a bitter separation battle...
that raged through the courts for years.
Foolishly, I tried to help them both.
2001
ATTACK ON WORLD TRADE CENTRE
Then, when it was finally over, and the world was engulfed in disaster...
THE DOMINION POST
Obituaries
Fortune founded
savvy and concrete
my father suddenly died.

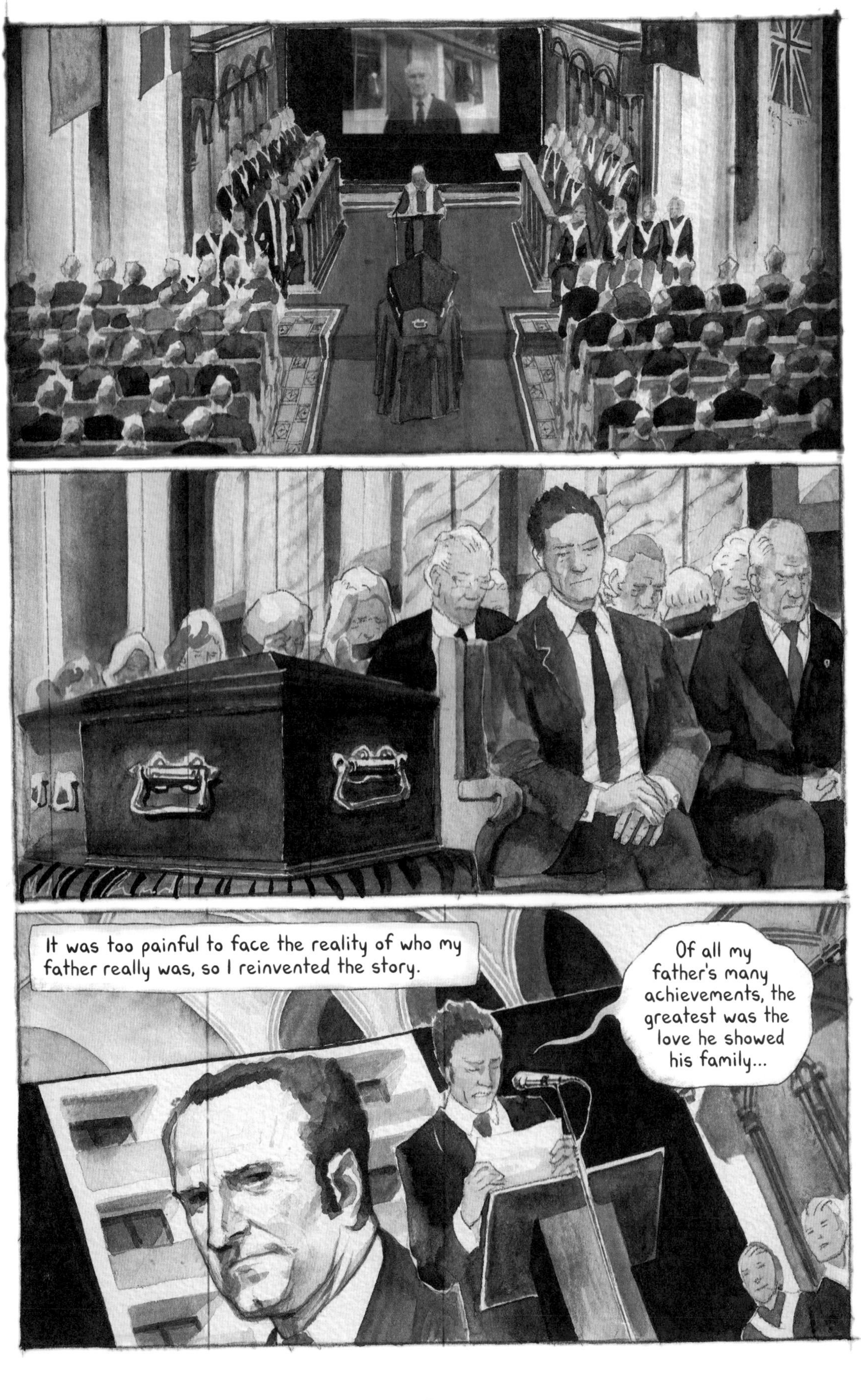
It was too painful to face the reality of who my father really was, so I reinvented the story.
Of all my father's many achievements, the greatest was the love he showed his family...

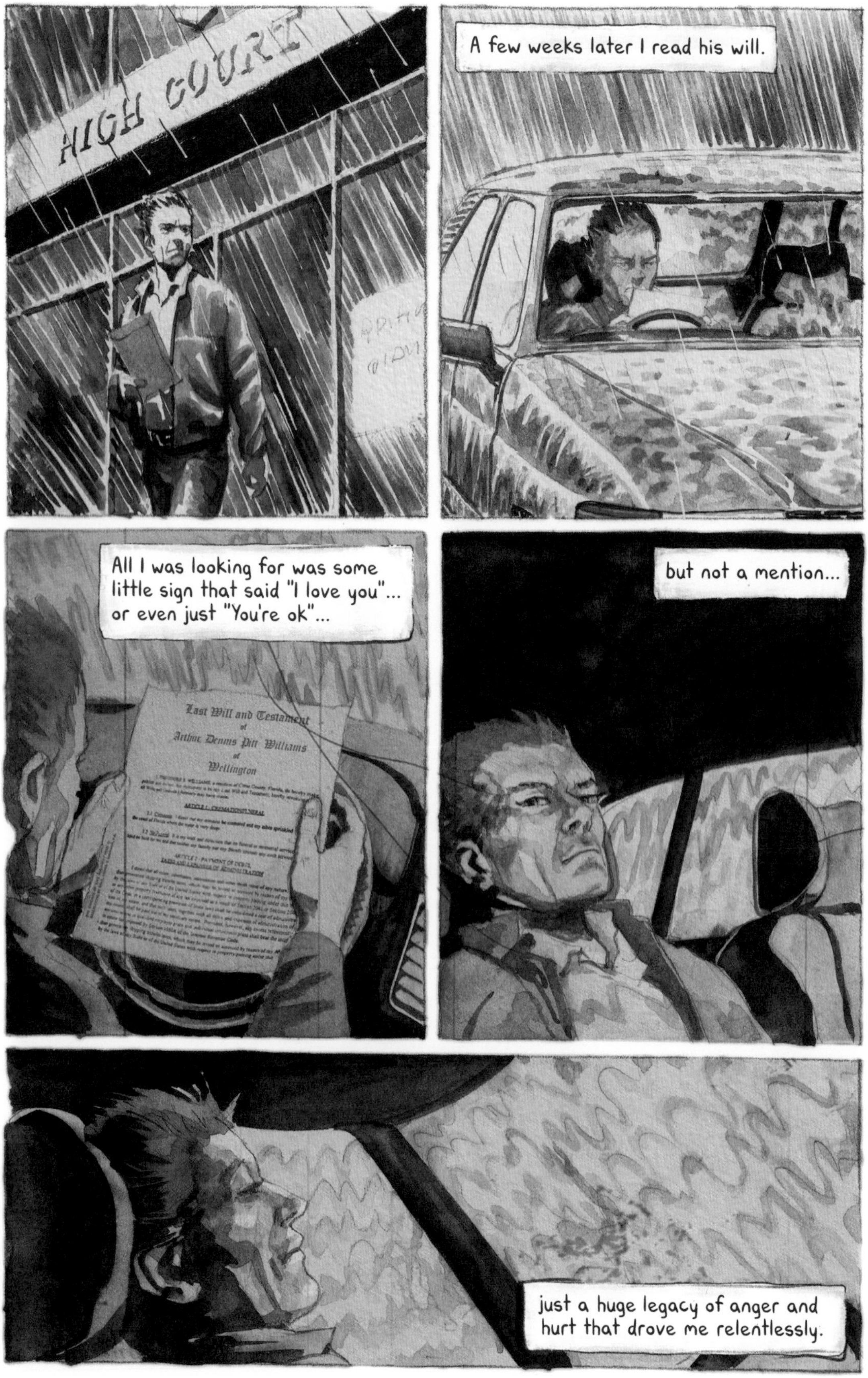
HIGH COURT
A few weeks later I read his will.
All I was looking for was some little sign that said "I love you"... or even just "You're ok"...
Last Will and Testament
of
Arthur Dennis Pitt Williams
of
Wellington
but not a mention...
just a huge legacy of anger and hurt that drove me relentlessly.

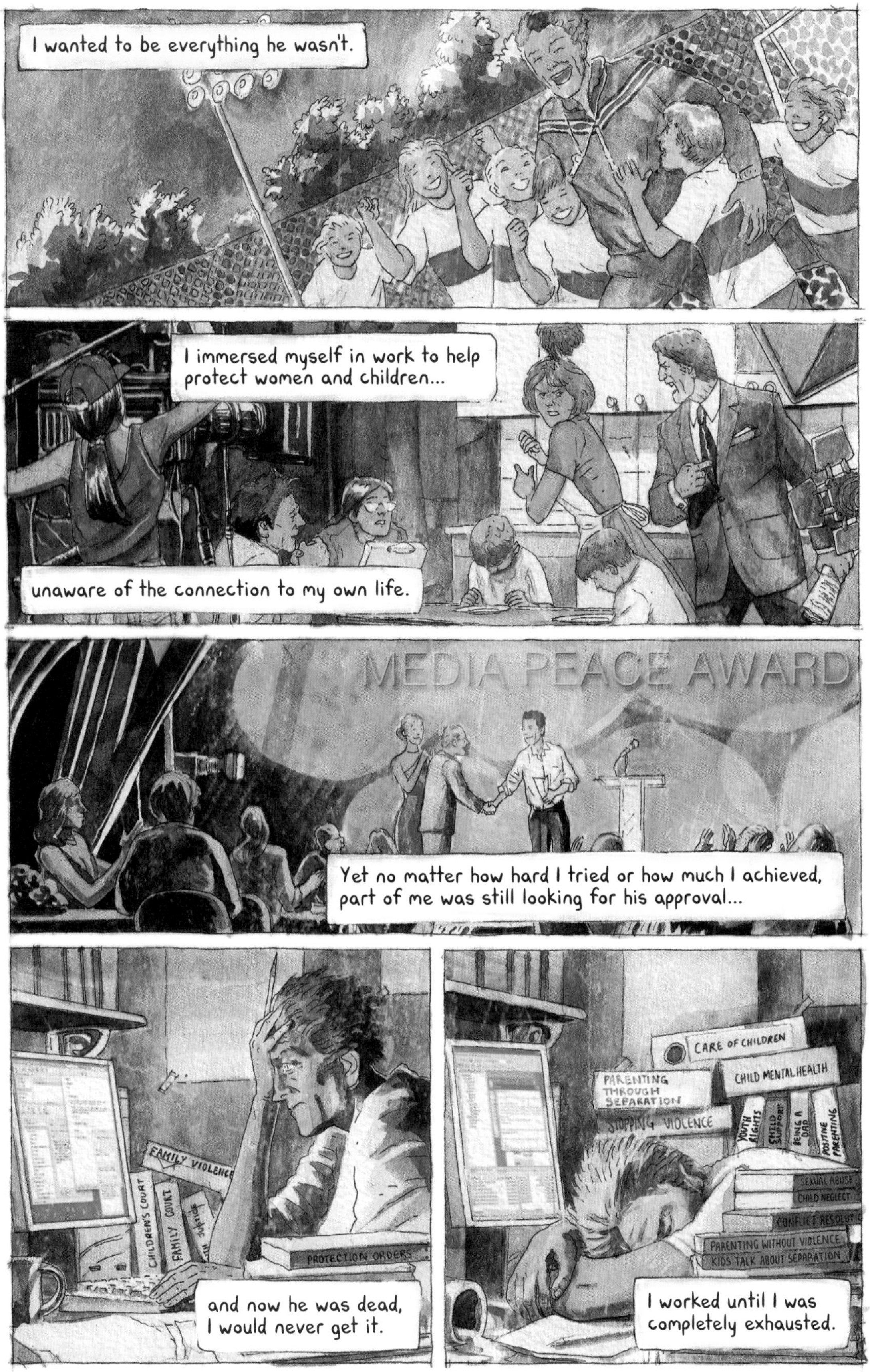
I wanted to be everything he wasn't.
I immersed myself in work to help protect women and children...
unaware of the connection to my own life.
MEDIA PEACE AWARD
Yet no matter how hard I tried or how much I achieved, part of me was still looking for his approval...
FAMILY VIOLENCE
CHILDREN'S COURT
FAMILY COURT
PROTECTION ORDERS
and now he was dead, I would never get it.
CARE OF CHILDREN
PARENTING THROUGH SEPARATION
CHILD MENTAL HEALTH
STOPPING VIOLENCE
YOUTH RIGHTS
CHILD SUPPORT
BEING A DAD
POSITIVE PARENTING
SEXUAL ABUSE
CHILD NEGLECT
PARENTING WITHOUT VIOLENCE
KIDS TALK ABOUT SEPARATION
I worked until I was completely exhausted.

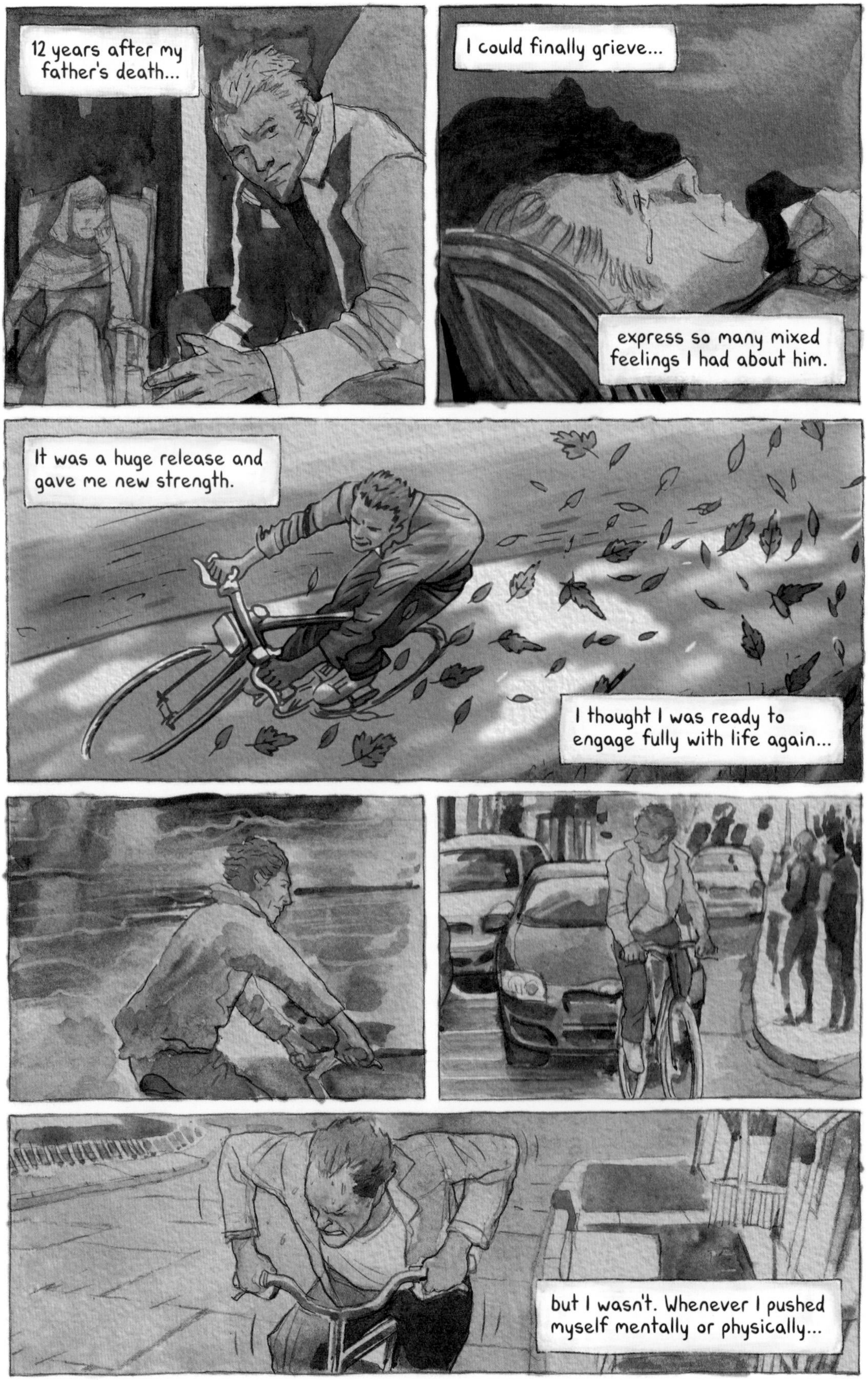
12 years after my father's death...
I could finally grieve...
express so many mixed feelings I had about him.
It was a huge release and gave me new strength.
I thought I was ready to engage fully with life again...
but I wasn't. Whenever I pushed myself mentally or physically...

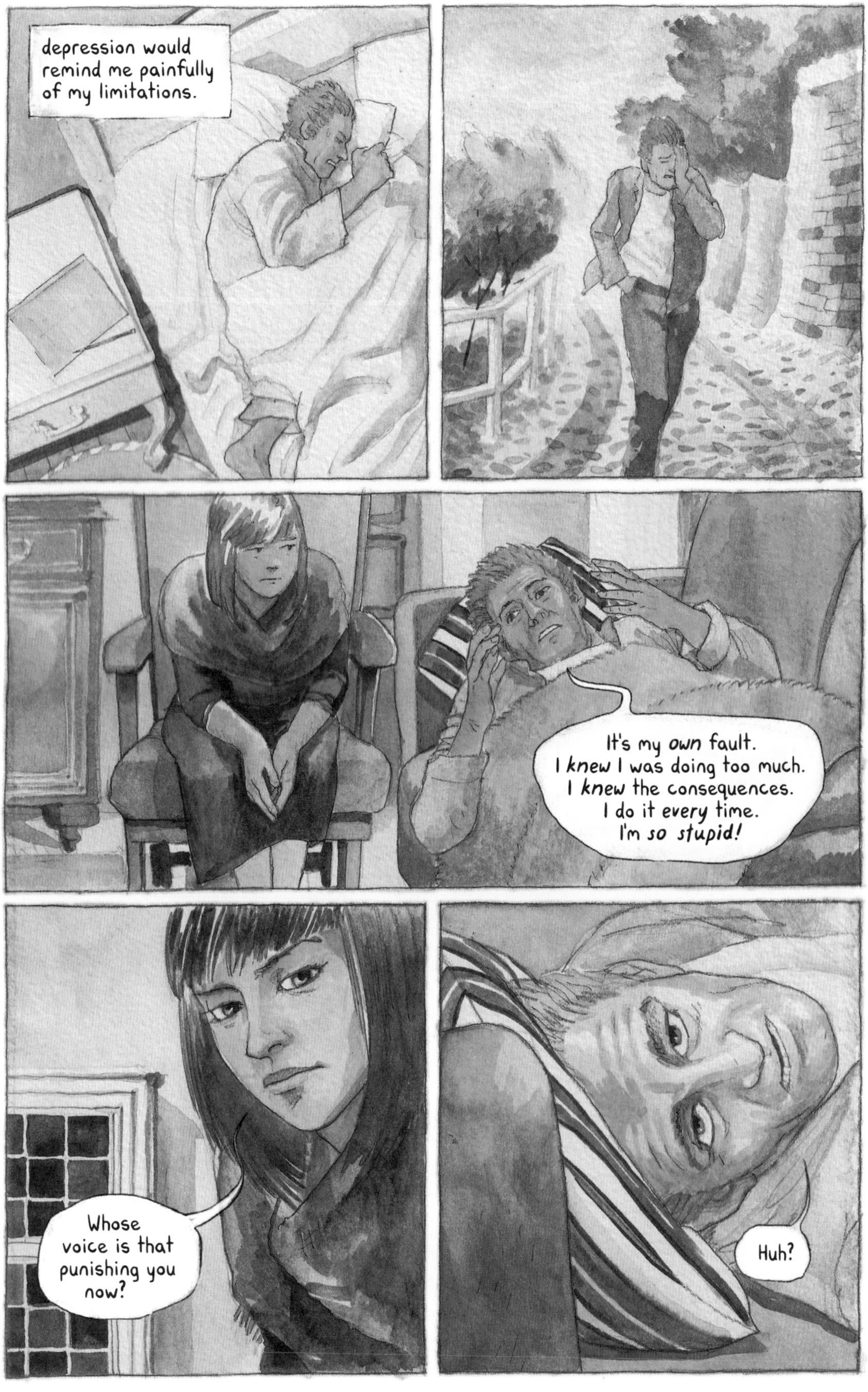
depression would remind me painfully of my limitations.
It's my *own* fault. I *knew* I was doing too much. I *knew* the consequences. I do it *every* time. I'm *so stupid!*
Whose voice is that punishing you now?
Huh?

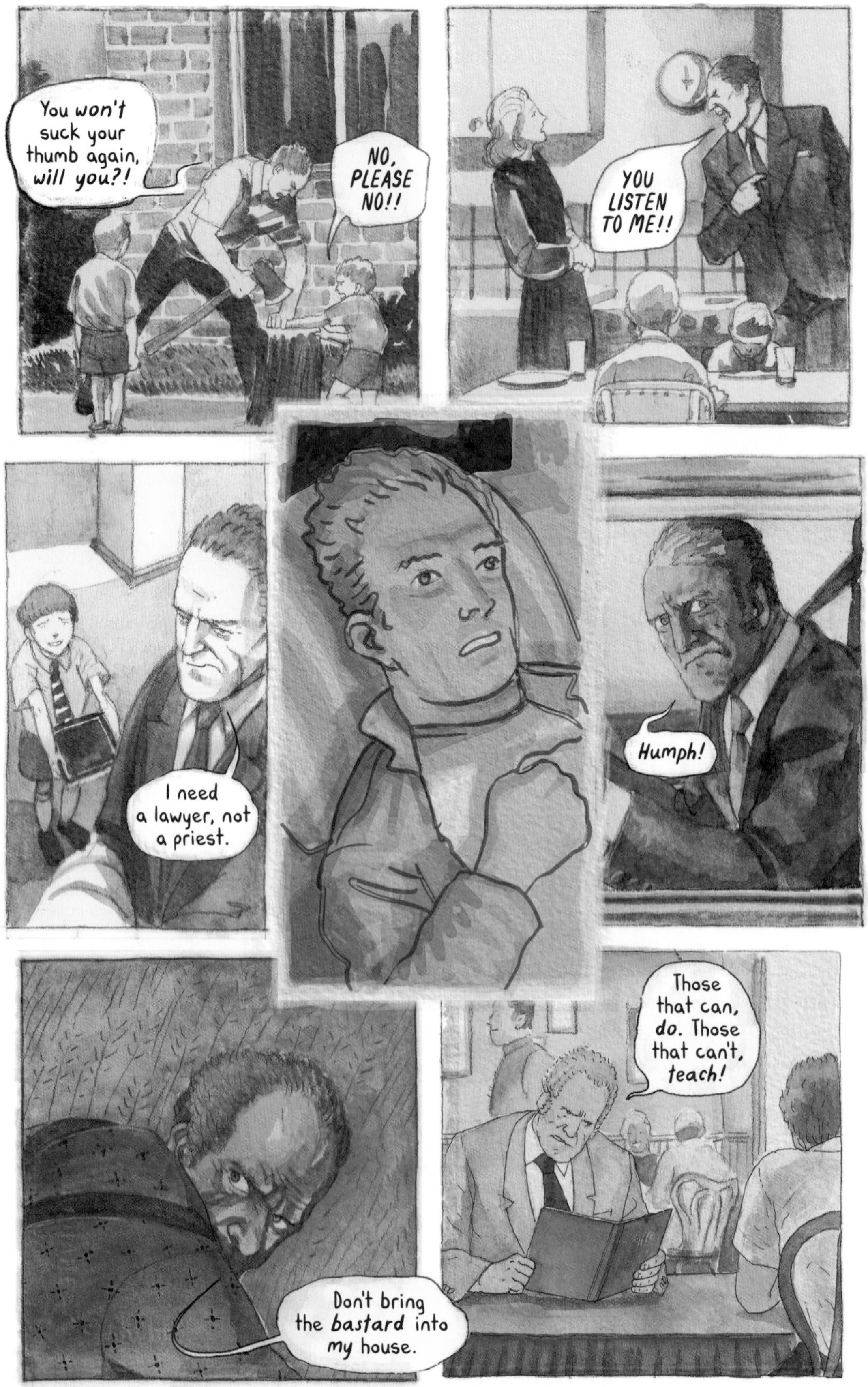
You won't suck your thumb again, will you?!
NO, PLEASE NO!!
YOU LISTEN TO ME!!
I need a lawyer, not a priest.
Humph!
Those that can, do. Those that can't, teach!
Don't bring the bastard into my house.

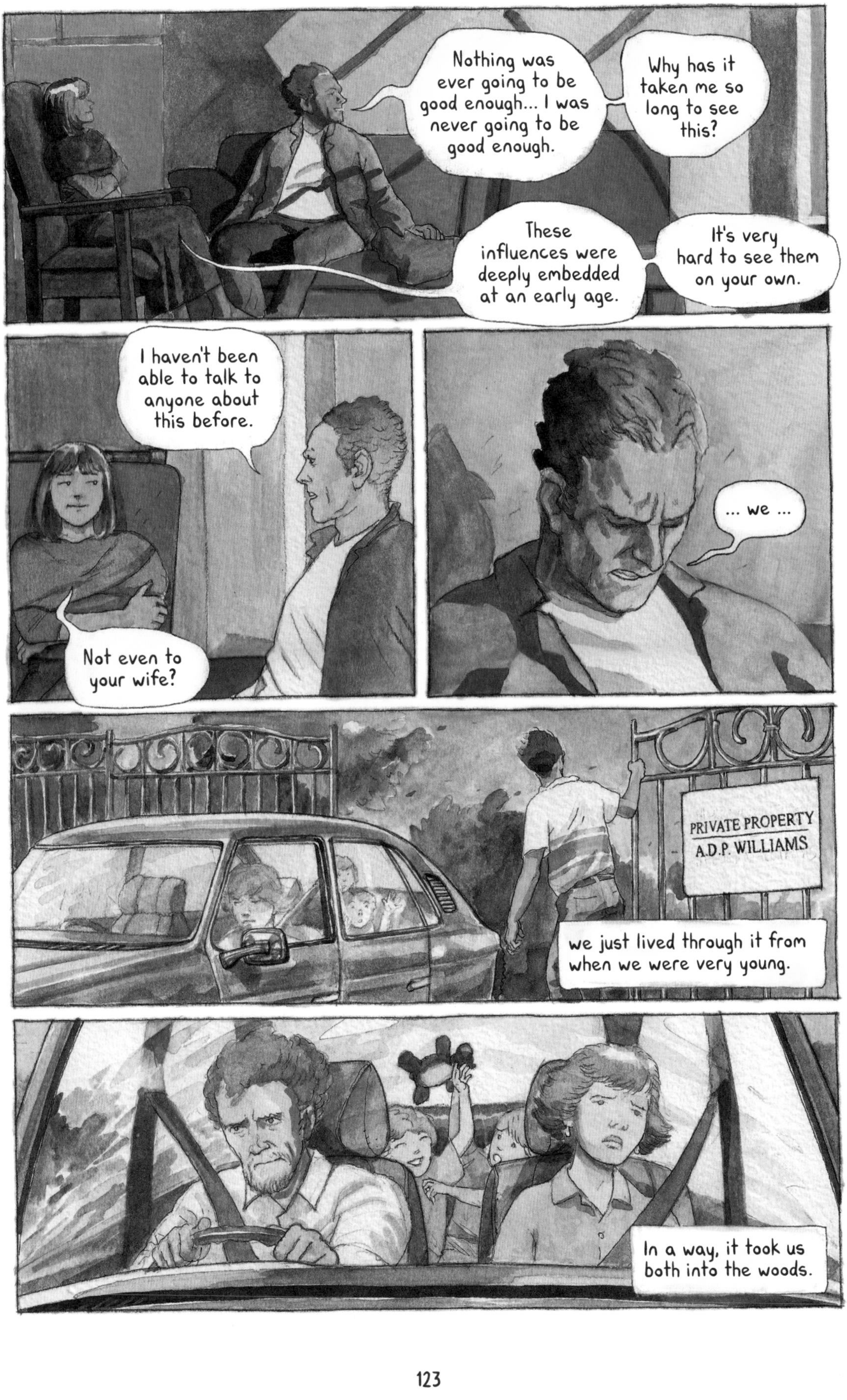
Nothing was ever going to be good enough... I was never going to be good enough.
Why has it taken me so long to see this?
These influences were deeply embedded at an early age.
It's very hard to see them on your own.
I haven't been able to talk to anyone about this before.
Not even to your wife?
... we ...
PRIVATE PROPERTY
A.D.P. WILLIAMS
we just lived through it from when we were very young.
In a way, it took us both into the woods.

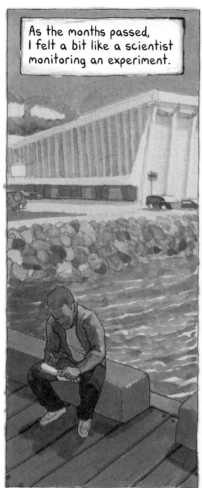

As the months passed, I felt a bit like a scientist monitoring an experiment.

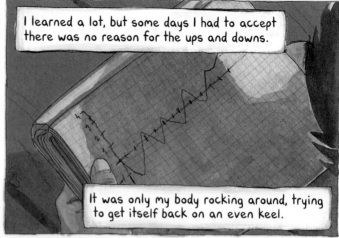

I learned a lot, but some days I had to accept there was no reason for the ups and downs.

It was only my body rocking around, trying to get itself back on an even keel.

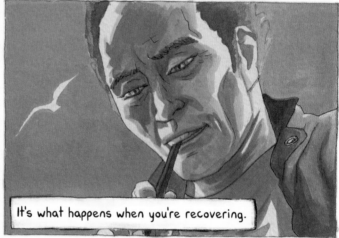

It's what happens when you're recovering.

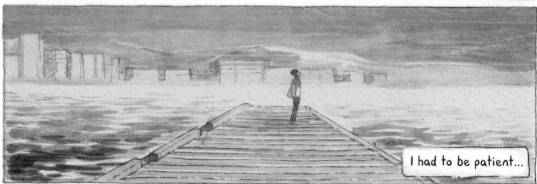

I had to be patient...

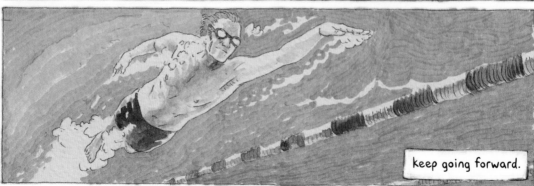

keep going forward.

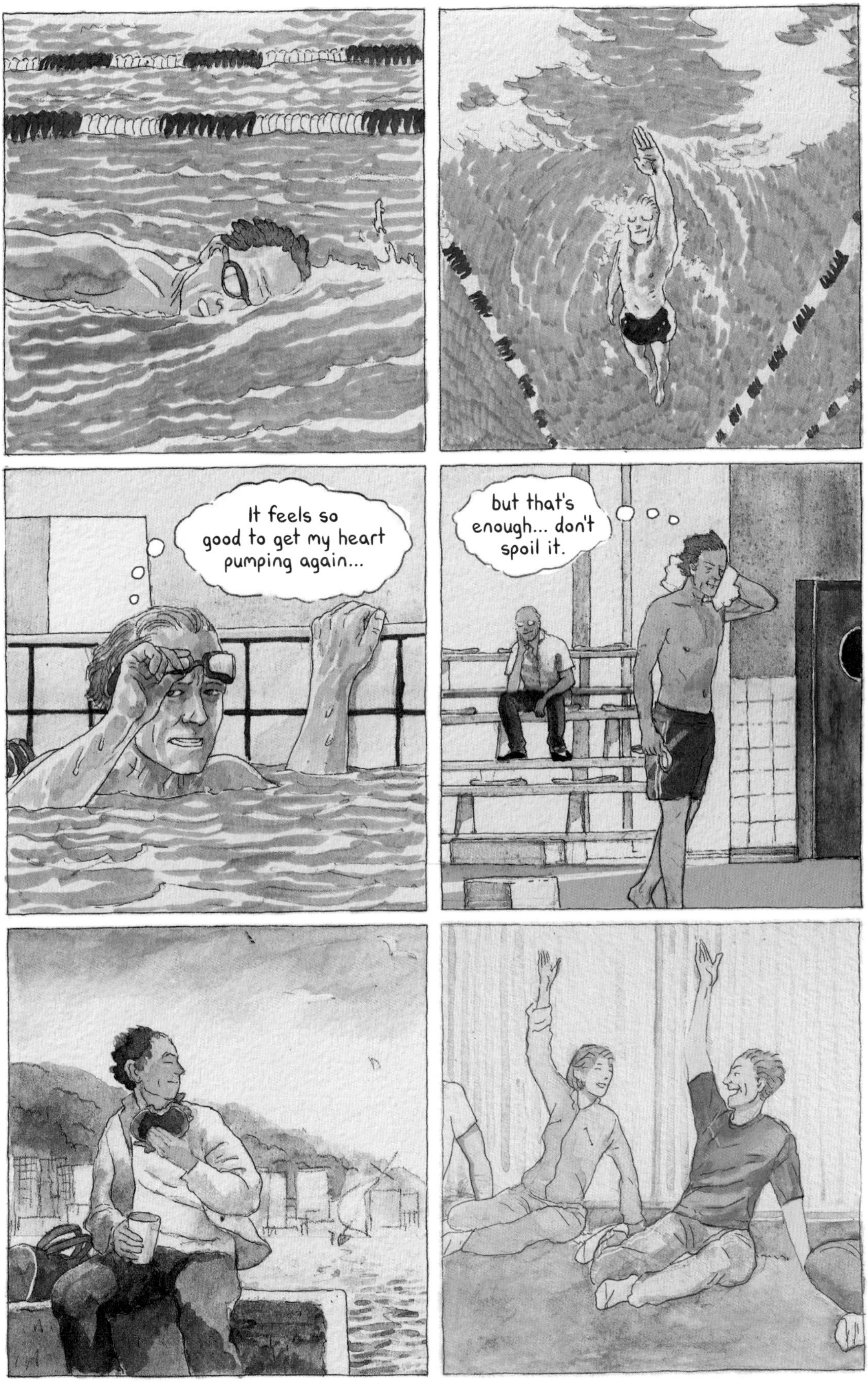
It feels so good to get my heart pumping again...
but that's enough... don't spoil it.

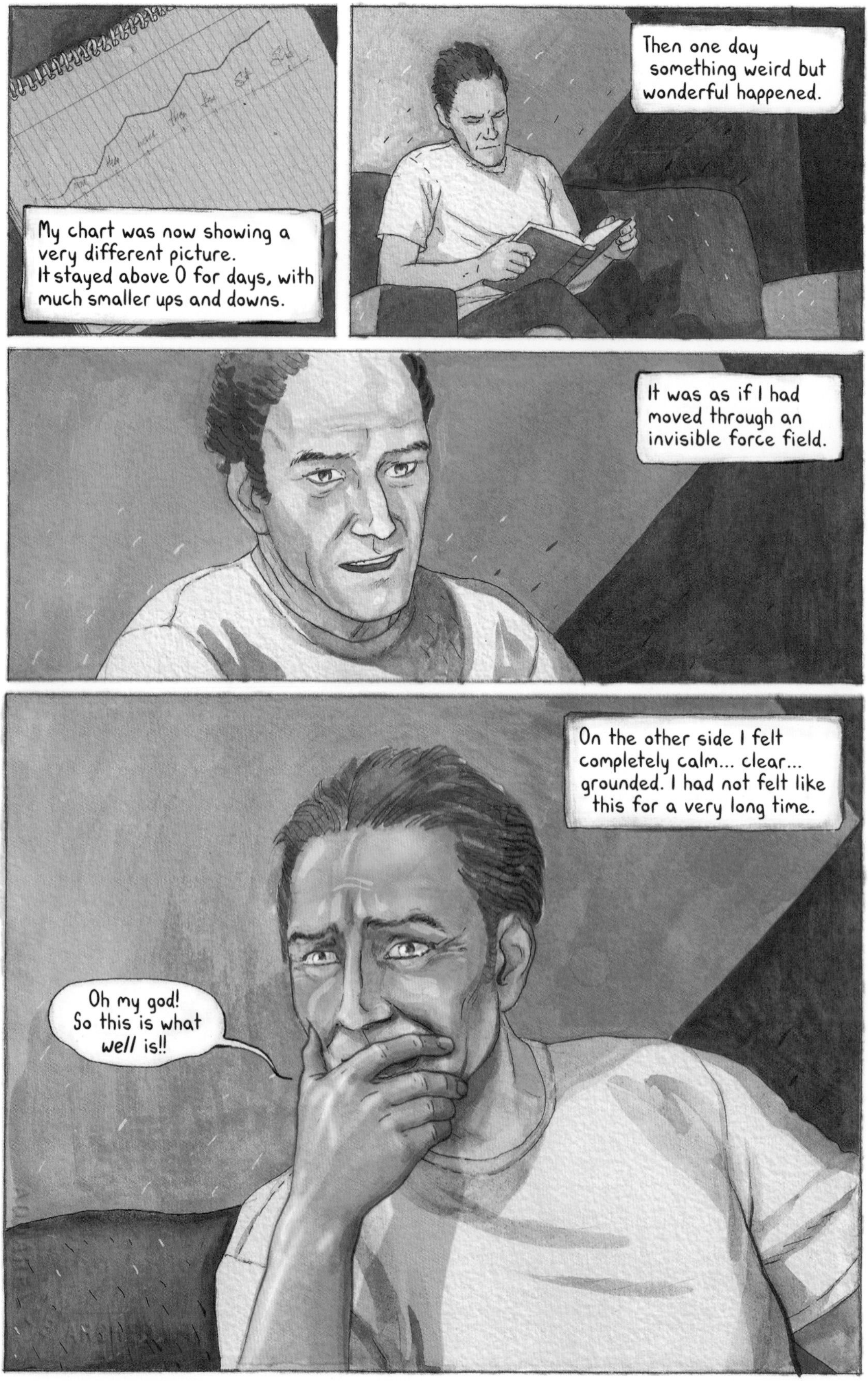
My chart was now showing a very different picture. It stayed above 0 for days, with much smaller ups and downs.
Then one day something weird but wonderful happened.
It was as if I had moved through an invisible force field.
On the other side I felt completely calm... clear... grounded. I had not felt like this for a very long time.
Oh my god! So this is what *well* is!!

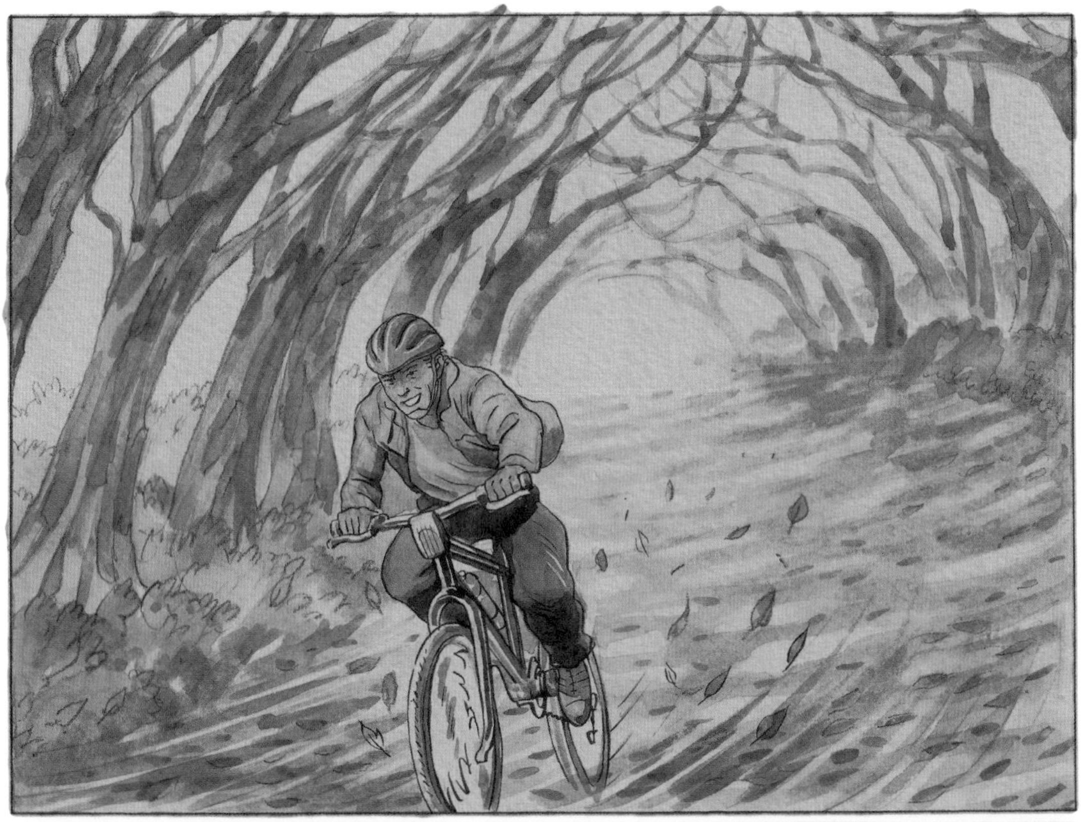

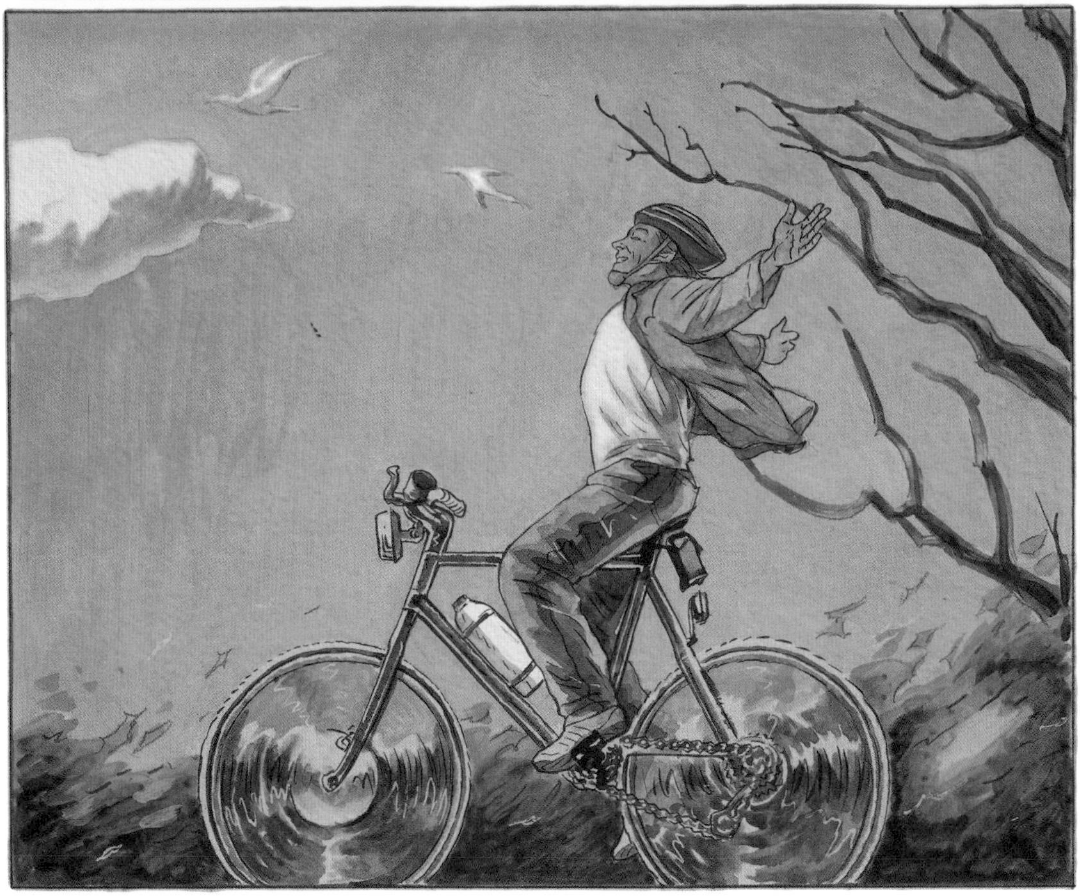

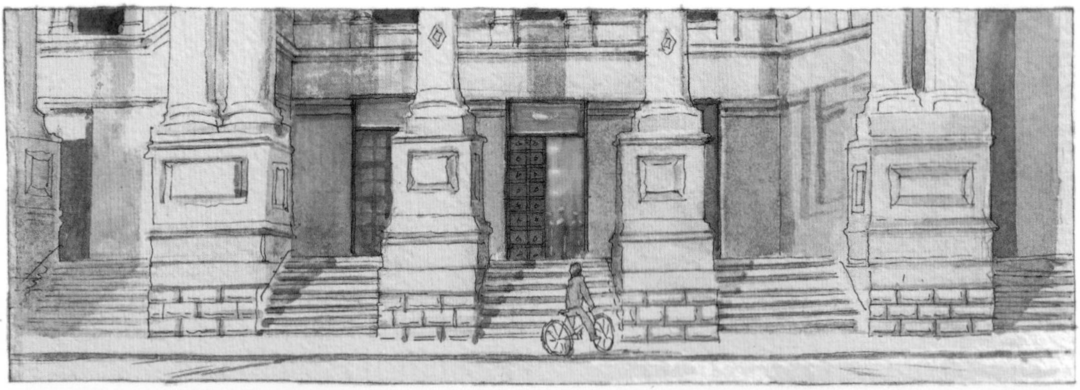

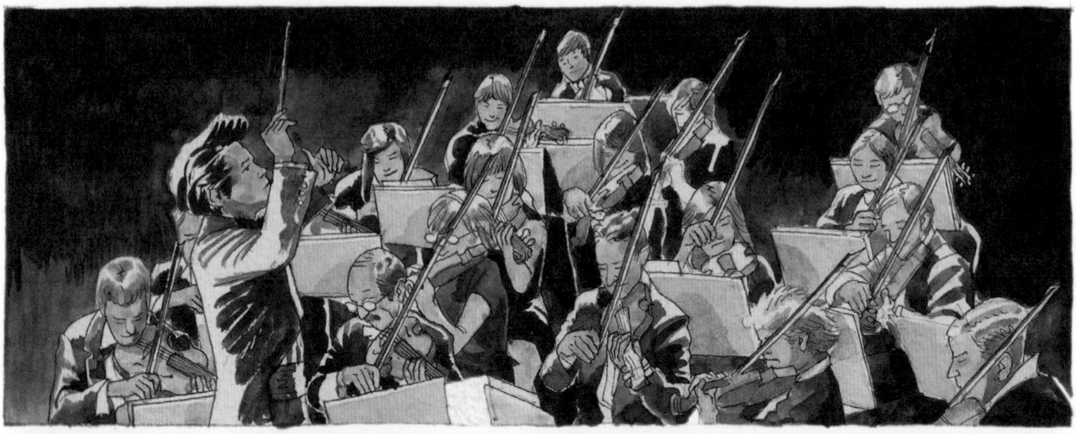

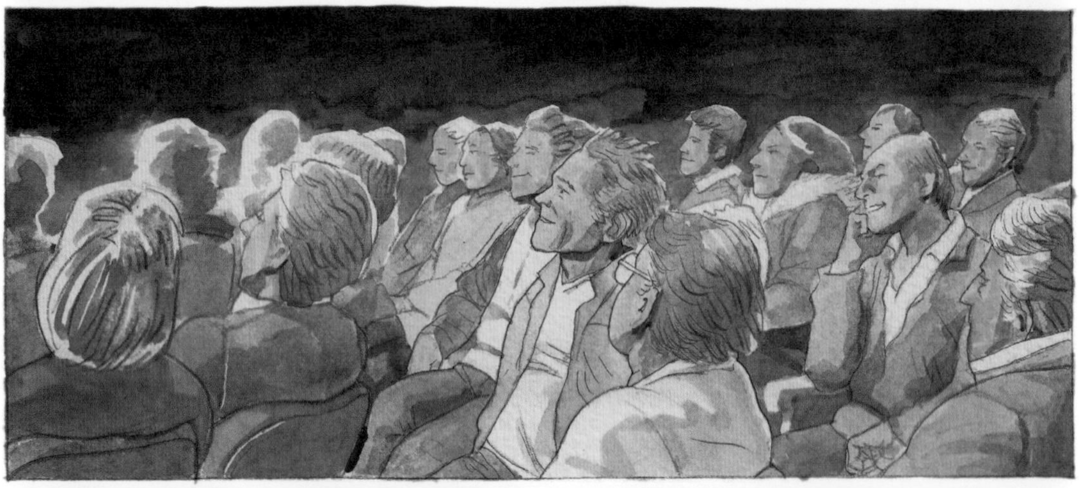

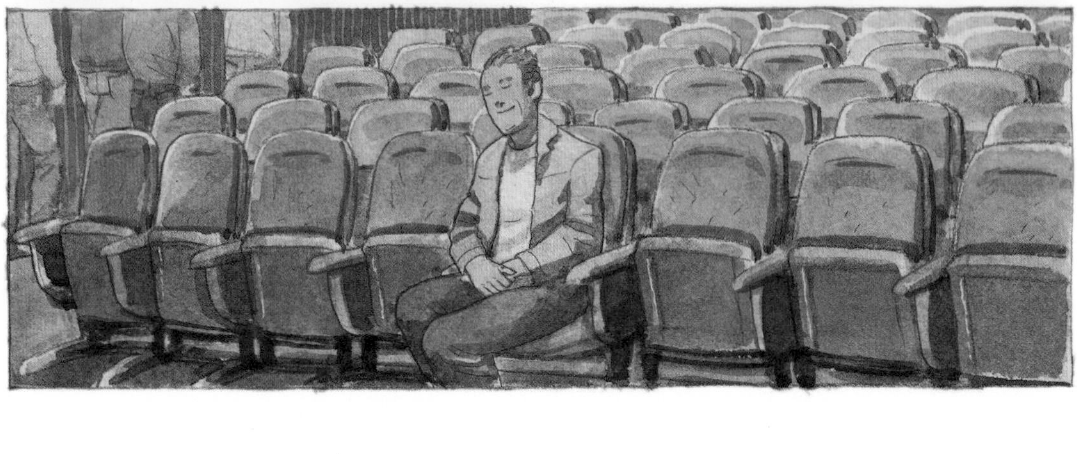

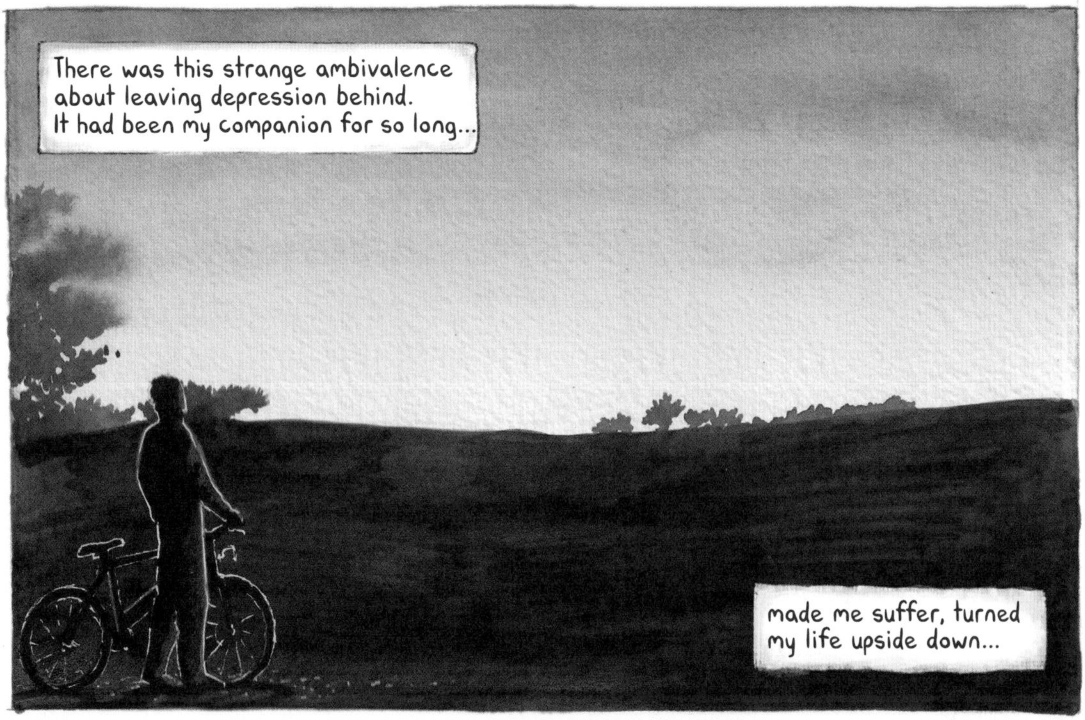
There was this strange ambivalence about leaving depression behind. It had been my companion for so long...
made me suffer, turned my life upside down...

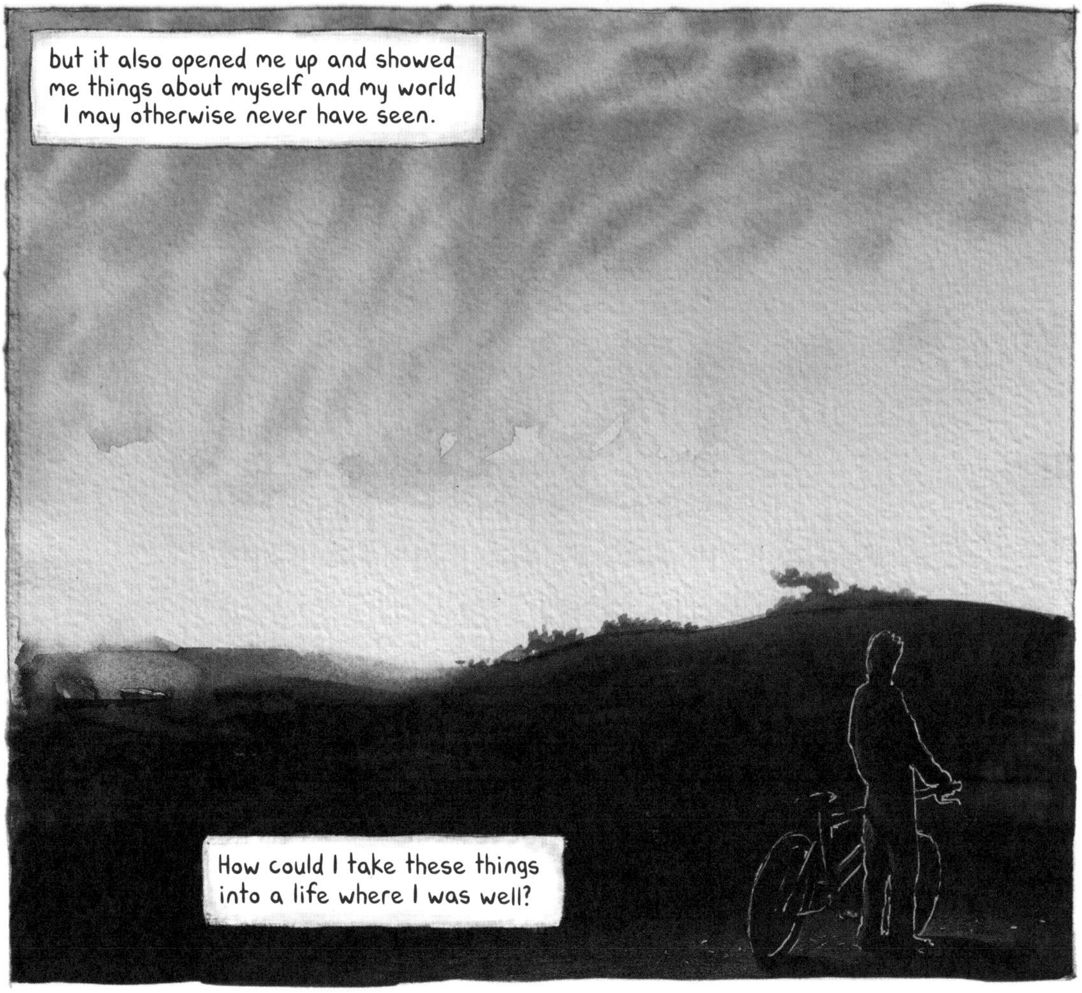
but it also opened me up and showed me things about myself and my world I may otherwise never have seen.
How could I take these things into a life where I was well?

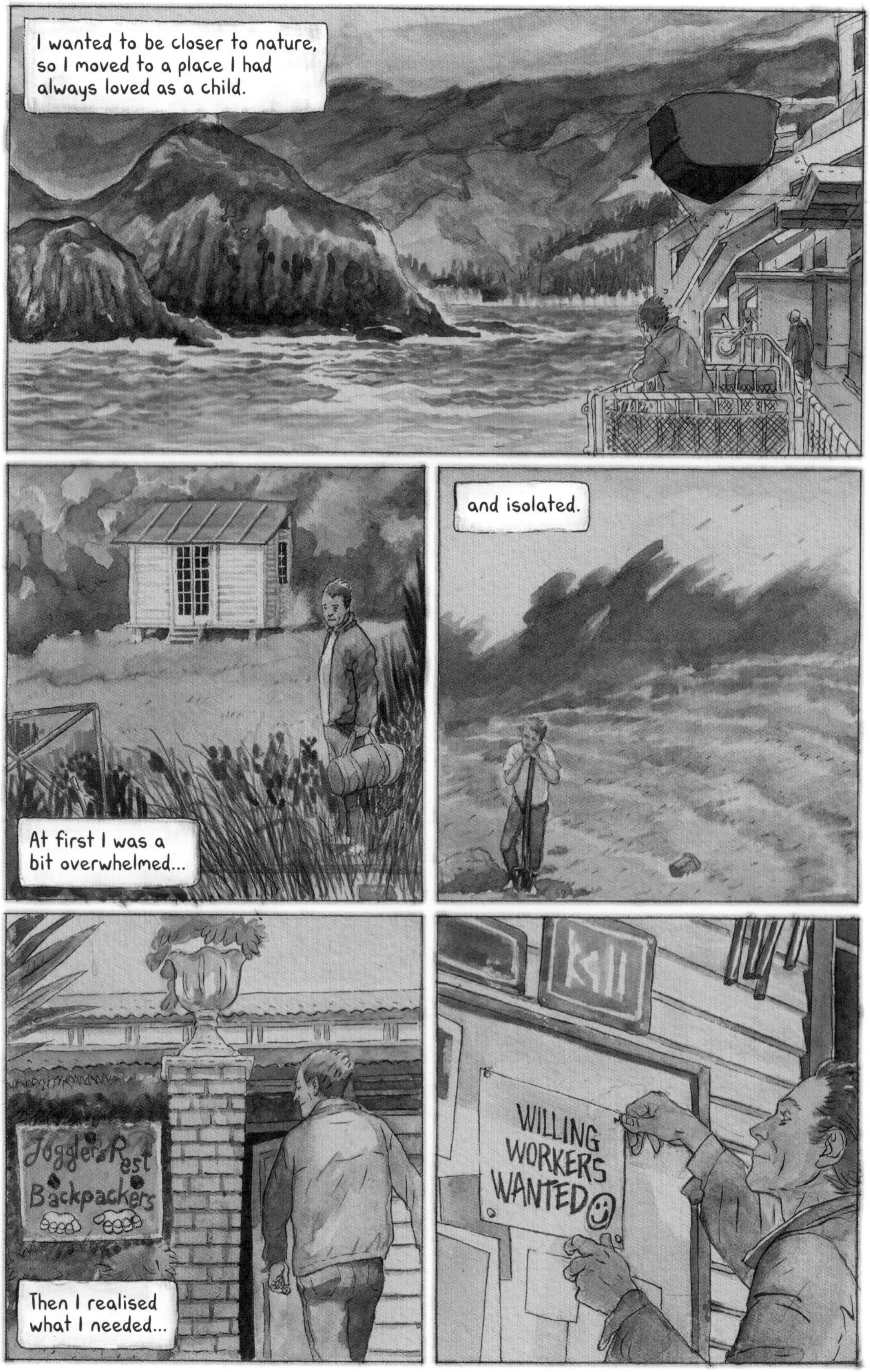
I wanted to be closer to nature, so I moved to a place I had always loved as a child.
At first I was a bit overwhelmed...
and isolated.
Joggler's Rest Backpackers
Then I realised what I needed...
WILLING WORKERS WANTED

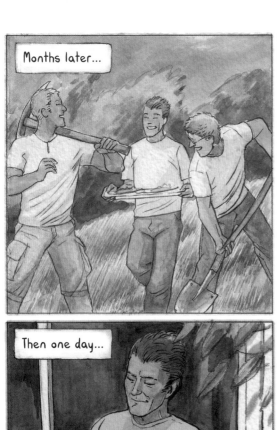

Months later...

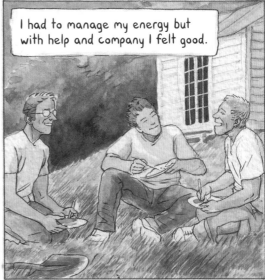

I had to manage my energy but with help and company I felt good.

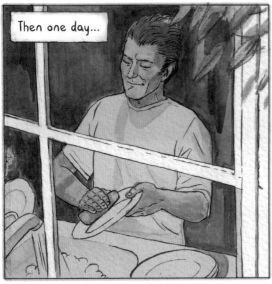

Then one day...

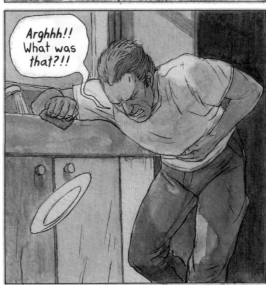

Arghhh!! What was that?!!

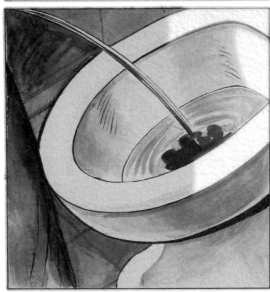

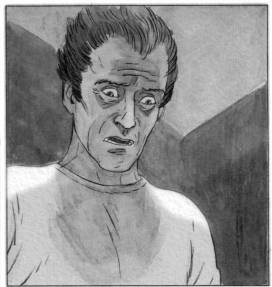

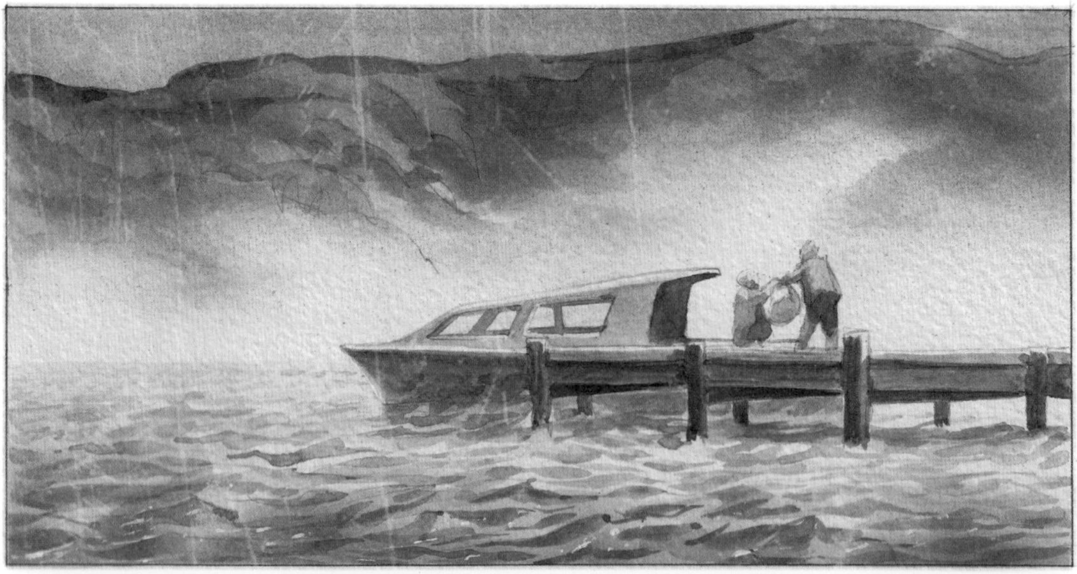

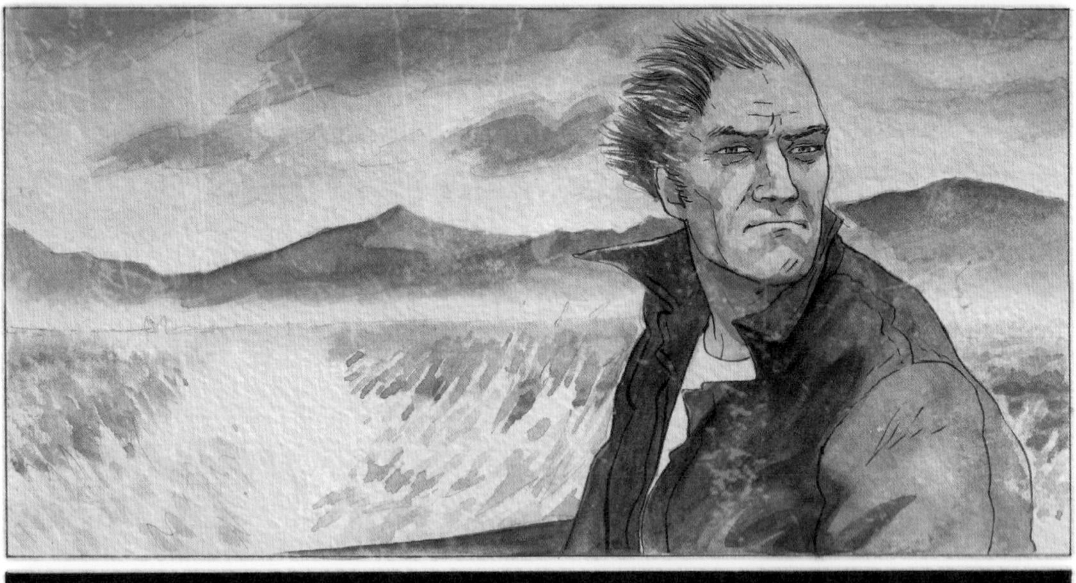

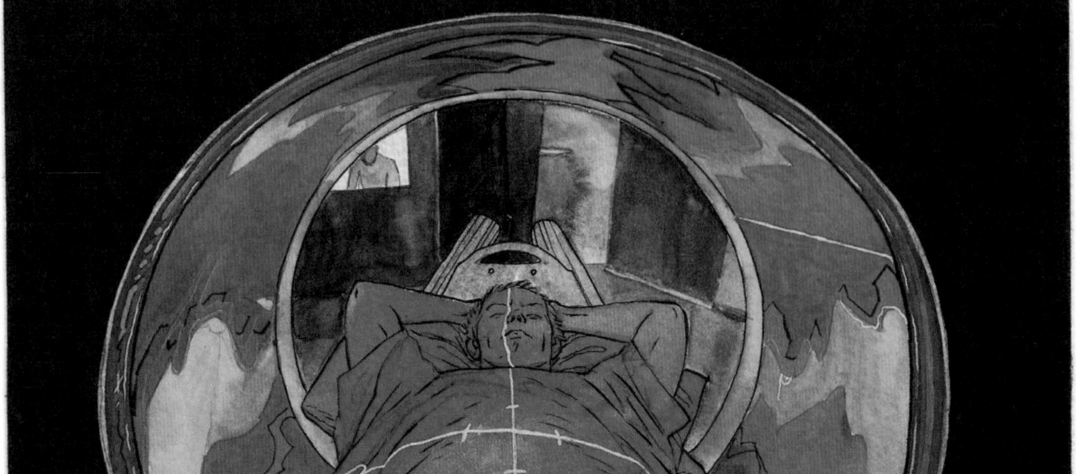

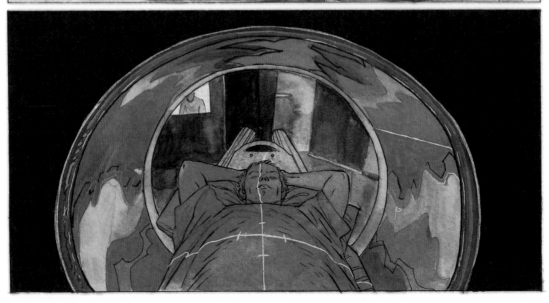

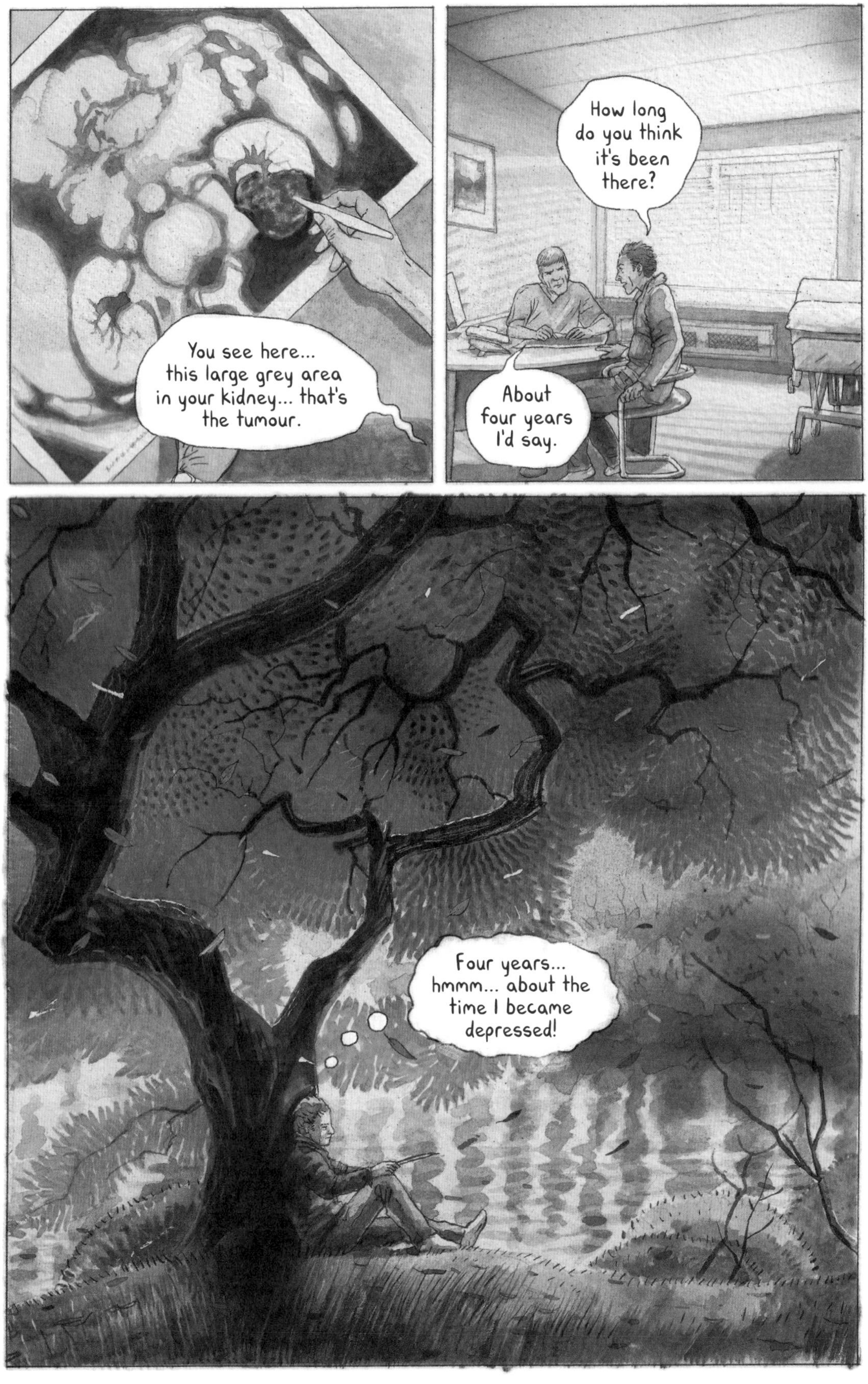
You see here... this large grey area in your kidney... that's the tumour.
How long do you think it's been there?
About four years I'd say.
Four years... hmmm... about the time I became depressed!

I'm pleased to tell you the operation was successful.

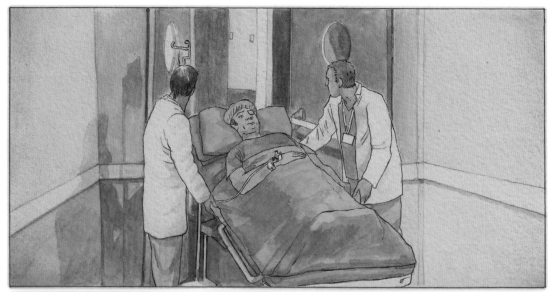

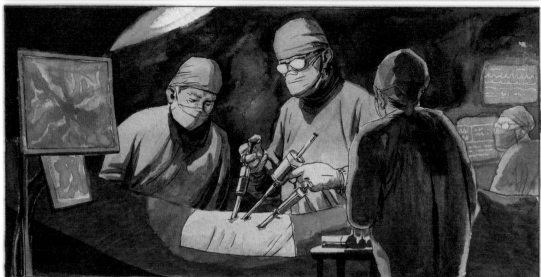

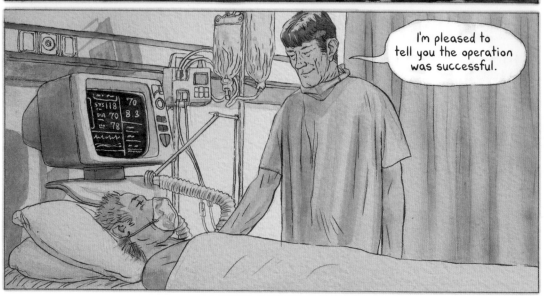

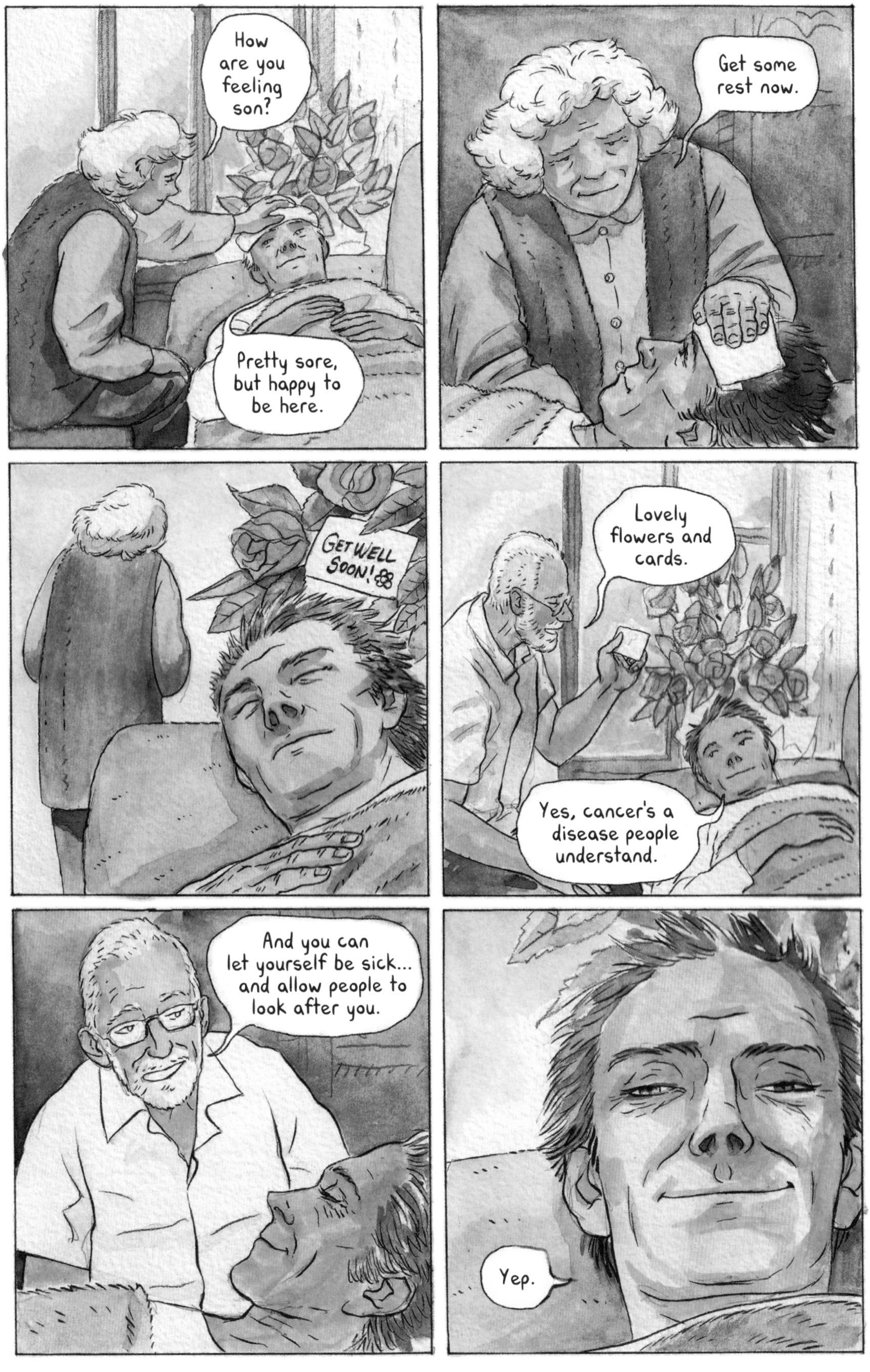
How are you feeling son?
Pretty sore, but happy to be here.
Get some rest now.
GET WELL SOON!
Lovely flowers and cards.
Yes, cancer's a disease people understand.
And you can let yourself be sick... and allow people to look after you.
Yep.

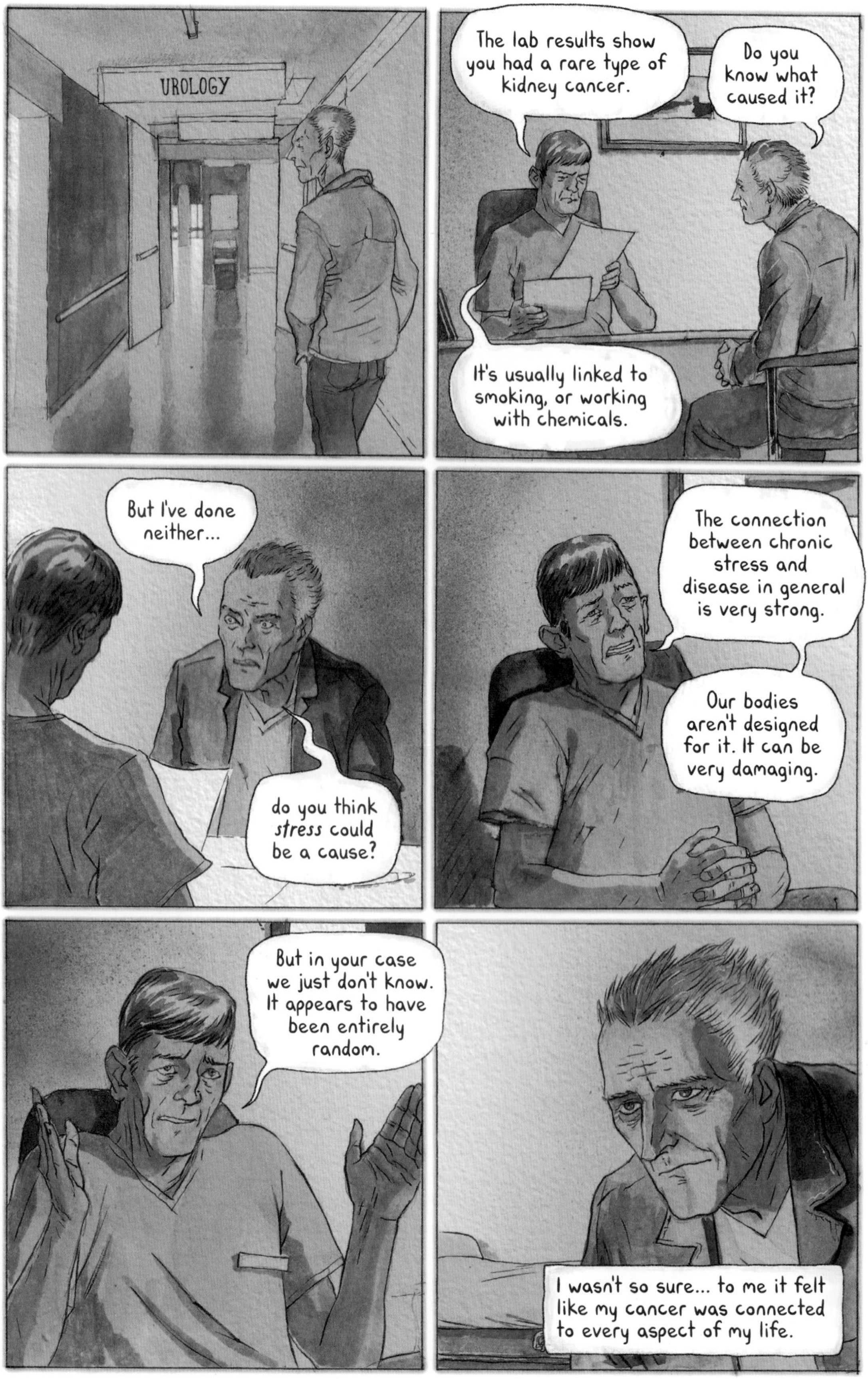
UROLOGY
The lab results show you had a rare type of kidney cancer.
Do you know what caused it?
It's usually linked to smoking, or working with chemicals.
But I've done neither...
do you think *stress* could be a cause?
The connection between chronic stress and disease in general is very strong.
Our bodies aren't designed for it. It can be very damaging.
But in your case we just don't know. It appears to have been entirely random.
I wasn't so sure... to me it felt like my cancer was connected to every aspect of my life.

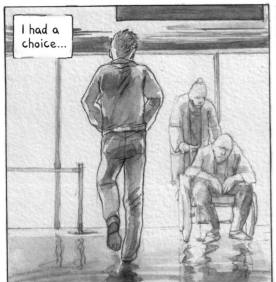

I had a choice...

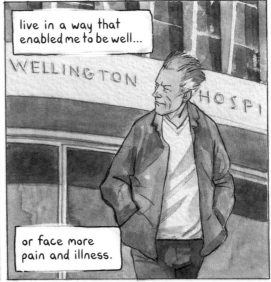

live in a way that enabled me to be well...

or face more pain and illness.

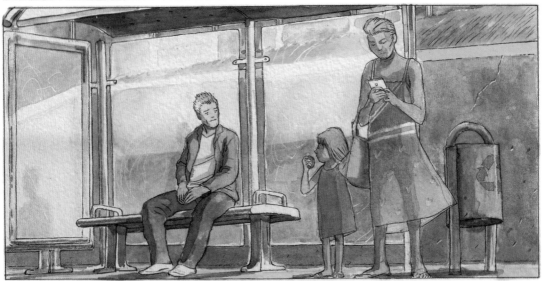

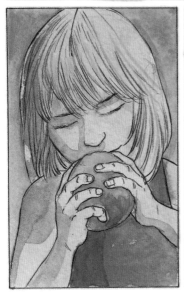

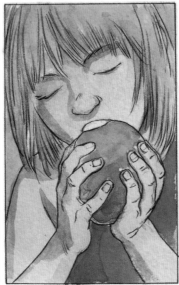

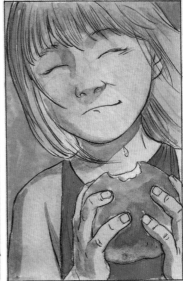

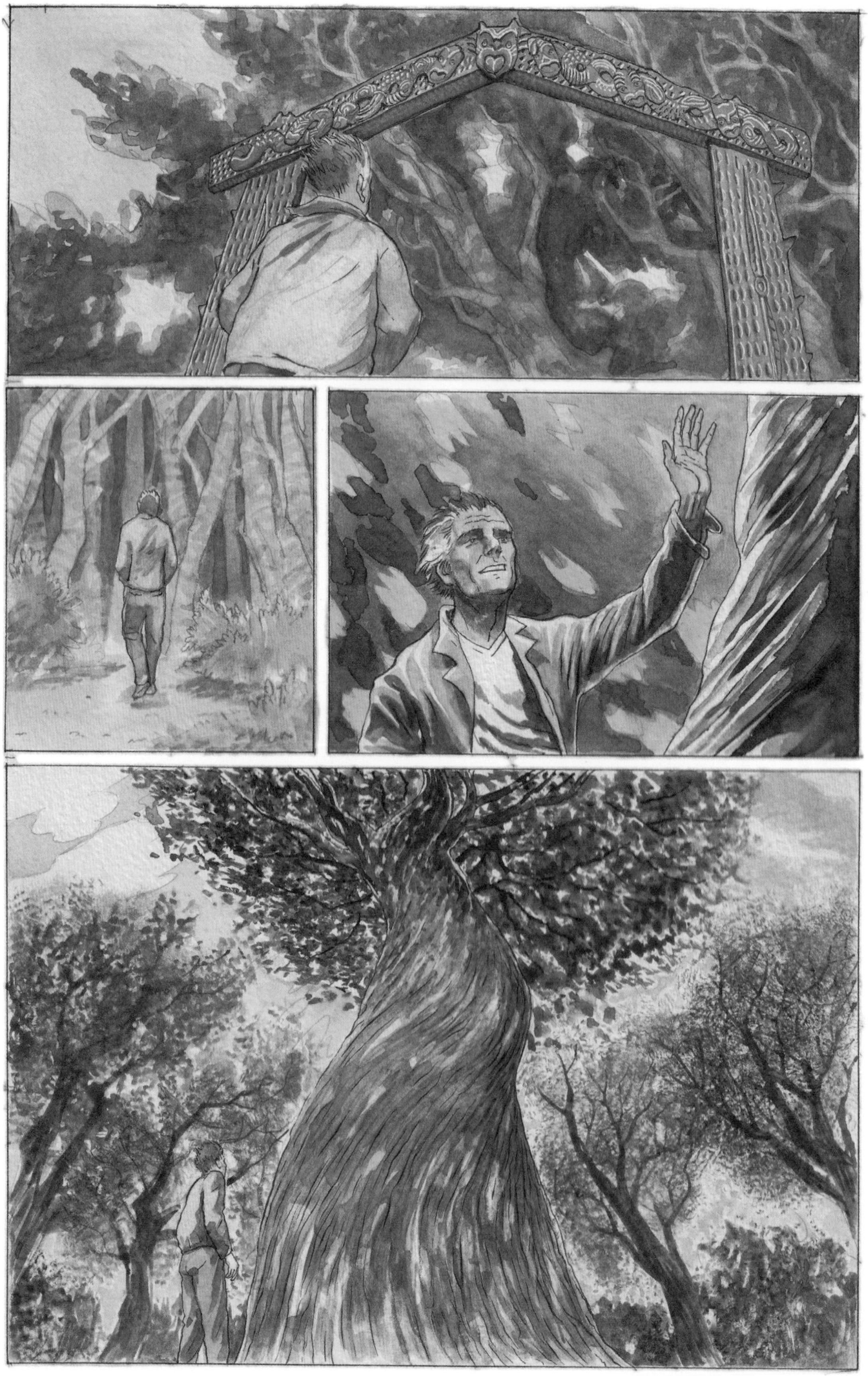

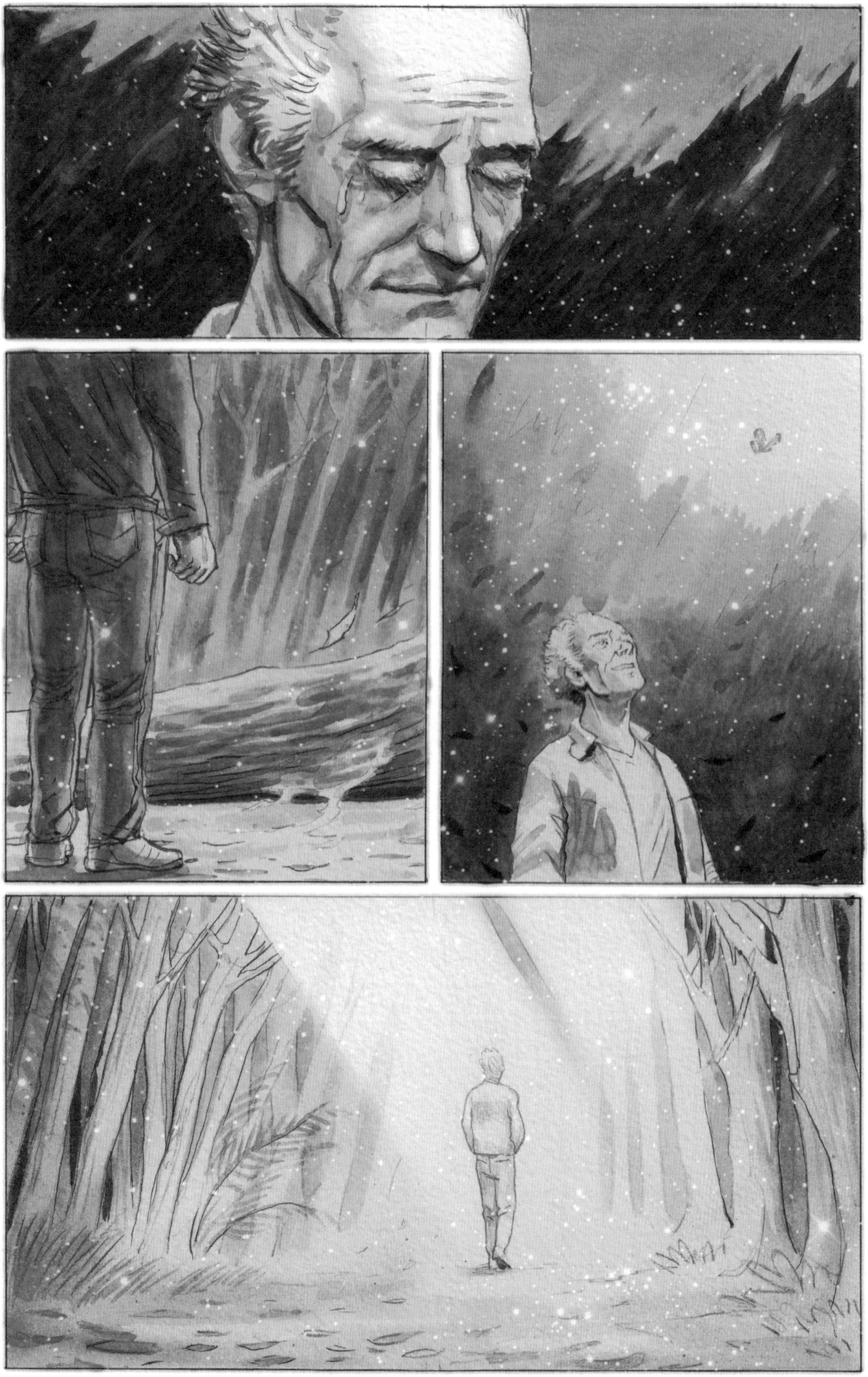

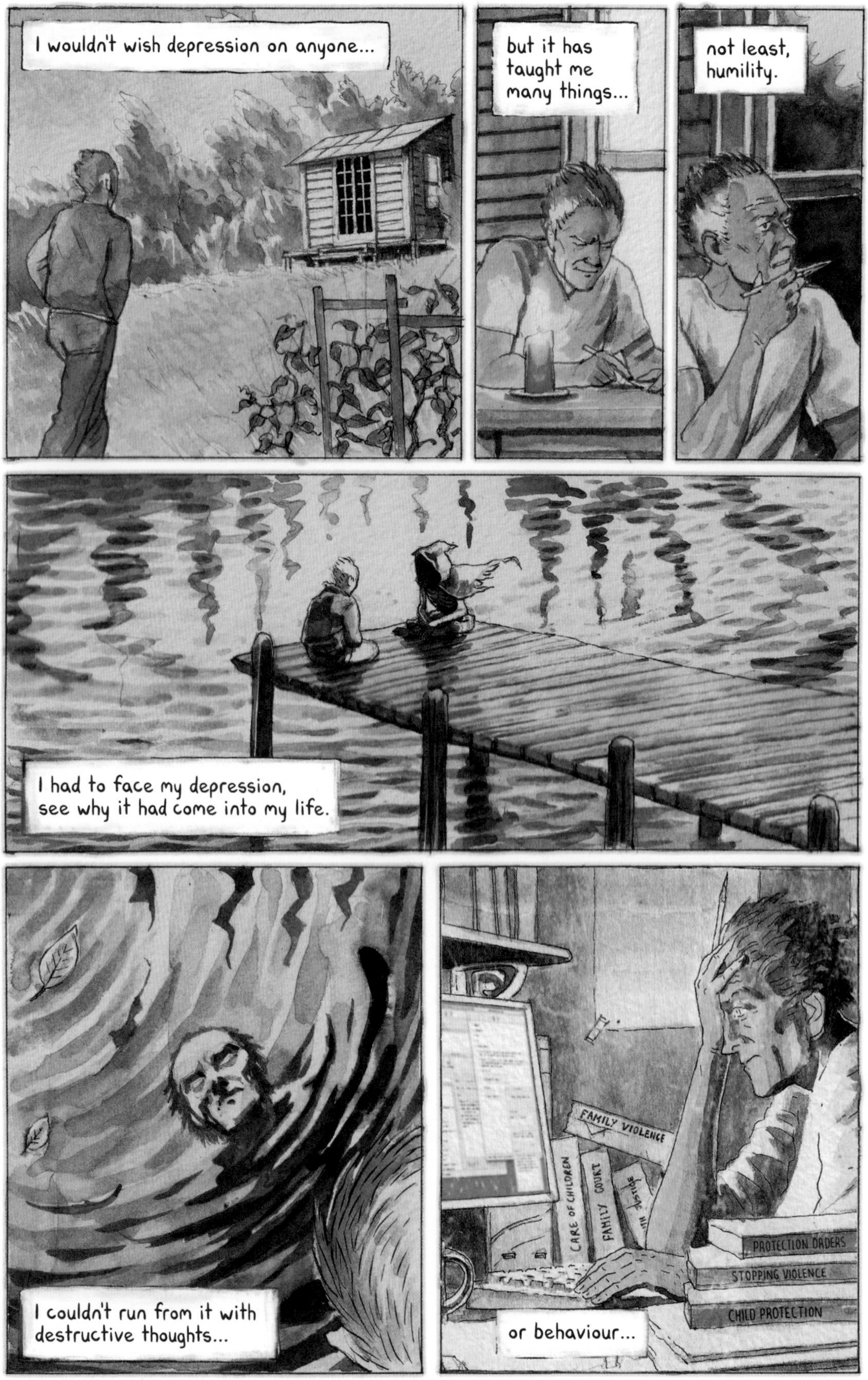
I wouldn't wish depression on anyone...
but it has taught me many things...
not least, humility.
I had to face my depression, see why it had come into my life.
I couldn't run from it with destructive thoughts...
FAMILY VIOLENCE
CARE OF CHILDREN
FAMILY COURT
PROTECTION ORDERS
STOPPING VIOLENCE
CHILD PROTECTION
or behaviour...

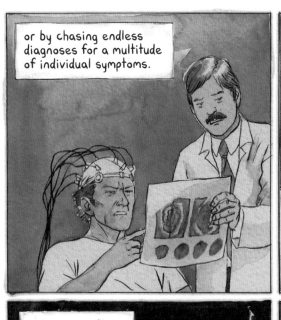

or by chasing endless diagnoses for a multitude of individual symptoms.

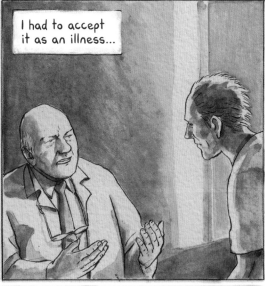

I had to accept it as an illness...

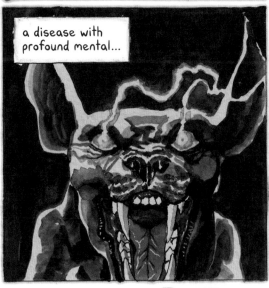

a disease with profound mental...

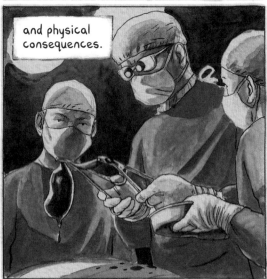

and physical consequences.

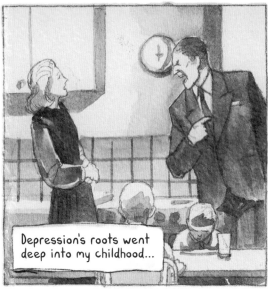

Depression's roots went deep into my childhood...

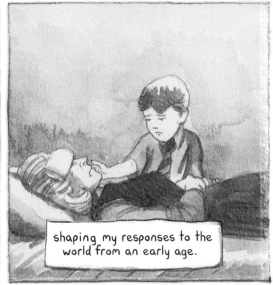

shaping my responses to the world from an early age.

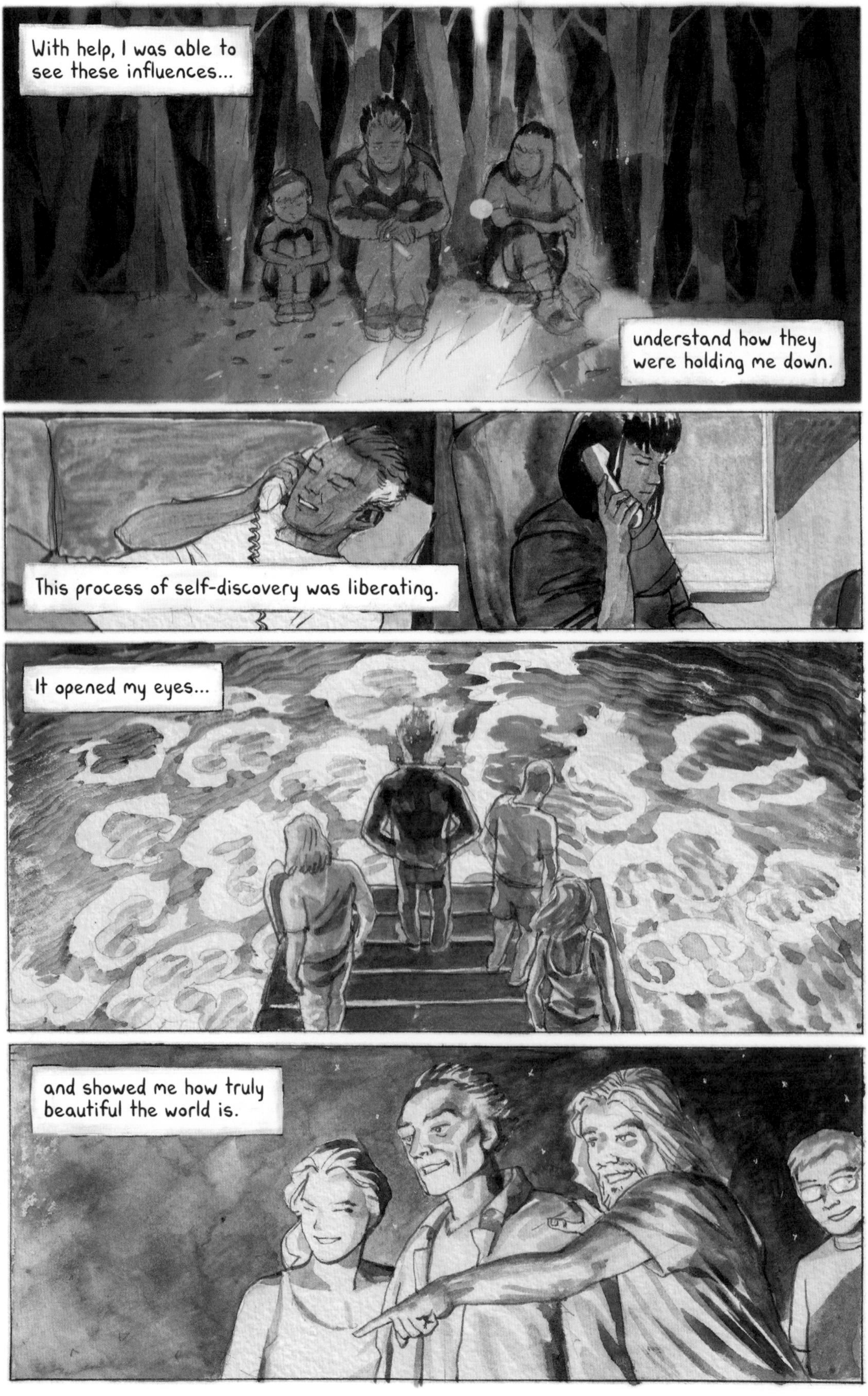
With help, I was able to see these influences...
understand how they were holding me down.
This process of self-discovery was liberating.
It opened my eyes...
and showed me how truly beautiful the world is.

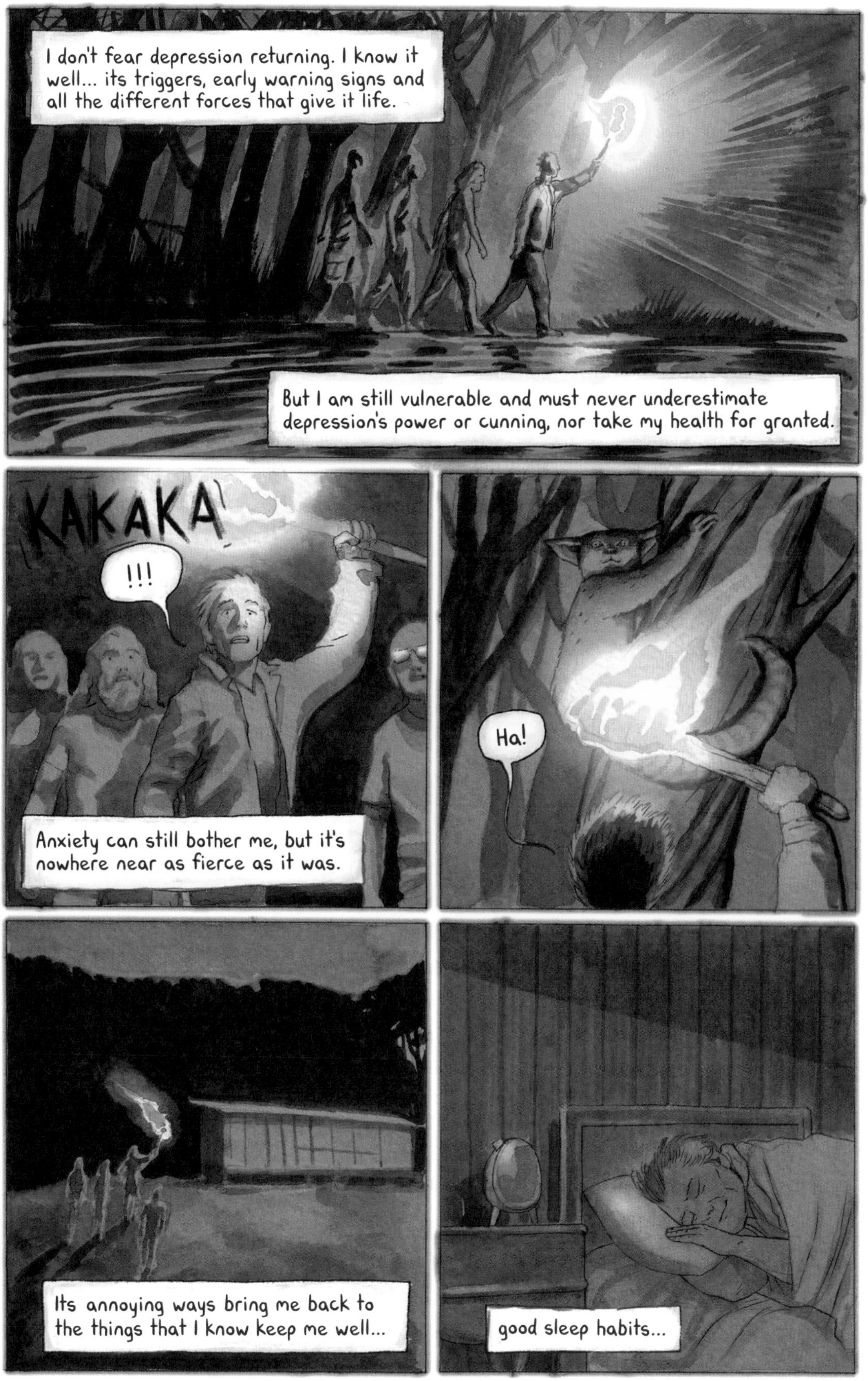
I don't fear depression returning. I know it well... its triggers, early warning signs and all the different forces that give it life.
But I am still vulnerable and must never underestimate depression's power or cunning, nor take my health for granted.
KAKAKA
!!!
Anxiety can still bother me, but it's nowhere near as fierce as it was.
Ha!
Its annoying ways bring me back to the things that I know keep me well...
good sleep habits...

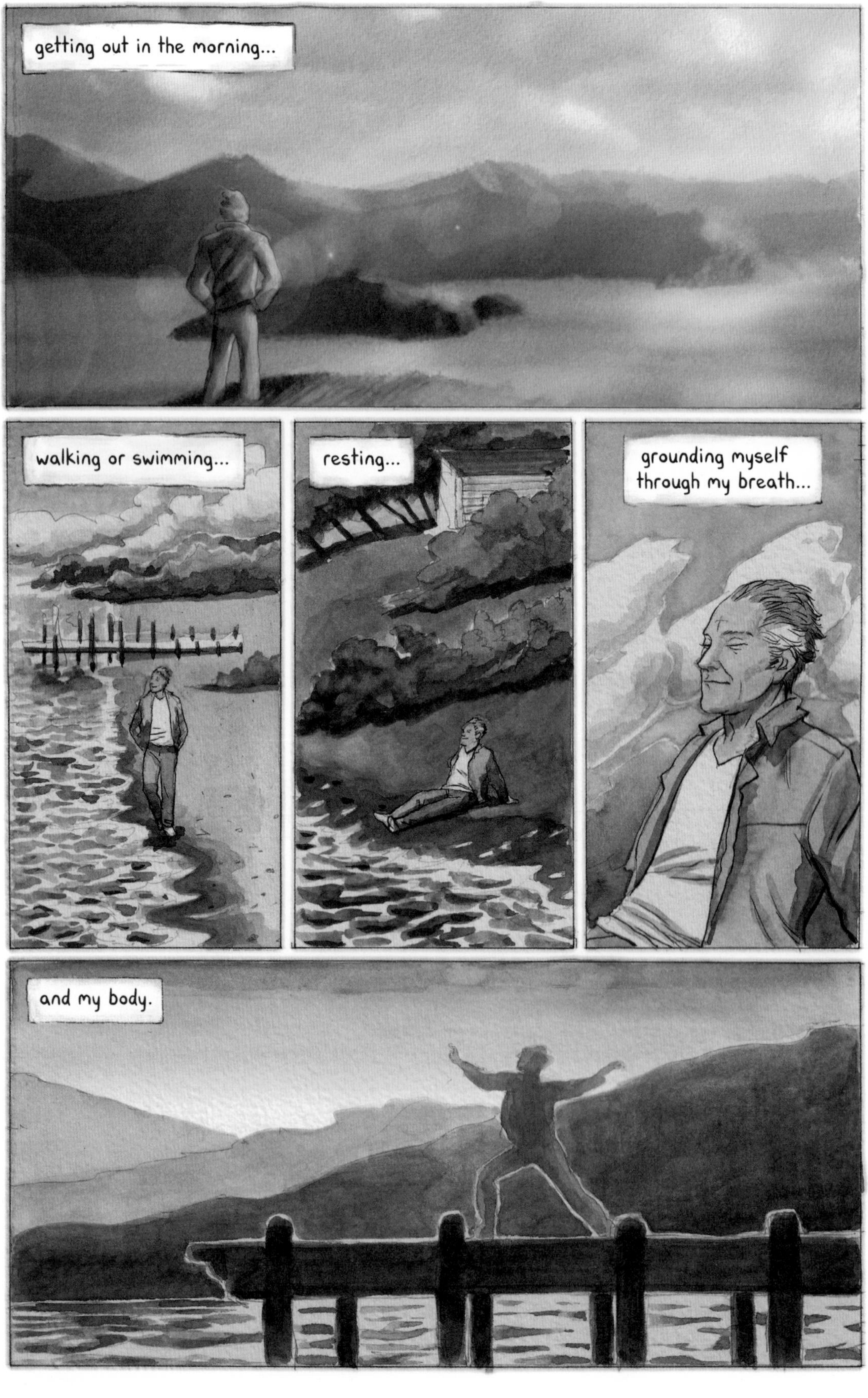
getting out in the morning...
walking or swimming...
resting...
grounding myself through my breath...
and my body.

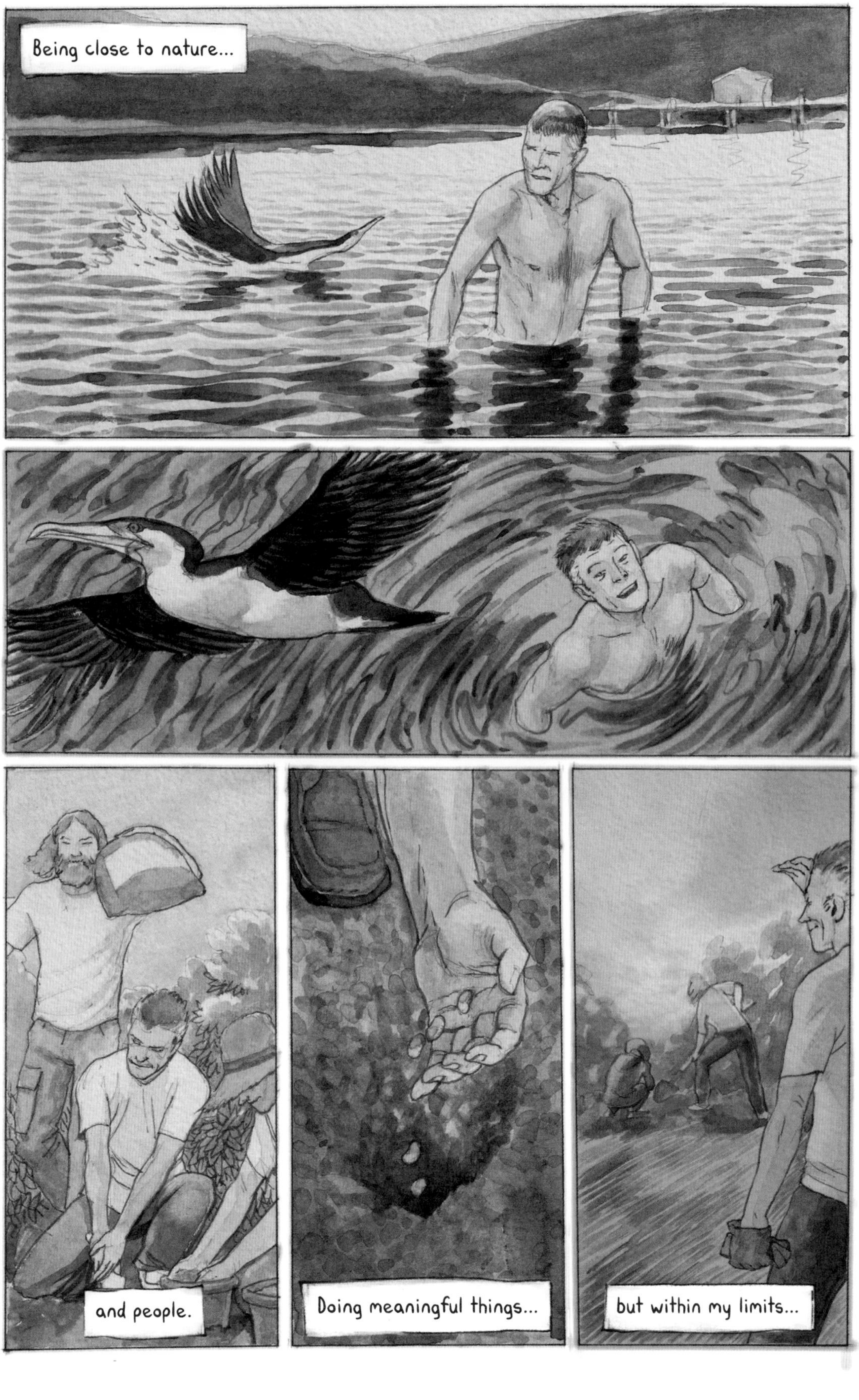
Being close to nature...
and people.
Doing meaningful things...
but within my limits...

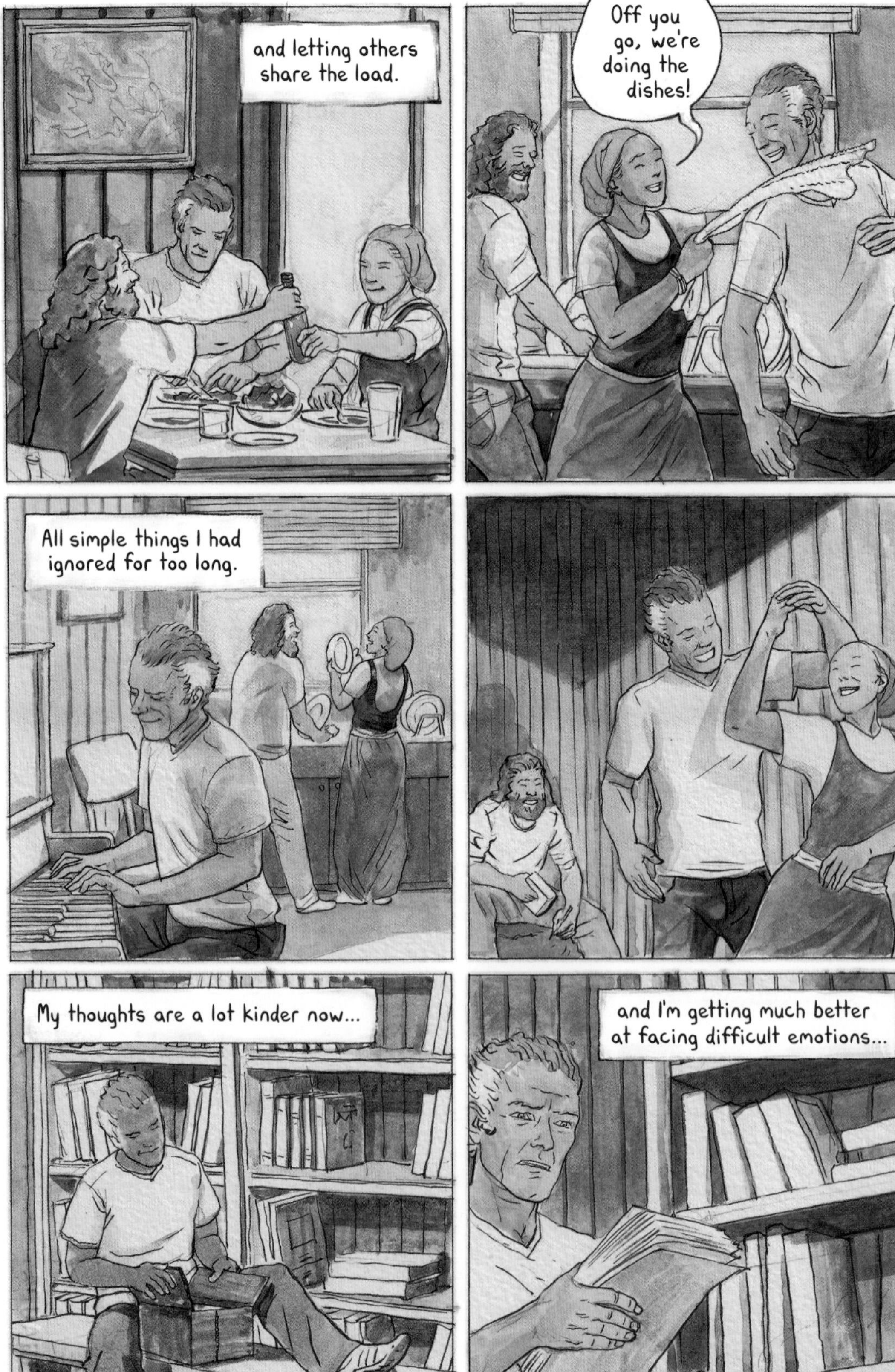
and letting others share the load.
Off you go, we're doing the dishes!
All simple things I had ignored for too long.
My thoughts are a lot kinder now...
and I'm getting much better at facing difficult emotions...

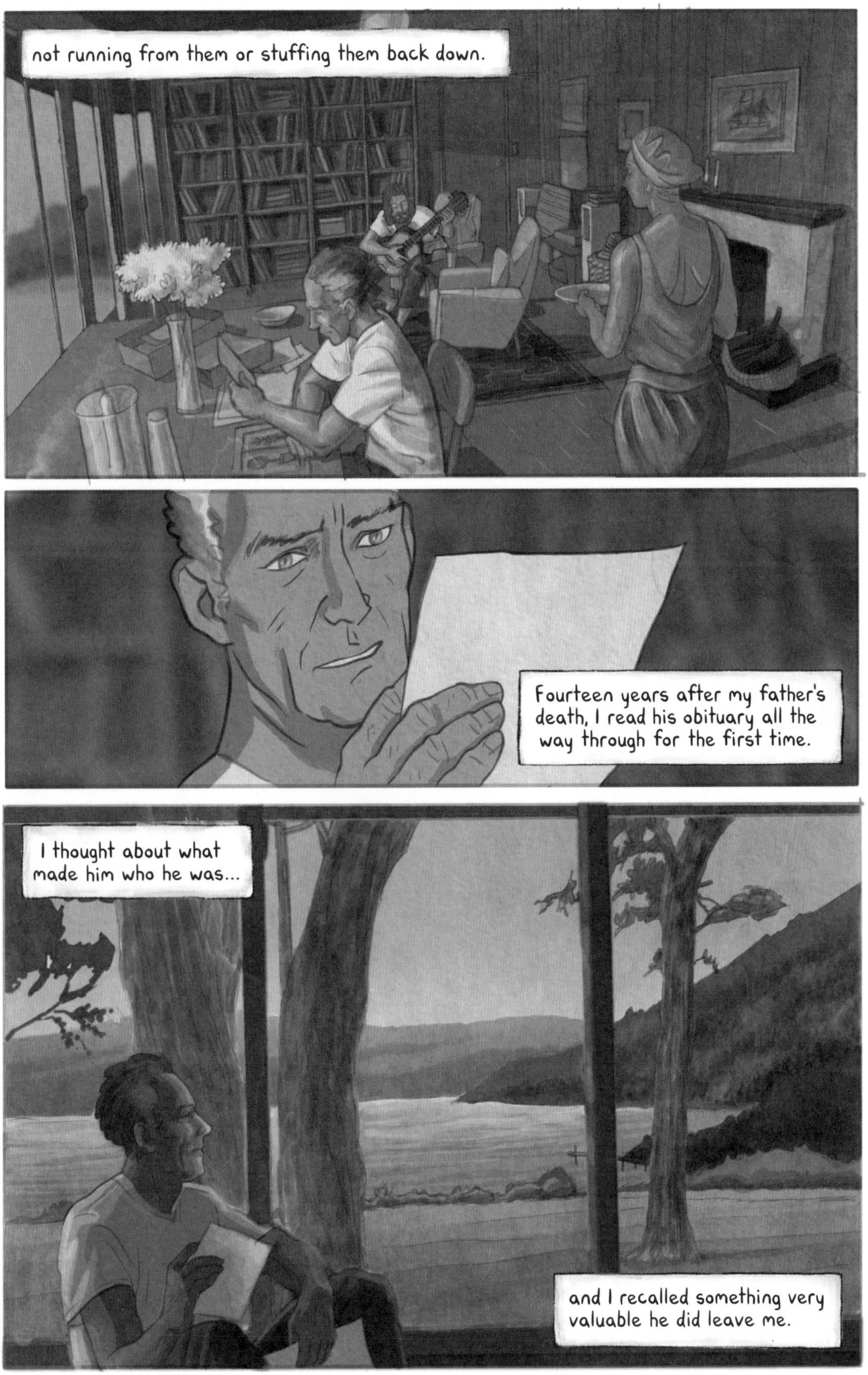
not running from them or stuffing them back down.
Fourteen years after my father's death, I read his obituary all the way through for the first time.
I thought about what made him who he was...
and I recalled something very valuable he did leave me.

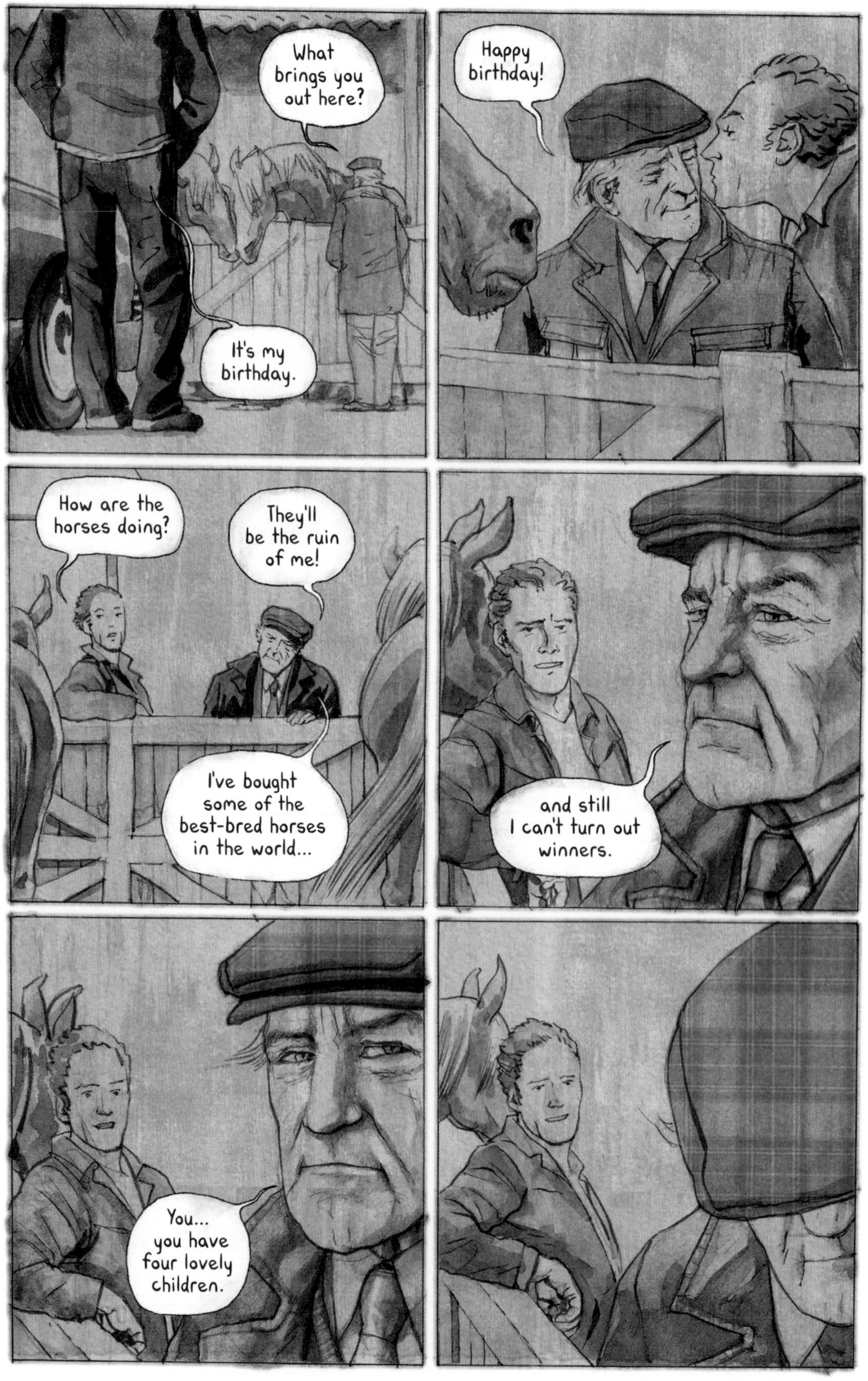
What brings you out here?
It's my birthday.
Happy birthday!
How are the horses doing?
They'll be the ruin of me!
I've bought some of the best-bred horses in the world...
and still I can't turn out winners.
You... you have four lovely children.

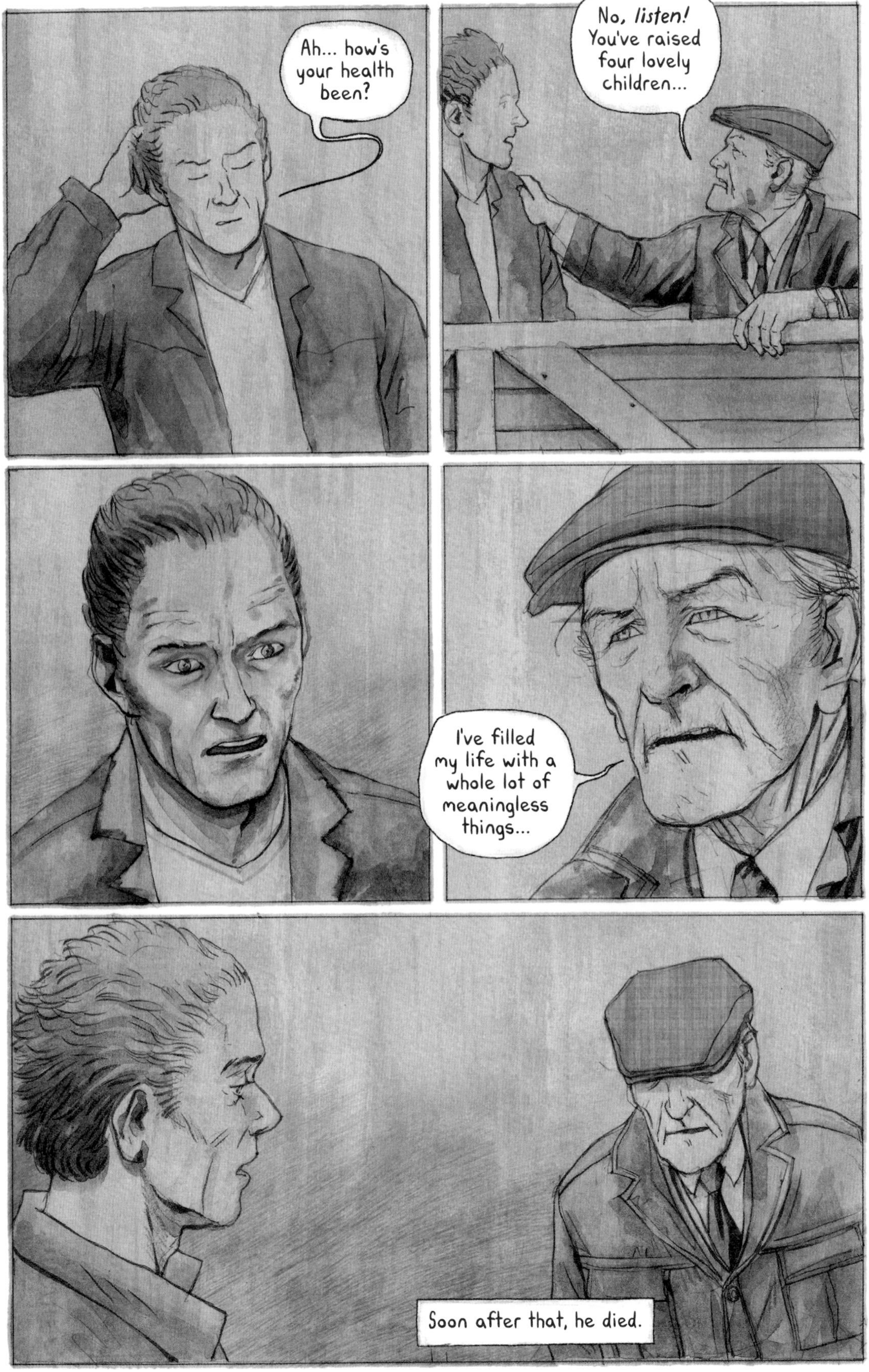
Ah... how's your health been?
No, *listen!* You've raised four lovely children...
I've filled my life with a whole lot of meaningless things...
Soon after that, he died.

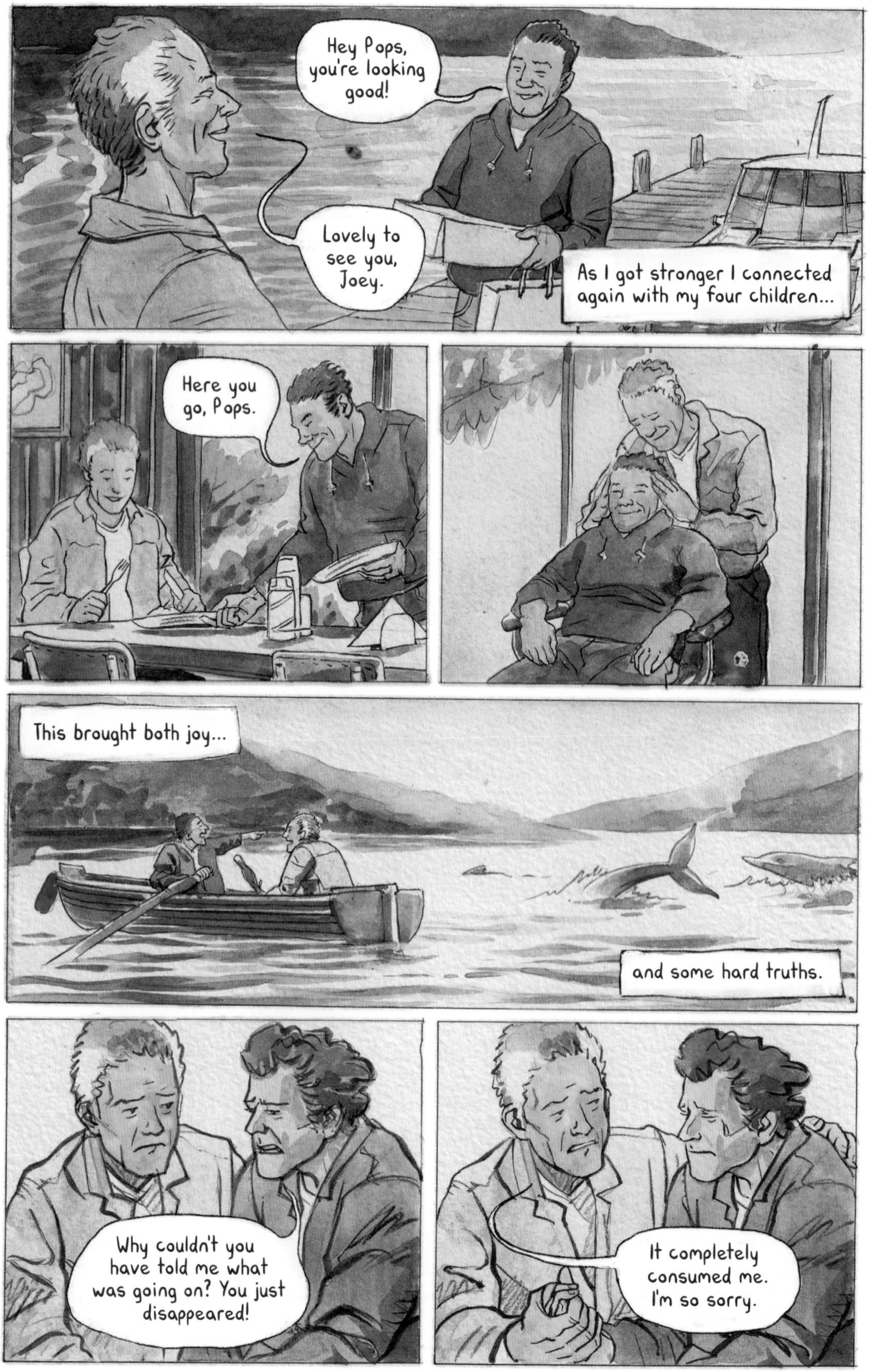

Hey Pops, you're looking good!
Lovely to see you, Joey.
As I got stronger I connected again with my four children...
Here you go, Pops.
This brought both joy...
and some hard truths.
Why couldn't you have told me what was going on? You just disappeared!
It completely consumed me. I'm so sorry.

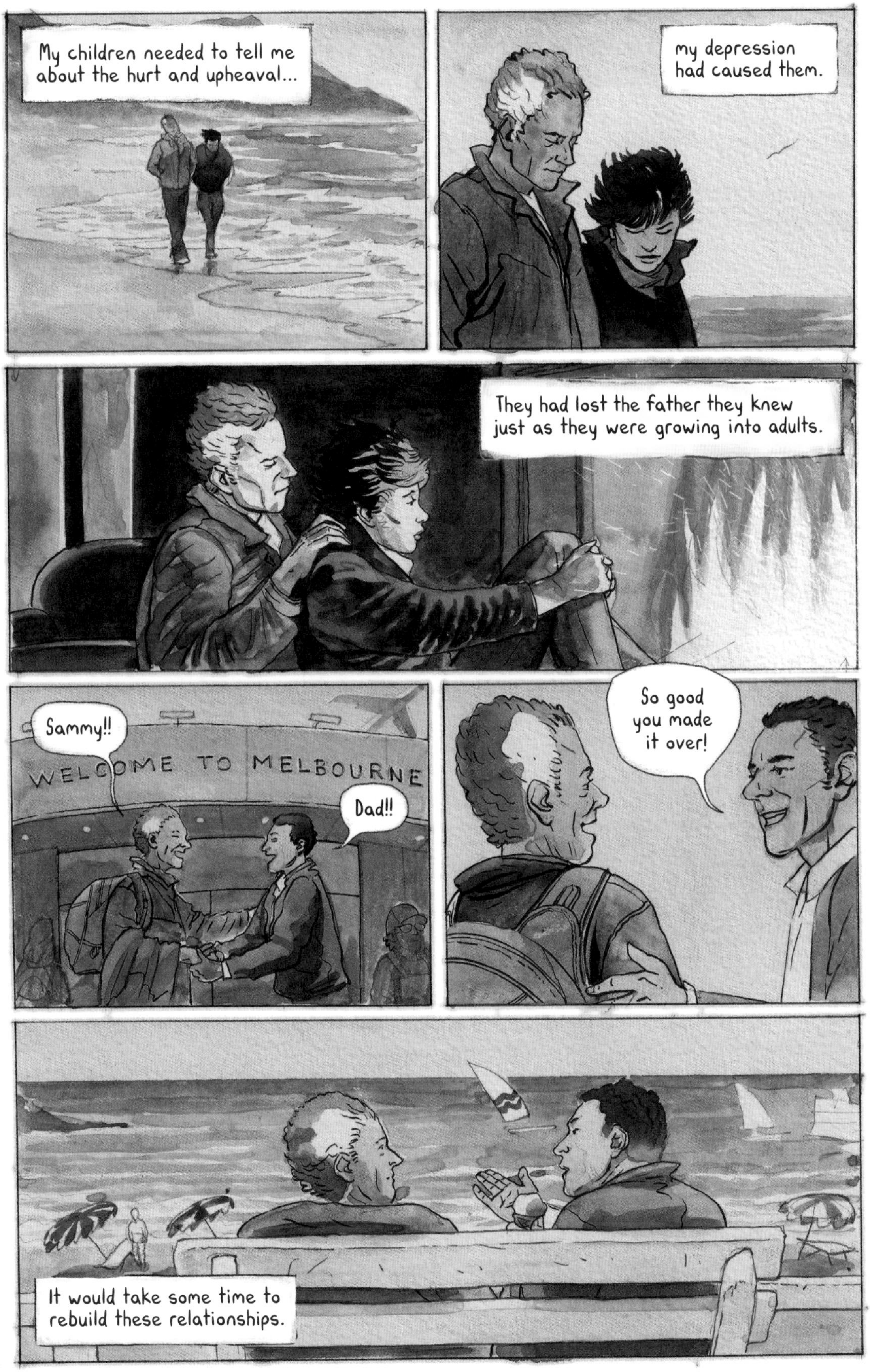
My children needed to tell me about the hurt and upheaval...
my depression had caused them.
They had lost the father they knew just as they were growing into adults.
WELCOME TO MELBOURNE
Sammy!!
Dad!!
So good you made it over!
It would take some time to rebuild these relationships.

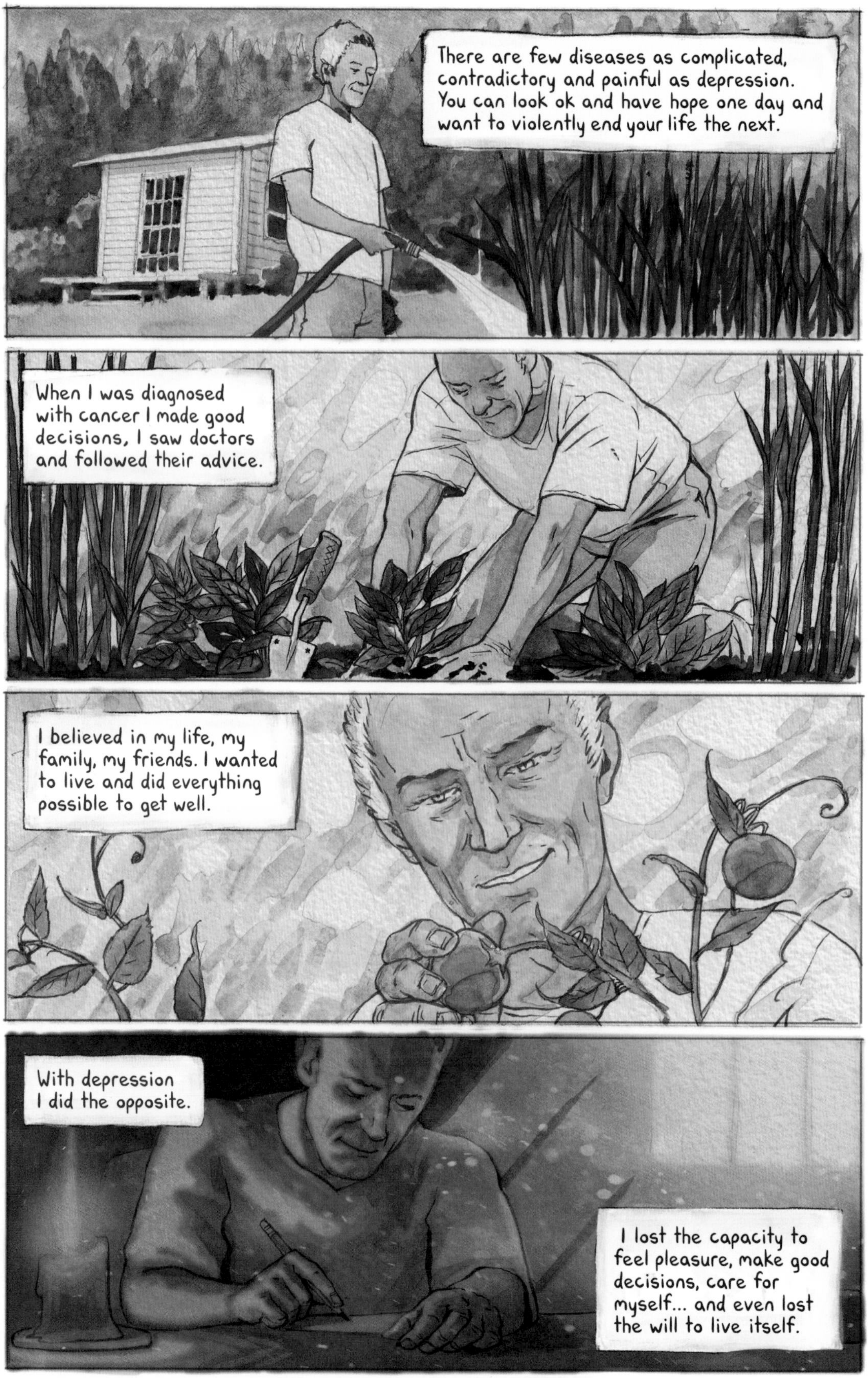
There are few diseases as complicated, contradictory and painful as depression. You can look ok and have hope one day and want to violently end your life the next.
When I was diagnosed with cancer I made good decisions, I saw doctors and followed their advice.
I believed in my life, my family, my friends. I wanted to live and did everything possible to get well.
With depression I did the opposite.
I lost the capacity to feel pleasure, make good decisions, care for myself... and even lost the will to live itself.

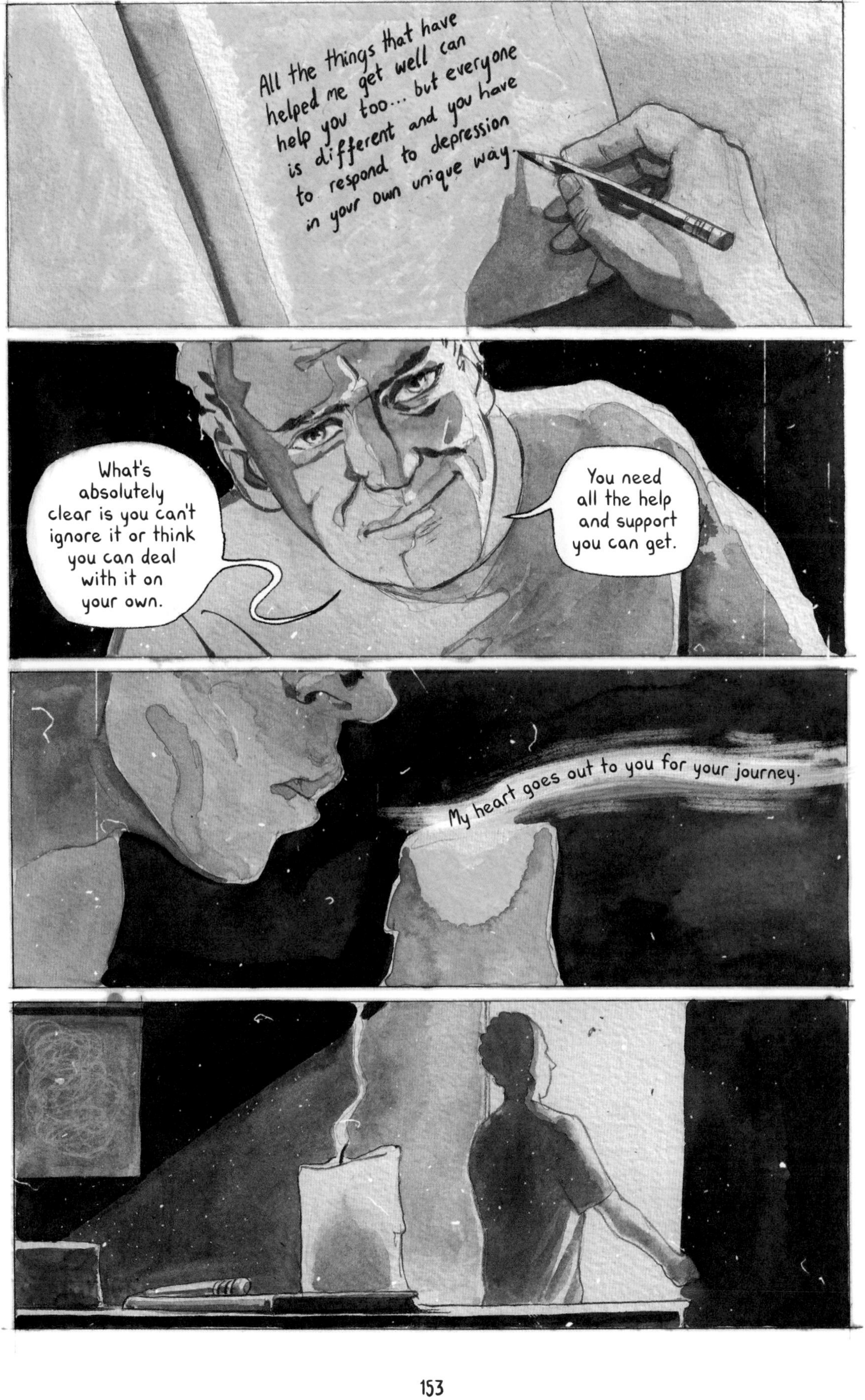
All the things that have helped me get well can help you too... but everyone is different and you have to respond to depression in your own unique way.
What's absolutely clear is you can't ignore it or think you can deal with it on your own.
You need all the help and support you can get.
My heart goes out to you for your journey.

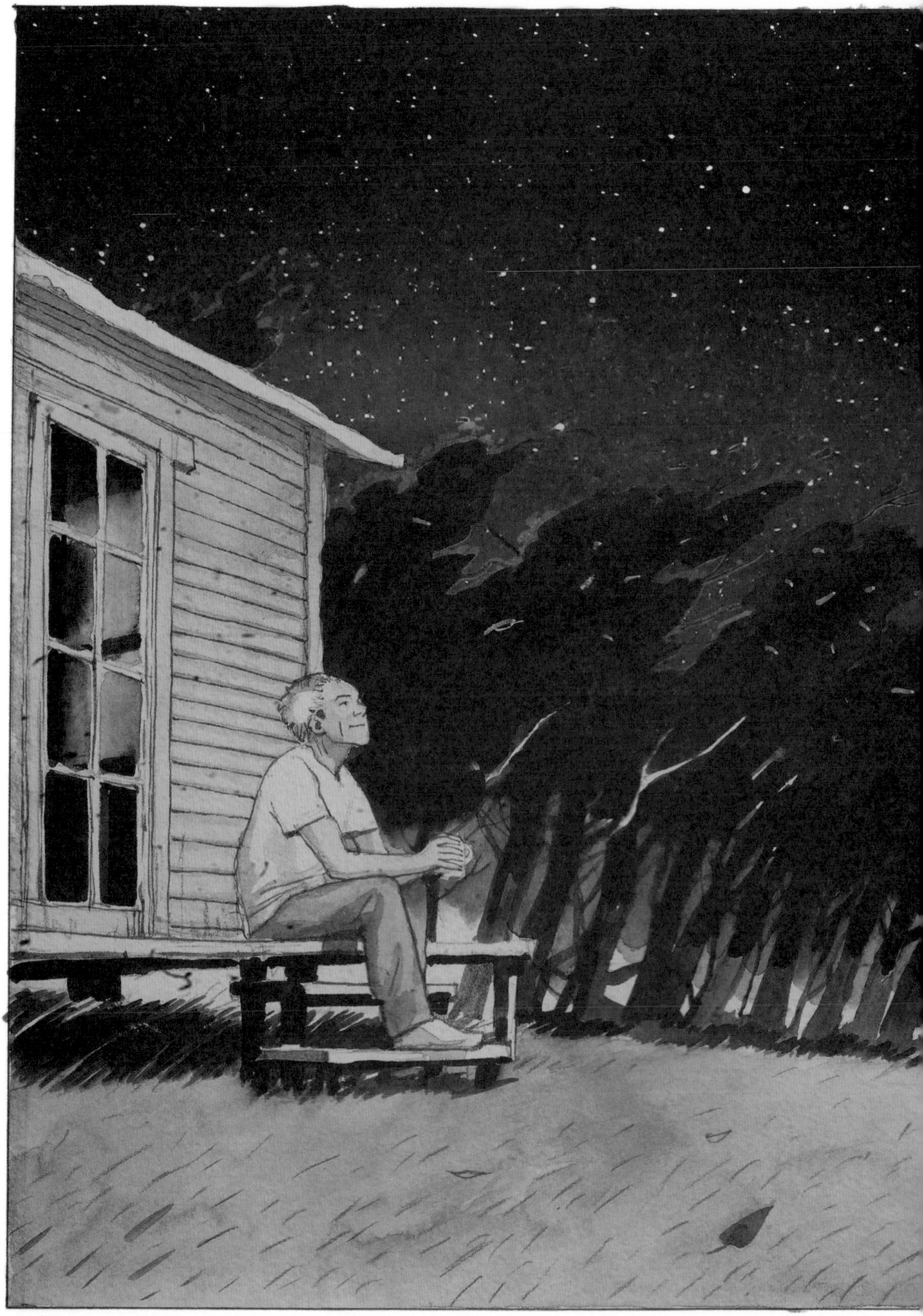

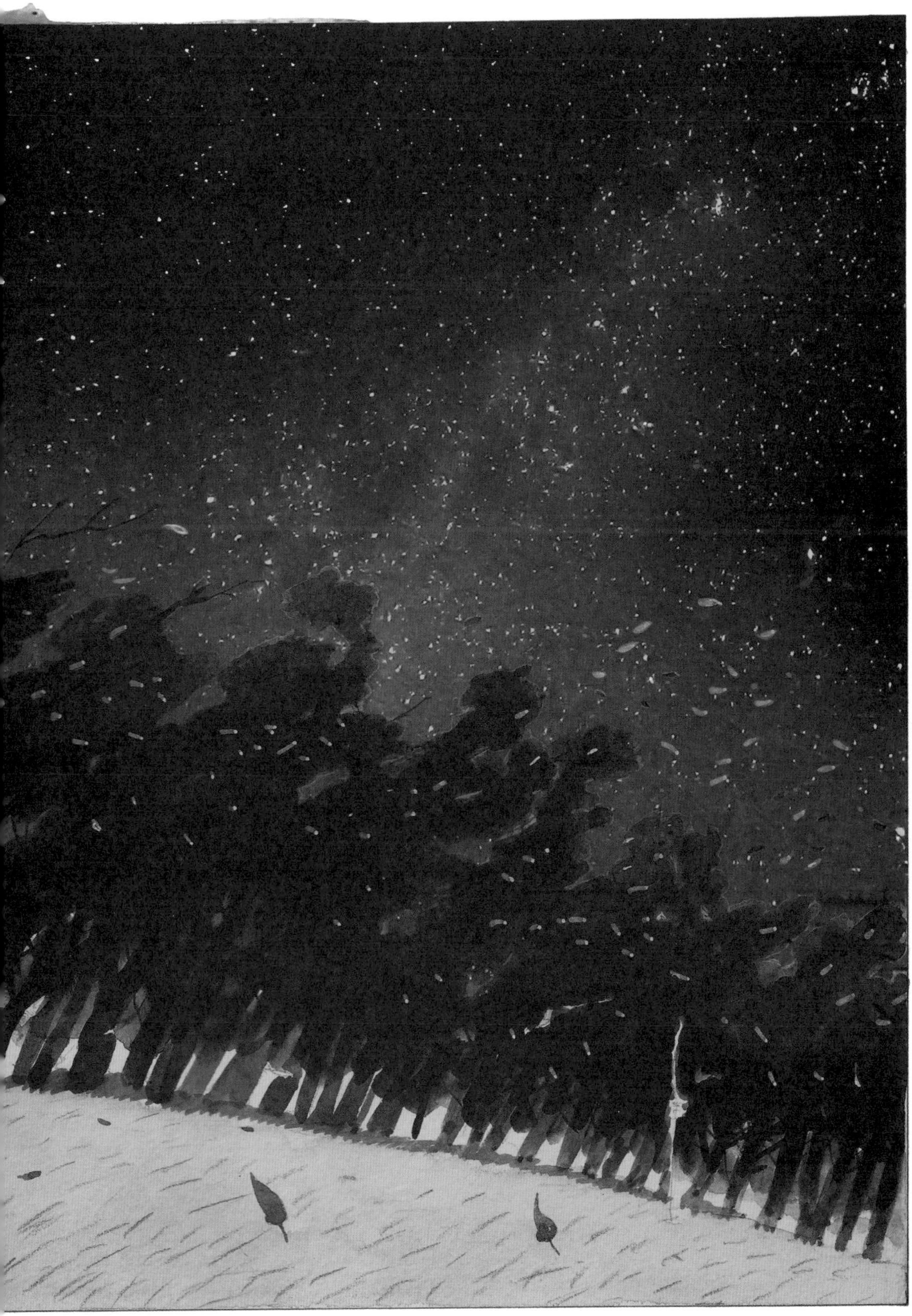

OUT OF THE
WOODS

For further resources about
depression and anxiety go to:
www.outofthewoods.co.nz

Thank you

My sincere appreciation and love to all the people who have helped me get well and supported me in the creation of this book...

My children: Helen, Joe, Henry and Sam; my sisters Bronwyn and Rebecca; my brothers Arthur and Martin; my mother Ngaire; and Louise. Without my family's support I could not have written this book.

My friends who supported me in so many ways: Julia and Paul, Dan and Anna, Stuart and Neil, Yolande, Helen, Catherine, Paul and Clare, James and Diana, Sharon and Geoff, Andrea and Richard, Paul and Janette, Elizabeth, Pip, Carina, Philip and Trish, Theresa, Maggie, Kevin and Jane, Don and Julia, Averil, Otti, Jackie and Phil, Stephen, Carrie, Tore, Annie, Nic, Andy, Noel, Mel and John, Ann, Phillip, and Trace.

My WWOOFer friends who shared my life while I was writing the book, for their inspiration and good company.

The professionals who in no small measure helped me get well:
Alisa Hirschfeld, Dr. Chris Kalderimis, Dr. Tim McLeod, Mr Andrew Kennedy-Smith, and Professor John Nacey.

The professionals who so generously commented on drafts of the book:
Dr. Ben Beaglehole, Dr. Tony Marks, Dr. Simon Bainbridge, Patricia Gerbarg MD, Professor Shaun Holt, and Dr. Bronwyn Sweeney.

Stephanie Houpt at the Otago Medical School Library for library assistance.

Jessie Leov for typing.

Cassie McCracken for publishing assistance.

Mitch Marks for copy editing, comic expertise, and support.

The team at Cato Brand Partners: Cam, Andy, Matt, Mike, Michaela, John, Melissa, Ruth and Belinda, for their design work.

Pippa Keel for lettering and artwork revisions.

Tom Barclay for lettering and assistance in getting the book to print.

My long time colleague, friend and editor, James McLean, who said 'yes!' on day one, and never tired of giving me his invaluable creative guidance. I could not have made the book without his professional and personal support.

And, finally, Korkut – a man whose artwork sang out so powerfully when I was looking for an illustrator. He has given his all, amidst political and social turmoil in his region, a full teaching load, the birth of his first child, and his mother's illness. I have shared his life and he mine, and the book reflects this strong partnership. It has been an honour to work with Korkut and I owe him my utmost gratitude.

Brent Williams
Author

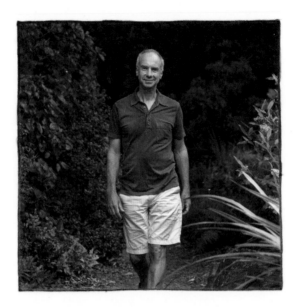

Brent Williams was born in Wellington, New Zealand, in 1958. He built his career in community law, creating services and resources to help vulnerable people - particularly children, young people, and victims of family violence.

In his resource work Brent used comics, re-enactments, and documentaries to tell stories of people asserting their legal rights. However, in his late forties he found he could no longer do this work. It was like he had hit an insurmountable wall. That wall was depression and anxiety.

Denial, shame, and a misguided belief he had to fight these illnesses on his own made Brent's situation worse. Not until he really acknowledged that he was ill, and accepted help, could his recovery begin.

Out of the Woods is an honest account of what Brent experienced and learned in his journey out of depression and anxiety.